HOMBURGER AND BONNER'S

Medical Care and Rehabilitation of the Aged and Chronically Ill

HOMBURGER AND BONNER'S

Medical Care and Rehabilitation of the Aged and Chronically Ill

THIRD EDITION

Charles D. Bonner, M.D.
Medical Director and
Director of Rehabilitation,
Youville Hospital,
Cambridge, Massachusetts

LITTLE, BROWN AND COMPANY
BOSTON

Copyright © 1964, 1974 by Freddy Homburger and
Charles D. Bonner

First Edition Copyright 1955, by Freddy Homburger

Third Edition

Library of Congress catalog card No. 73–2032

ISBN 0–316–10200

Printed in the United States of America

To my family unit:
Wife, Frances J. (M.D.)
Daughters, Carol Elaine and Dale Denise

A man produces only to the extent that he is
respected, encouraged, morally supported,
understood, and loved.
For these blessings I thank you all.

Preface

The privilege and opportunity of writing and compiling this third edition have been graciously conferred on me by my coauthor of the second edition, Dr. Freddy Homburger. Our association began many years ago, when we coauthored many articles; and I was also a contributor to his first edition. I thank him for his trust and continuing friendship.

It is the intent of the third edition, as of earlier ones, to exclude those diseases that are well covered in the specialized textbooks and that are well covered medically by physicians because they are of more day-to-day interest. I wish to highlight the areas where physician and allied health personnel have failed to accept their responsibilities in the care of chronically ill patients.

To attain that goal, I have added several new chapters that directly relate to problems besetting the target population. Several chapters have been completely written by new contributing authors. All remaining chapters have undergone extensive revision and updating.

During my years of responsibility in a rehabilitation and chronic disease hospital that receives its patients by referral from many hospitals—teaching and otherwise—in the Boston area, I have had the opportunity to assess many aspects of the medical care and rehabilitation of the aged and chronically ill. In this book, I attempt to address the weak points of this care.

Each chapter is presented in a way that, I hope, will provide a wealth of practical information illustrated by specific, detailed explanations and many photographs. Topics as simple as applying an Ace bandage properly and the successful use of a crutch or cane have an equal share with such things as the newer physical therapy techniques and discussion of the sexual problems of the patient with a spinal cord injury.

The care of the aged and chronically ill is still wanting in many areas, and I feel it can always be improved. This is not to say that progress has not been made since the last edition, but it comes slowly and painfully. Many physicians and allied health personnel, as well as patients and families, continue to need assistance and concrete advice regarding the comprehensive management of chronically ill patients. These patients are entitled to and must get better care. I have attempted to address myself to these issues, and if any, or many, patients become able to enjoy and live better lives through the information herein contained, I will have been amply rewarded.

C. D. B.

Acknowledgments

Rarely can an author become an island unto himself, and this author is no exception. I am indebted to many individuals who, by their advice, contributions, and faith have helped make this third edition a reality.

First, I thank Dr. Freddy Homburger, co-author of the second edition, for giving me the opportunity to prepare this edition. Through the years, I have been privileged to have his collaboration in scientific endeavors as well as his friendship. I trust the current edition will confirm for him his confidence and trust.

Second, I express my appreciation to others who have contributed advice and services in a multitude of ways. Margaret Johnson, R.P.T., Cheryl Ehrenkranz, R.P.T., Frances Physic, R.N., Faith Copley, M.S.W., Cynthia Marks, O.T.R., Stephanie Thomas in the photostating section of Youville Hospital, plus James Holzer, B.S., and Lawrence Lentz, B.S., of the Youville Hospital Public Relations and Audio-Visual departments.

Third, I acknowledge my debt to Lewis A. Miller, Editor of *Patient Care*, for allowing us to reproduce the material in Chapter 18.

And last, but not least, I owe a profound debt of gratitude to Mrs. Alison Curry, my secretary, for the long hours of typing, reading, and re-reading the multiple drafts until the final page of the final draft was done.

Contributing Authors

ALBERT SCHILLING, M.D.
Associate Professor of Medicine, Boston
University School of Medicine
CHAPTER 1

HENRY A. SCHLANG, M.D.
Assistant Professor of Medicine, Boston
University School of Medicine
CHAPTER 1

MAUREEN O'BRIAN FLAHERTY,
R.N., M.S.
Formerly Coordinator, Medical-Surgical
Nursing, Boston College
CHAPTER 10
CHAPTER 17

SUSAN B. O'SULLIVAN,
R.P.T., M.S.
Instructor, Physical Therapy, Sargent
College of Allied Health Professions,
Boston University
CHAPTER 11

KATHERINE LAQUE SHINE,
O.T.R., B.S.
Formerly Supervisor of Occupational
Therapy, Youville Hospital, Cambridge
CHAPTER 12

BARBARA BAKER FINGER, M.A.
Supervisor, Speech Therapy, Youville
Hospital, Cambridge
CHAPTER 13

AMY GOON, M.S.W.
Director of Social Service, Youville
Hospital, Cambridge
CHAPTER 14
CHAPTER 17

PATRINA MANDELLA
Dietitian, Youville Hospital, Cambridge
CHAPTER 15

SUZANNE VAN AMERONGEN, M.D.
Psychiatric Consultant, Youville Hospital,
Cambridge
CHAPTER 16

Contents

HOMBURGER AND BONNER'S

Medical Care and Rehabilitation of the Aged and Chronically Ill

Philosophical Basis for the Good Management of the Aged and Chronically Ill

People throughout the world are easily aroused by a great number of problems. Often they are provoked into such actions as the waging of wars to decide ideological or territorial conflicts; they resort to violence and rioting to protest social injustices; or they will organize concerted rescue missions for the victims of famines or disasters; reforms are instituted and sometimes even revolutions are undertaken to correct the exploitation of minorities. Yet, strangely, little action is provoked by the plight of the aged, who often remain neglected, victimized, and abandoned.

The problems confronted, in part, by the aged and chronically ill are to a large extent those produced by a poorly planned, disinterested, thoughtless society—a society which, as a by-product of enlightened medicine, has prolonged life expectancy while increasing the incidence of chronic ailments.

With such emphasis upon the saving of lives, no matter what the cost (coronary-care units, widespread cardiopulmonary resuscitation usage, heart transplants, etc.), it is unfortunate that no one has built into the planning the necessary ingredients to make those saved lives productive, dignified, and livable.

In 1972, 3,400 delegates gathered in Washington, D.C. for the White House Conference on Aging. Throughout the conference ran the theme that a basically youth-oriented, urbanized, and fast-paced American society has failed to provide an integrated role for the elderly. Statistics cited revealed that one fourth of persons aged 65 and over live below the poverty level, 40 percent of couples and more than 60 percent of single persons live below the Bureau of Labor Statistics moderate budgets of $4,489 and $2,301, respectively; and, despite increases in Social Security, the benefits still fall almost $300 below the poverty threshold. Housing costs have risen more than 25 percent since 1967 and actually have outstripped the general increase in the cost of living. Added to this is the fact that Medicare and Medicaid programs have been cut back in a number of states at the same time that premium costs have nearly doubled.

Statistical trends continue. One in ten Americans is now a senior citizen. Approximately three-fifths of the 9.9 percent of the population who are over 65 years of age live in metropolitan areas. Thirty percent live alone while 7 percent are in institutions. Health continues to be a major concern, and although modern medicine has made great strides for some, dedication to finding relief for the problems of the chronically ill is often wanting. It is still very difficult to find qualified physicians and allied health personnel who will work in facilities involved primarily in long-term care. Therefore, the need still exists to state that more enlightened management than prevails today is required and must be made available to these chronically ill older people in order to keep them well, self-sufficient, and respected for as long as possible.

It should no longer happen that aged persons, paralyzed by a stroke, be simply put to bed and allowed to become permanent invalids. It should no longer happen that the misguided efforts of their own uninformed families prevent such patients from taking part in the daily activities of living and from becoming self-sufficient. It should no longer happen that elderly patients with fractured hips be immobilized for long

1

periods of time without restorative surgery and without rehabilitation exercises, thus needlessly becoming permanently crippled. It should no longer happen that an aged paraplegic, whose spine was injured in a fall, be placed in a nursing home to linger on without any rehabilitation measures. It should no longer happen that urological, ophthalmological, and other surgery be denied these patients merely because of their advanced age. Yet, these examples of poor practice and mismanagement still occur, because the proper attitude toward chronic disease is not being emphasized in medical teaching.

What, then, are the main pillars of the modern effective management of chronic illness that will maintain patients in functional condition and reduce to a minimum their dependence and immobilization? First and foremost, patients, families, ancillary medical personnel, and, above all, the attending physician himself must realize that much can be done for the majority of elderly, incapacitated persons. One requisite is up-to-date knowledge of the treatment and rehabilitation aspects of the disorders being faced. For instance, it is necessary to know that most stroke patients who are able to understand simple commands can be retrained to dress, feed, and bathe themselves, handle their own toilet, and walk; that paraplegics can respond to bladder, wheelchair, and gait training, and that some can eventually become employable; and that patients with fractured hips need exercises to maintain strength in their arms and the unaffected leg. It is equally necessary to know where the services so desperately needed by these patients can be obtained and what the various paramedical personnel— the physical, occupational, and speech therapists, especially—are able to provide for them. One should also be familiar with some of the simple, basic techniques designed to protect patients from secondary complications or at least know where to find this information when it is needed.

A reasonable amount of daring is required in the care of some of these patients, since in many instances generally accepted, conservative methods of management do not provide the patients with the motivation, activity, defect repair, and security that are indispensable to achievement of their goals. Indeed, better management methods demand new approaches, new mechanisms of action, new equipment, new therapies—even new and daring thoughts.

Those caring for these unfortunate people must have faith—faith in their own ability to handle patients and their problems in the most effective manner possible. They must have faith in their own knowledge and skill, even though the treatment they propose may conceivably differ from currently accepted methods. Above all, they must have faith in their patients, faith that they will have, or will develop, the motivation, will make the effort, and will achieve their ultimate goals—activity and independence.

Courage and determination are required in order to set high goals for a rehabilitation program, even though it would be easier to follow the path of least resistance by lowering these aims. How far the patient will progress toward achievement of his program is never predictable, yet each one must be given the opportunity to *attempt* full rehabilitation before he is left to live out his life in useless inactivity. Finally, two intangibles assume the greatest importance in the care of chronically ill patients. These are love and understanding, both of which assist immeasurably in promoting good readjustment and eventual rehabilitation of the patient beset by physical and emotional problems.

When all these factors—awareness of the problem, and knowledge, daring, faith, love, and understanding—are intelligently applied to the problems of chronically ill people, it becomes possible to redeem the individual destined to oblivion; it becomes possible for many a difficult case, given up as hopeless by others, to return to an active and useful role in society. Thus, the elderly hemiplegic can return to his work, the partially immobilized patient can enjoy limited activity; the hip-fracture patient can walk again, the paraplegic can become self-sufficient; and no one will be denied the opportunity for necessary surgical repair solely on the basis of advanced age.

I
Specific Problems

1
Cancer

All too often, rehabilitation of the cancer patient is equated with measures taken following surgical excision of an organ, e.g., laryngectomy. A much broader focus is needed, in concept and practice. This concept of rehabilitation is succinctly stated in the *National Cancer Plan,* as its seventh program objective: "to restore patients with residual deficits as a consequence of their disease or treatment to as nearly a normal functioning state as possible." In this context, rehabilitation may be practiced as a continuing process of comprehensive care for the cancer patient (and his family), aimed at achieving as much function, as much physical and emotional comfort, and as normal social and occupational living as can be achieved under the changing conditions imposed by his disease. Thus, management of the cancer patient is concerned not only with his survival, but with the quality of survival. It addresses itself not only to the initial phase of cancer when curative measures are attempted, but to the continuing management undertaken for the patients who have not been cured.

THE CANCER PROBLEM

It was estimated that 650,000 new cases of cancer would be diagnosed in the United States in 1972. More than 52,000,000 Americans now living will probably develop cancer, according to the present rate, one person out of four. In 1972, it was estimated that there would be 345,-000 cancer deaths. Cancer is second only to heart disease as a cause of death in the United States. In children, it is second only to accidents as a cause of death. In American women, ages 35 to 54, it is the commonest cause of death.

Cancer occurs at all ages, from infancy to old age. The majority of cancer patients are in their years of greatest productivity, with family, social, and community responsibilities. The loss due to disability and death is enormous.

Of the 650,000 new cancer patients, it is estimated that one out of three will be cured. This includes 118,000 patients with skin cancer, of whom 95 percent will be cured. Treating and rehabilitating cancer patients involves not only the one out of three who may be cured, but controlling and trying to rehabilitate the majority who are not cured.

Cancers are characterized by proliferation of abnormal cells growing into tumor masses. The cancer cells differ from their normal counterparts in their microscopic appearance and their function. Cancer cells may originate in any body tissue and invade locally by direct extension. They can also spread to other parts of the body (metastasize) via blood or lymphatic vessels. These metastatic cells can then grow in the tissues where they have lodged. All cancers are malignant in their potential to cause death if not cured or controlled.

Cancer is a group of diseases with the above general characteristics; within this group are hundreds of different cancers. Each is characterized by a specific cancer cell, originating in a specific organ. Table 1, depicting cancer incidence by site, refers to broad categories in each of which many different types of cancer are represented. To compound the problems of pre-

TABLE 1. INCIDENCE OF CANCER BY SITE AND SEX

	Male	Female
Skin	23%	13%
Oral	3%	2%
Breast		23%
Lung	18%	5%
Colon & Rectum	11%	13%
Other Digestive	11%	7%
Prostate	11%	
Uterus		14%
Urinary	6%	3%
Leukemia & Lymphomas	7%	6%
All Others	10%	14%

vention, diagnosis, and treatment of this multiplicity of diseases, each cancer may initially present as a minute primary focus, or as an extensive tumor confined to the primary site, or as spreading regionally. In these localized presentations, the potential for cure by surgery or radiation therapy is relatively high. The malignancy may be of diffuse involvement, such as in the leukemias, or the cancer may have metastasized widely. In such instances, cure cannot be achieved by local measures.

Cancers cause specific symptoms, disability, and eventually death by a variety of mechanisms. The invasive and destructive characteristics of primary and metastatic tumors may lead to hemorrhage, obstruction, pain, or loss of function. Direct and indirect effects of the tumors may cause anorexia, inanition, infection, neurological deficits, and hormonal, fluid, or electrolyte disturbances. The course of the disease may be characterized by slow or rapid growth, local confinement or widespread metastases; it may become an acute, rapidly fatal disease or a chronic impairment. The course is not invariably downhill. Spontaneous remissions and exacerbations of symptoms are not rare. Complicating secondary illnesses occur frequently and are treatable. Some cancer patients have a chronic course, with little disability from their cancer, and die of another cause.

GOALS IN THE TOTAL CARE OF THE CANCER PATIENT

The *National Cancer Plan*, in its sixth and seventh objectives, outlines as goals of treatment:

Objective 6: to cure as many patients as possible and to maintain maximum control of the cancerous process in patients not cured.

Objective 7: to restore patients with residual deficits as a consequence of their disease or treatment to as nearly a normal functioning state as possible.

In general, the total care required to attain these goals involves measures aimed at: (1) prevention, (2) cure, (3) control and palliation, and (4) rehabilitation.

Comprehensive care involves treating not only the direct manifestations of the cancer, but its secondary effects and complications. Therefore, throughout the course of the disease, at one time or another, benefit may be achieved by measures that are curative, preventive, controlling and palliative, rehabilitative, or supportive. By carefully following the condition of the cancer patient, by treating problems as they arise, and anticipating others that may occur, the doctor may benefit the cancer patient as much as is feasible under the changing situations imposed by his disease and his environment. At times the goals are high, e.g., cure and complete rehabilitation. At other times the situation dictates more limited goals, e.g., control, palliation, and partial rehabilitation. Finally, the goals may be limited to physical and emotional support, with concern for the family as well as the patient.

PREVENTION

The ideal way to control cancer is to prevent it. This requires knowing what causes a specific cancer and being able to remove it from the human environment or to minimize the exposure. For example, it has been demonstrated that cigarette smoking is a major factor in causing lung cancer. It is also known that some people develop more than one cancer in a lifetime. Therefore, preventive measures can be undertaken even for the patient who already has cancer. For example, if surgery has been undertaken for cure in a patient with lung cancer, if he stops smoking, he may have a lesser chance of developing a second lung cancer. Even more significant, if this is applied to his family and friends, and if some of them stop smoking, they will have a better chance of not developing lung cancer. Another example is skin cancer which is related to overexposure to sunlight in some people. When these patients are cured by surgery or radiation therapy, avoiding further exposure to the sun may prevent their developing new skin cancers.

Unfortunately, the causes of very few human cancers are known, thus the ability to prevent most of them is limited. The principles of preventive medicine, however, are applicable in the comprehensive care of cancer patients. Preventive measures may be undertaken by anticipating events that are likely to occur during the course of disease, whether caused by the cancer directly or indirectly, by complications of the disease, or by side effects of therapy. For example, if a patient has extensive destruction of a weight-bearing bone, the femur, that is in imminent danger of fracture, radiation therapy to the involved femur may arrest the destruction and prevent fracture. Another example is seen in Hodgkin's disease, when successful treatment by radiation or chemotherapy with rapid tumor destruction may cause hyperuricemia and renal failure. Prophylactic Allopurinal therapy will prevent the hyperuricemia and its consequences. A wide variety of measures are available to prevent or ameliorate complications throughout a cancer patient's course. With this outlook, preventive measures may significantly affect cancer control and rehabilitation.

CURE

Once cancer has developed, the ideal is to cure the patient and achieve total rehabilitation. Cure may be achieved, depending on the type of cancer and its extent when first diagnosed. For example, the great majority of patients with skin cancer are cured, whereas cures are achieved in only a minority of patients with lung cancer. Cancer of the cervix is highly curable in its earliest stages, whereas cures are less frequent when there is extensive local spread. Earlier diagnosis of cancer of the cervix is achievable by routine screening with Papanicolau smears, resulting in earlier treatment and a higher cure rate.

Cure is achieved in most instances by surgery, i.e., by totally removing the primary cancer and its regional spread, if localized. Certain cancers, e.g., localized cancer of the cervix, are cured by radiation therapy. Chemotherapy, the third major form of cancer treatment, rarely achieves cure. There are exceptions, however. The majority of women with choriocarcinoma are cured with chemotherapy, even if the tumor has metastasized. Some patients with acute leukemia may be cured by chemotherapy. In some instances, cures are achieved by a combination of two or three treatment modalities. For example, a higher cure rate is achieved in Wilms' tumor by combined radiation therapy, surgery, and chemotherapy.

In addition to the initial efforts to cure the presenting tumor, curative measures may have a continuing role in the management of the cancer patient. For example, the patient, who may be cured of his first cancer, may also have a second coexisting malignancy or may subsequently develop one. Curative measures are indicated also for coexisting nonmalignant diseases and for disease complicating the cancer or resulting as a side effect of therapy. These principles also apply in the total management of the patient who has not been cured of his initial cancer. For example, a woman with incurable Kaposi's sarcoma of the skin that has run an indolent course for twenty years and is not life-threatening may develop localized cancer of the cervix that is highly curable. Or a patient with Hodgkin's disease may develop pulmonary tuberculosis that can be cured.

CONTROL AND PALLIATION

For the majority of cancer patients, those in whom cure cannot be achieved, the goal is maximum control of the cancer and its complications. In some instances, treatment may result in apparently total reduction of all discernible and measurable tumor, with complete disappearance of all symptoms, and the patient is able to function normally. This complete response may last for months or years. In other situations a partial response is attainable. When these patients relapse, another complete or partial response may be again achieved. Under those circumstances, survival may be prolonged, and the quality of survival is good. In other patients, in whom objective tumor responses have not been achieved, significant improvement in symptoms (palliation) and function may be obtained by specific antitumor therapy or by symptomatic treatment. In these cases, survival may not be lengthened, but the quality of survival is improved. In all these patients, direct or indirect complications of the cancer or therapy may arise, and nonrelated disease may occur. Diagnosis and treatment of the secondary events may result in their cure, control, or palliation.

The therapeutic modalities for specific antitumor effects include surgery, radiation therapy, chemotherapy, and hormone therapy in some cancers. Surgery has a continuing role in managing the advanced cancer patient by relieving obstruction, arresting hemorrhage, draining abcesses, stabilizing fractures, or relieving intractable pain by neurosurgical procedures. Generally, these are local measures for localized complications. In some cancers, e.g., breast or prostate, ablative surgery (oophorectomy, adrenalectomy, hypophysectomy, or orchiectomy) may result in marked regression of widely metastatic tumor. Significant antitumor effect may also be obtained by administering hormones: androgens or estrogens in breast cancer, estrogens in prostate cancer, and progesterone in endometrial cancer. Radiation therapy is a potent tool in the control of tumor and its complications, particularly for localized problems, in arresting hemorrhage, relieving obstruction, healing ulcerating tumors, and relieving pain. Dramatic improvement is frequently obtained by radiation therapy for brain metastases, obstruction of the superior vena cava, and compression of the spinal cord. Chemotherapy, with its potential for systemic antitumor effect, is an effective means for controlling the cancers that are sensitive to the various agents available. Some cancers are highly sensitive to specific agents and others moderately sensitive, so that complete or partial responses are obtained with single agent chemotherapy. The skillful use of combination chemotherapy (several drugs with different modes of action) has achieved more complete responses and longer survival in several cancers, e.g., acute lymphocytic leukemia and Hodgkin's disease. In some situations, localized chemotherapy may achieve local control, e.g., intrapleural instillation for malignant pleural effusion.

Thus, in cancer patients who have not been cured, the skillful use of surgery, radiation therapy, and chemotherapy may afford effective control and certainly significant palliation.

REHABILITATION

Cancer may cause a variety of acute or chronic disabilities stemming from the disease or its complications or arising secondary to treatment. The disabilities may be physical or psychological, and frequently the two combine. These disabilities may occur early or may appear with multiple manifestations throughout the course of the chronic illness. Disability may occur in cancer patients who are cured as well as in those who are not. The disability may be temporary and completely reversible or permanent. Rehabilitation, as part of comprehensive care, aims at restoring as much function, achieving as much physical and emotional comfort, and returning the patient to as normal a social and occupational a life as is possible under the conditions imposed by his disease. Rehabilitation, whether total or partial, permanent or temporary, affects not only the patient, but his family and his society.

Thus, the goal of rehabilitation is to restore the cancer patient to function at his optimal level physically, emotionally, socially, and vocationally. Ideally, rehabilitation is an integral part of his comprehensive care. Rehabilitation care should be developed concomitant with specific cancer therapy. It should be offered not only to the patient who is potentially curable, but to the larger number of patients who have not been cured. Concomitant with efforts to maintain maximum control or palliation, worthwhile rehabilitation should be sought throughout the patient's course.

Obviously, the results of rehabilitation treatment depend on the problems imposed in the individual patient. It has been stated that 80 percent of unselected cancer patients are improved by rehabilitation treatment. One-third become fully independent and are restored to full function or become fully independent with residual permanent disability, needing further training (e.g., the amputee or the laryngectomy patient). The remainder of the patients who improve by rehabilitative measures experience varying degrees of physical and psychological benefit.

The actual and potential disability occurring after curative therapy may result from the psychological impact of the disease on the patient and his family, as well as from the therapy undertaken for cure. For example, in the woman who has had a radical mastectomy for breast cancer, rehabilitative measures are taken for several actual or potential difficulties. The patient and her husband are assisted in their emotional adjustment to her disease and to the operation. Exercises are undertaken to maintain range of motion and function of the arm and shoulder. The patient is instructed in arm care, positioning, and active exercises to help prevent lymphedema. To restore physical and cosmetic balance, the patient is advised in the selection of a breast prosthesis.

Many patients who have been treated for cure may have no residual physical disability and may require mainly psychological support and careful follow-up. In others, the curative therapy involves radical surgery with major functional, cosmetic, and psychological disabilities. For example, radical surgery for head and neck cancers may require a prolonged, complicated rehabilitative regimen involving plastic surgical and orthodontic reconstruction and the provision of prostheses to compensate for the multiple functional and cosmetic deficits. Psychological support is a major requirement for these patients, to assist them to adjust to the disfigurement, to the functional deficits, and to the difficult return to family and occupation.

For patients who cannot be cured when they are first evaluated, the need for rehabilitation may be as great, albeit the challenge is greater. For example, one may consider two men with cancer of the rectum, the one potentially curable, the other incurable. In the first, abdominoperineal resection and colostomy are done. Rehabilitation is started prior to the operation by explaining what the therapy involves and how the patient will be able to adjust to the function of his colostomy. Postoperatively, the patient is instructed in the self-care of his colostomy. Regular follow-up and instruction help initiate a program of good care, confidence, and adjustment to the colostomy. Instruction of the family is helpful. In the second patient, whose cancer is not curable, the situation may be that at operation liver metastases were found. However, the rectal tumor was partially obstructing, but resectable. Accordingly, an abdominoperineal resection and colostomy were done to prevent the complication of obstruction and perineal spread. In spite of his limited survival, which may be just for one or several years, the patient might be able to return to his home, family, and occupation. Accordingly, he will benefit from the same colostomy rehabilitation program and perhaps receive benefit from chemotherapy and other measures indicated for his comprehensive management for the duration of his life.

Another example of comprehensive care and rehabilitation for the patient who is not cured may be a woman with breast cancer, in whom radical mastectomy for cure was done four years previously. The rehabilitative measures for the mastectomy patient were followed with successful return to her normal living as a wife and mother. Careful, periodic follow-up examinations were normal, until four years after mastectomy, when x-rays revealed bone metastases, although the patient was asymptomatic. Fairly good control of her metastases was obtained by hormonal measures and later with chemotherapy. Three years later, however, she developed a pathological fracture of the femur. Active orthopedic management involved internal fixation of the fracture, postoperative radiation therapy, and re-

habilitation to the point of her being able to walk and return home. The alternative to this management would have been immobilization in bed with traction, pain, medications, confinement in the hospital, later in a nursing home, and the complications of prolonged immobilization in bed.

Thus, comprehensive management of the cancer patient involves ongoing assessment of the need and the potential for rehabilitative measures. It is applicable not only to the patient who may be cured, but to those who are not cured. It aims to overcome the initial shock of sudden disability and the consequent fear, depression, and withdrawal. Even when life expectancy is limited, rehabilitation to functioning at maximum potential is valuable to the patient, his family, and the community, even if the results are partial and temporary.

REFERENCES

Cancer Facts and Figures. New York: American Cancer Society, 1972.

J. E. HEALEY, JR., ed. *Ecology of the Cancer Patient.* Washington, D.C.: Interdisciplinary Communication Associates, Inc., 1970.

National Cancer Plan. Bethesda, Md.: National Cancer Institute, 1972.

Rehabilitation of the Cancer Patient. M. D. Anderson Hospital, Houston, Texas. Chicago: Year Book, 1972.

P. REUBIN, ed. *Clinical Oncology for Medical Students and Physicians, a Multidisciplinary Approach* (3rd ed.) New York: American Cancer Society, 1971.

2
Arthritis

In the minds of most people, the term *arthritis* has become identified with any disease that causes pain in or around a joint, and when such pains are dull and persistent, people immediately suspect that they are suffering from rheumatism. Since a host of diseases can cause pain in the muscles, tendons, bursae, and joints, it is often difficult both to determine the exact nature of the underlying cause and, accordingly, to treat and to cure or control the disease. Do-it-yourself medication for such aches and pains at any age is therefore ill advised, and it may readily be seen that when symptoms of arthritis or rheumatism persist, a competent physician should be consulted without delay. This offers two distinct advantages: (1) the disease may possibly be arrested, and (2) lost motion and function may be restored.

ARTHRITIS

In the strict sense of the word, *arthritis* signifies any inflammatory change of any joint. In actual practice, the concept of arthritis embraces an even wider range of pathological conditions. Anyone with painful symptoms in the neighborhood of a joint is usually told, at one time or another during the illness, that his or her trouble is "arthritis." Anything from myositis, bursitis, or neuritis to osteomyelitis or metastases from malignant lesions may thus be falsely labeled *arthritis*, either deliberately to satisfy the patient's curiosity as to the cause of the pain by giving it a casual, acceptable label, or unintentionally by including in the diagnosis of arthritis some of the conditions listed above, which may occasionally present real problems of differential diagnosis.

This chapter on arthritis includes rheumatoid arthritis, osteoarthritis, which is better called *osteoarthrosis* because it is a degenerative and not an inflammatory disorder, and gouty arthritis. These three separate entities have in common that they manifest some of their most striking and incapacitating symptoms in joints. Apart from that they are, in fact, entirely different diseases with distinctly separate etiology, pathogenesis, and pathology. Rheumatoid arthritis is a manifestation of a systemic disease; the osteoarthroses are probably the end results of a combined effect of metabolic anomalies and gradual degeneration through use and aging; and gouty arthritis is the result of an error in metabolism.

RHEUMATOID ARTHRITIS

The term *atrophic arthritis* is often used synonymously with rheumatoid, inflammatory, chronic proliferative arthritis, and arthritis deformans, to distinguish this condition from the hypertrophic osteoarthroses. Rheumatoid arthritis is an extremely prevalent and always chronic disorder that may occur at any time of life and takes many forms according to the patient's age, the location of the affected joints, and many other factors. As is often the case in medicine, where least is known about a disease the most intricate classifications and morphological descriptions have been devised and will no doubt become totally obsolete once the true nature of the disease has become apparent. The classification of the New York Rheumatism Association lists the following subtypes under the heading of rheumatoid arthritis (atrophic, chronic infectious):

1. Adult type
2. Juvenile type (Still's disease)
3. Ankylosing spondylarthritis (Strümpell-Marie, etc.)
4. Psoriatic arthritis

In the light of the concept of diseases of adaptation and responses to stress conceived by Hans Selye, it becomes possible that all these varied manifestations are adaptive responses of the organism to various stresses and that other types of joint responses, such as the arthritis of serum sickness and lupus erythematosus, may fall under the same classification of disease. Various joint, skin, and other connective-tissue manifestations may merely represent symptoms of a broad type of body response to certain unspecific stresses.

These manifestations may take the form of vague muscle pains and stiffness or inflammation of specialized structures, such as bursae, tendon sheaths, and joint synovial membranes, and may eventually progress to fibrosis and irreversible changes in such structures.

The cause of rheumatoid arthritis, however, remains unknown, despite years of study. It may possibly result from the action of a variety of triggering mechanisms. Some investigators speculate that microorganisms may play a major role in its development. Among the organisms under investigation are viruses, pleuropneumonia-like organisms (*Mycoplasma*), streptococci, and organisms of the psittacosis-lymphogranuloma-venereum-trachoma group (*Bedsonia*).

It is postulated that a microorganism sets off the disease process, with the tissue at the joint responding in an inflammatory manner, primarily at a cellular level. During this process, gamma globulin may be produced as an antibody to the microorganisms, subconstituents of the microorganisms, or even to local altered connective-tissue constituents. The 7-S gamma globulin may become altered in its combination with these microorganisms or constituents.

DIFFERENTIAL DIAGNOSIS AND SPONTANEOUS COURSE

Rheumatoid arthritis affects women twice as often as men, but age is no aid in the diagnosis, since the disease may attack at any age. The onset of rheumatoid arthritis may be insidious or rapid. In the first case the diagnosis may be difficult in early stages, and in the second instance it is often hard to differentiate the disease from acute rheumatic fever. Prodromal symptoms such as fatigue and weakness may precede by weeks or months the involvement of joints. Eventually the polyarticular, usually symmetrical, involvement of joints appears and the disease becomes more typical. The proximal interphalangeal joints of the fingers are often first affected with involvement of the metacarpophalangeal joints, knees, wrists, feet, shoulders, elbows, and hips following in order of frequency.

During the typical active stage of the disease a positive diagnosis can usually be made with considerable accuracy. Swelling and pain in several joints, accelerated sedimentation rate of red blood cells, mild hypochromic anemia, sometimes with moderate leukocytosis, and typical x-ray findings of affected joints are usually present.

A number of diagnostic serological tests are based on the presence of a "rheumatoid agglutinating factor" in the serum of patients with rheumatoid arthritis. Three commonly used tests of this nature are: the *Waaler-Rose procedure*, which employs sheep cells; the *Fraction II test* of Heller et al., in which tanned sheep cells coated with Cohn fraction II are used; and the *latex fixation test* of Singer and Plotz, in which latex particles coated with human gamma globulin are used. Positive results are obtained in over 70 percent of patients with rheumatoid arthritis, but false-positive findings occur in about 5 percent of normal subjects. This indicates that these tests cannot substitute for sound clinical judgment.

The course of the disease, which is nearly always progressive, may be foretold to some extent, although it is characterized by alternations between periods of active progression and spontaneous remission.

With simple medical and orthopedic measures as the only treatment, Short and Bauer found that of 250 patients with rheumatoid arthritis, 200 of whom they followed for 5 years, 15 percent were in remission, 38 percent were somewhat improved, 13 percent were the same, and 34 percent were worse. These figures must be kept in mind when evaluating any form of treatment.

In order to evaluate the rate of progression or the effect of therapy, it is well to record the patient's status at regular intervals, using the classification of Steinbrocker et al. (see Table 2). Guesswork is thus reduced to a minimum, and therapy may be evaluated in a quantitative fashion.

CONVENTIONAL THERAPY

Because little is known about rheumatoid arthritis and because it is a severe and crippling chronic disease, innumerable methods of treatment have been suggested and used at one time or another, with varying degrees of success. The spontaneous course of the untreated disease is so capricious that one must admit that many spontaneous remissions occur in a patient's lifetime, regardless of therapy.

The goals of any antiarthritic therapy are the reduction of pain in the affected joints and the prevention of the crippling irreversible lesions. There is today no known treatment that can eradicate the cause of the disorder.

The coexistence of pain with articular changes that limit joint mobility creates a vicious circle, because immobilization results in further stiffening, painful osteoporosis from disuse, and muscular atrophy: all phenomena that in turn render

motion ever more difficult. Although it is common practice, based on no well-controlled evidence, to recommend rest for the arthritic patient, exercise is, in fact, perhaps the most important single therapeutic agent for the sufferer, and one that not only will sometimes retard the crippling manifestations of the disease but also will prevent the occurrence of the secondary complicating disorders just mentioned. In order to render exercises possible, analgesia is extremely important.

Salicylates are the old stand-by in the therapeutic armamentarium and should be used freely and in amounts as needed, up to tolerance. The tolerance of patients for salicylates is variable. Some will do well on large doses of aspirin, but others will have gastrointestinal difficulties with such medication. It is sometimes possible to improve tolerance by the simultaneous use of antacids, and many salicylate preparations are on the market that contain such agents in addition to the salicylate.

The mechanism of action of salicylates, apart from their analgesic effects, is quite obscure, but there is evidence that in some respects they may imitate certain effects of ACTH and therefore are perhaps more than just analgesics in the management of rheumatoid arthritis. There are many other useful analgesics, including codeine (0.015 gm., repeated as necessary), acetaminophens, such as Tylenol, phenacetin, propoxyphene HCl (Darvon), and Percodan, which (until a perfect analgesic is found) must be used only when joint pains are intolerably severe.

It is impossible to give a dosage schedule for salicylates that would suit most patients. Doses recommended in standard texts vary from 0.3 to 0.5 gm. of sodium salicylate after meals and before bed, to 0.9 gm. every three hours. Doses of as high as 12 gm. per day have been given in some cases without undesirable side effects. On the other hand, with such high doses hemorrhagic complications may occur before tinnitus or gastric discomfort arise as warning signs of overdosage. That dose is the best which affords the

TABLE 2. CRITERIA FOR CLASSIFICATION OF THE STAGES OF SEVERITY AND DEGREES OF RESPONSE TO THERAPY OF PATIENTS WITH RHEUMATOID ARTHRITIS

A. Classification of Rheumatoid Progression

Stage	Roentgenologic Signs	Muscle Atrophy	Extraarticular Lesions (Nodules, Tenovaginitis)	Joint Deformity	Ankylosis
I	Osteoporosis; sometimes no destructive changes	0	0	0	0
II	Osteoporosis; slight cartilage or subchondral bone destruction may be present	Adjacent	May be present	0	0
III	Osteoporosis, cartilage destruction, bone destruction	Extensive	May be present	Subluxation, ulnar deviation and/or hyperextension	0
IV	Same as stage III, with bony ankylosis	Extensive	May be present	Same as stage III	Fibrous or bony ankylosis

B. Response of Rheumatoid Activity to Therapy

Grade	Systemic Signs	Signs of Joint Inflammation	Signs of Extraarticular Activity	Remaining Impairment of Joint Mobility	Articular Deformity	Erythrocyte Sedimentation Rate	Roentgenologic Signs
I Complete remission	0[a]	0[a]	0[a]	Due only to irreversible changes	Due only to irreversible changes	0[a]	No progression
II Major improvement	Elevated erythrocyte sedimentation rate and/or vasomotor imbalance permissible	Only minimum[a] residual joint swelling (no new sites)	Minimum[a] (no new sites)	Only consistent with minimum residual activity	Due only to irreversible changes	May be elevated	No progression
III Minor improvement	Decreased[a]	Only partially[a] resolved (no new sites)	Decreased[a] (no new sites)	In relation to residual inflammation	May be present	May be elevated	No progression
IV Not improved	Undiminished[a]	Same[a] or worse	Same or new sites or exacerbation[a]	Same, better or worse	Present or not	Any rate	Changes indicative of progression

[a] Indicates criteria required to be present.
SOURCE: Steinbrocker et al., *JAMA* 140:659–662, 1949.

patient reasonable comfort and does not cause toxic symptoms. This varies from case to case and must be determined by trial and error. Underdosage is, however, as poor medical practice as overdosage. The physician cannot merely prescribe a standard dose and hope for the best. He has to devote considerable time and effort to the patient with rheumatoid arthritis so that the best possible schedule of individual medication can be obtained.

Often, when a patient states that taking a lot of aspirin has not helped, it is well to determine whether or not the patient has achieved the desired salicylate level. He may be taking enteric-coated aspirin, which is not fully absorbed, or a compound which contains other drugs. A daily dosage to maintain a salicylate plasma level of 15 mg. percent, or just below the toxic level, is optimal.

Since tinnitus from high doses of aspirin may be insidious, particularly in older patients, the patient should check his own hearing periodically with a watch. When tinnitus occurs, the daily dose should be decreased by decrements of 0.6 or 0.9 gm. (10 to 15 grains) until the undesirable symptom disappears.

Since rheumatoid arthritis is a systemic disorder in which joint involvement is merely the most striking manifestation, numerous general measures have been advocated for its management. There is no conclusive evidence that any of these measures is more than a factor in the nature of psychotherapy. This holds true also for rest cures, spa treatment, changes of climate, diets, vitamin regimens, and such hormone therapies as desoxycorticosterone and vitamin C, pregnenolone, testosterone, and progesterone.

OTHER FORMS OF THERAPY

When results with salicylates are unsatisfactory, a trial of indomethacin (Indocin) might be considered. Its value in rheumatoid arthritis is still highly controversial, and it has often been given for nonspecific conditions where diagnosis has not been clearly established.

Dosage should start at 25 mg. a day and build up to a maintenance level of four a day over a two-week period. It should be taken with milk or food and should not be prescribed for children, pregnant women, psychotics, and other highly emotional patients.

The more common side effects include nausea, vomiting, diarrhea, dizziness, morning headache, and transient BUN elevations. Some patients are able to eliminate the headache by taking the medication with coffee. More severe complications include peptic ulceration, gross hematuria, tachycardia, and hepatitis, although the latter two have not been clearly implicated.

PHENYLBUTAZONE

Phenylbutazone (Butazolidin) alone or in combination with aminopyrine was studied by Stephens et al. (1952) and by Steinbrocker and his coworkers (1952) in the United States, a considerable literature on the substances having previously been accumulated in Europe. Their observations on more than 300 patients lasted from 3 to 455 days and therefore cannot be considered as adequate trials for these drugs in the long-term management of arthritis. The drugs were given by mouth in doses ranging from 200 to 1600 mg. per day, and in some cases intramuscular injections of up to 1500 mg. per day were used. Striking improvement followed therapy in a significant number of cases, particularly in patients with spondylarthritis, and somewhat less frequently in subjects with peripheral joint involvement. The incidence of toxic reactions, however, was high—up to 44 percent of the patients had some type of reaction, including skin rashes, depression of bone marrow and circulating blood elements, marked sodium retention with formation of edema, liver dysfunction, and severe gastrointestinal difficulties. This experience with phenylbutazone in rheumatoid arthritis shows that it should be used only in certain well-selected special situations.

Bimonthly blood counts and urinalysis must be made while the patient is on this drug. Some patients have been helped by short courses during a flare-up in the disease, while others have improved with phenylbutazone when all other therapeutic modalities have been ineffective. Maintenance doses of 100 to 200 mg. per day, used with the necessary precautions, should be adequate. It should be discontinued in one week if the patient does not improve.

Most experts reserve this drug for the treatment of gouty arthritis and ankylosing spondylitis, where a diagnostic trial of four to five days will usually bring dramatic relief of pain.

Butazolidin alka, which contains antacids, will help to prevent one of the more common side effects: peptic ulceration. Oxyphanbutazone (Tandearil) may be used in similar circumstances but has no special merit over the parent compound.

CHLOROQUINES

Chloroquine and its analogues are capable of exerting significant antirheumatic action for short periods of time; prolonged medication, however, results in sustained benefits without unpleasant side effects in only a minority of patients.

It appears that hydroxychloroquine (Plaquenil) has a smaller incidence of side effects than chloroquine phosphate (Aralen). Two ophthalmologic complications may occur: (1) pigmentary changes of the retina, which are completely irreversible, and (2) corneal changes, which are usually asymptomatic, manifested by halos around lights, or fuzzy vision. These latter are reversible when the drug is omitted.

The first condition is rare; the second occurs in about 10 percent of patients. A baseline ophthalmologic examination should be done at the outset and repeated every six months.

Other side effects are some blood dyscrasias, alopecia, and a lightening of hair color. Some patients show photosensitive reactions and should be warned to watch for hyperpigmentary changes on areas of the body which are exposed directly or indirectly to sunlight.

GOLD THERAPY

Gold salts were introduced into the therapeutic armamentarium for rheumatoid arthritis by European physicians in the late 1920s. Whether the rationale for this therapy was sounder than the reasoning that led Paracelsus to employ gold in the treatment of syphilis, or than that which prompted its use for a time in the treatment of tuberculosis, still remains to be seen. Gold is one of the most toxic therapeutic agents, with an incidence of lethal reactions of from 1 to 3 percent. Even though British antilewisite (BAL) provides a new means of hastening the excretion of gold salts in the presence of toxic manifestations, gold therapy is justifiable today only when given by those skilled in its use. Some physicians feel that injections of gold salts should be a last-resort measure that is best left to rheumatologists. Gold salts may be helpful during the first years of the disease, in its early, active, proliferative phase, and when the patient has not responded to a basic, conservative program. At least six months of failure on the basic program should precede the initiation of gold therapy. Generally, patients will respond to the following schedule: weekly injections of 10 mg. of gold sodium thiomalate (Myochrysine) or aurothioglucose (Solganal) the first two weeks; 25 mg. injections for the third and fourth weeks; and 40 to 50 mg. thereafter until a level of about 800 to 1,000 mg. total dose has been reached. Then the interval between injections may be gradually increased until the patient is being maintained on monthly injections of 50 to 75 mg. If a remission is to occur, it will happen within six months.

Patients should be warned about the possible side effects which take place in 40 percent of the cases so treated. These include malaise, giddiness, headache, vertigo, gastroenteritis, acute pulmonary edema, laryngeal edema, asthma, and cardiovascular collapse, focal reactions such as joint exacerbation, stomatitis, gastroenteritis, vomiting, diarrhea and abdominal pain, toxic nephritis, acute yellow atrophy, many forms of skin rashes (including severe exfoliative dermatitis), agranulocytosis, aplastic anemia, and peripheral neuritis.

Two misleading reactions may occur when a patient is on gold therapy:

1. If a rash occurs, determine whether it is pruritic before stopping treatment. The patient could be on another drug which causes the rash. If there is no itch, one can be reasonably sure that the gold is not to blame.

2. If a patient becomes flushed and warm all over and has palpitations and weakness within one half hour of the injection—and if these symptoms disappear as quickly as they arrived—this is not necessarily a serious reaction. This may be due to the proteins for colloidal suspension of the compound and can be eliminated by changing to another compound.

HORMONE THERAPY

Selye postulated several years ago that an excess of mineral corticoids (of the desoxycorticosterone type), as part of a "derailed" defense mechanism against continuous nonspecific stress, was the possible cause of diseases of adaptation, including arthritis; he thus tacitly implied that administration of glucocorticoids (such as cortisone) might be useful. This clue was not exploited further, and cortisone was introduced into the therapy of rheumatoid arthritis for entirely different and primarily empirical reasons that led to the same conclusions.

In their first preliminary report, Hench and his coworkers (1949) explained that they had been led to use Compound E (17-hydroxy-11-dehydrocorticosterone) in rheumatoid arthritis because Hench had been impressed since 1929 with the beneficial effects of pregnancy and jaundice upon arthritis and had reasoned that there must exist an "antirheumatic substance X" common to both pregnancy and jaundice. Many possible agents of this type were tested empirically, and it was finally conjectured that the agent sought might be an adrenal hormone. "This conjecture was strengthened by the knowledge that temporary remissions of rheumatoid arthritis are frequently induced by procedures which are known to be capable of stimulating the adrenal cortices, such as general anesthesia or surgical operations." Pregnancy and jaundice or their underlying causes may merely be two nonspecific stresses acting upon the pituitary-adrenal axis and stimulating it enough to influence favorably such a "disease of adaptation" as rheumatoid arthritis.

Hench and his associates were the first to use and report on cortisone in the treatment of rheumatoid arthritis. They treated fourteen patients, with moderately severe to severe chronic polyarticular rheumatoid arthritis of from 4½ months' to 5 years' duration, with doses of 100 mg. of cortisone acetate given intramuscularly daily for periods ranging from 6 days to 6 months. They observed rapid reduction of muscular stiffness, lessening of articular pain and tenderness, and significant improvement of articular and muscular function. They also noted that the patients lost their "toxicity" and had a sense of well-being and increased appetite. It soon became apparent also that in most cases the symptoms returned more or less rapidly and completely shortly after treatment was discontinued.

Neither cortisone, its derivatives, nor ACTH is the much sought antiarthritic substance X, but rather they interfere with the processes of inflammation, often blocking them completely. This antiinflammatory property is their greatest asset in the management of arthritis and also their greatest danger, since intercurrent inflammatory diseases such as pneumonia, appendicitis, or abscess formation may be completely masked in patients receiving cortisone. The antiinflammatory action also reduces the patient's resistance against infections, such as tuberculosis.

ACTH and cortisone have other physiological effects besides their antiinflammatory action, which must be kept in mind whenever these substances are given. The following are particularly important:

1. ACTH causes a stimulation of the adrenal cortex, with marked hypertrophy and with hyperadrenalism, simulating Cushing's disease. There is an increased excretion of nitrogen, potassium, and calcium, favoring the appearance of osteoporosis and hypokalemia. Diabetes and hypertension may occur. There may be marked retention of sodium and water. Obesity, hirsutism, acne, and Cushing's facies are other complications. When the adrenal glands are stimulated continuously for long periods of time by ACTH, there may be adrenal atrophy instead of hypertrophy, which cannot be maintained indefinitely, and the functional reserve of such glands is reduced. Under stress from various causes, such as infections, surgery, and so forth, such glands may not respond and fatal adrenal failure may occur unless it is anticipated and either prevented or treated as outlined below.

2. Cortisone in sufficient dosage will cause atrophy of the patient's adrenal glands and at the same time may cause all the symptoms of hyperadrenalism described above, by its own direct effects upon the target organs.

Since the advent of cortisone therapy, many related and less toxic compounds have been synthesized by several drug companies. These include hydrocortisone, prednisone, prednisolone, methyl prednisolone, prednisolone phosphate, prednisolone tertiary butyl acetate, triamcinolone, and dexamethasone. One advantage of these preparations is a marked reduction in all the side effects noted above so that in many instances on reasonable doses the patient experiences no changes in water, mineral, or carbohydrate metabolism. The minimal effective doses of these compounds are smaller than that of cortisone, 25 mg. of cortisone corresponding to 20 mg. of hydrocortisone, 5 mg. of the prednisone-prednisolone group, 4 mg. of triamcinolone and methyl prednisolone and 0.5 mg. of dexamethasone. The original cortisone and ACTH have few and specialized usages in recent years.

The use of triamcinolone must be closely supervised because it can cause a type of muscular atrophy which is seen more commonly in the quadriceps muscle of the thigh. This often makes walking difficult or impossible and cannot usually be controlled by physical-therapy exercises or anabolic agents.

Rules of Thumb for Hormone Therapy—Selection of Patients. Probably the first criterion in deciding when to use steroids is the failure of simpler measures. Rheumatoid arthritis may present itself in a variety of ways or degrees of severity. All such patients should receive immediate treatment with the use of conservative measures (basically salicylates and physical therapy) for as long as they are effective. Many patients will respond to this form of treatment, and pain, range of motion, and atrophy will be adequately controlled. However, if the disease cannot be controlled and it progresses with its crippling destruction, hormonal therapy is certainly indicated and should be tried. It does not offer a cure and is not a panacea, but there are certainly many thousands of patients today who have remained able to function on their own because of aggressive, intelligent use of steroids.

A thorough history, physical examination, and laboratory survey should precede the use of these agents. There are definite contraindications, such as active tuberculosis, severe diabetes mellitus, and malignant hypertension. There are further relative contraindications that must be assessed in relation to the severity of the disease and the rapidity with which irreversible joint destruction is taking place. These include hypertension, congestive heart failure, latent tuberculosis, peptic ulcer, chronic infection, and psychoses. Each case must of necessity be decided upon its own needs and merits because paradoxically these agents have at times been life-saving in some of these very instances noted as contraindications.

Techniques of Hormone Therapy. Once the decision has been made to proceed with steroids, the proper method must be chosen. If the active process involves one or few joints, it is best handled by local intraarticular injections. Excellent results in 85 to 90 percent of the joints treated have been seen in our series of cases over the past 20 years. Hydrocortisone or prednisolone tertiary butyl acetate have been used for these patients, and 72 percent of them have had remissions lasting longer than 8 weeks, with some complete and permanent remissions. The medication is instilled directly into the joint in doses ranging from 10 mg. (0.5 ml.) in small joints to 40 mg. (2 ml.) in joints such as the knee, ankle, shoulder, and wrist, and 100 mg. (5 ml.) in hip joints. Contrary to the usual manner of using isolated injections repeated only on return of symptoms, we believe the joint has to be treated aggressively by injecting the drug every other day for a course of 3 to 5 treatments. This usually suffices to create a long remission. Obviously this is done under strictest aseptic conditions utilizing autoclaved equipment and adequate antisepsis. Although a small number of joint infections due to intraarticular injection have been reported in the literature, the risk is small, provided caution is exercised. The actual procedure of injecting a joint is not difficult, and a thorough description of the technique and excellent illustrations are available in the 1960 edition of *Comroe's Arthritis and Allied Conditions.*

When the disease process involves multiple joints, intraarticular therapy becomes impractical and oral therapy is indicated. Usually oral treatment must be continued for a long period of time. The medication is first given in relatively high doses to suppress symptoms as soon as possible and then gradually reduced to minimum maintenance doses. Physical therapy should be used concomitantly. Joints that do not respond to oral therapy may be treated locally, as these routes of therapy complement each other.

These patients should be observed closely to ensure that mineral depletion, carbohydrate imbalance, protein depletion, hypertension, osteoporosis, peptic ulcers, or chronic infections do not develop. Because of the greater margin of safety of modern compounds, such complications are now rare.

The response to these agents occasionally seems to diminish after months or years of therapy. Their efficacy is sometimes restored by the administration of 20 to 40 units of Acthar Gel (repository corticotropin injection, U.S.P.) given 3 times per week during 1 month.

HISTIDINE

Recently it has been stated by Gerber that oral histidine, an amino acid found in most proteins, may be effective and harmless in producing clinical and laboratory improvement in patients with rheumatoid arthritis. Observations suggest that hypohistidinemia may participate in the pathogenesis of this disease by allowing gammaglobulin to aggregate and thereby become inflammatory. Histidine levels in rheumatoidarthritis patients are 28 percent less than in healthy persons. It is given as L-histidine in oral doses averaging 3 gm. per day. The patients' measured grip strength improved, walking time was reduced, and the sedimentation rate and anemia improved. Lesser amounts of other drugs were needed.

IMMUNOSUPPRESSIVE AGENTS

The use of chlorambucil, azathioprine, and cyclophosphamide is still in an experimental stage. These drugs seem to be effective in 30 to 40 percent of patients who fail on gold therapy. The first two seem to be relatively safe, but cyclophosphamide has a side effect incidence of 90 percent. At present, they are not commercially available and are used for investigative purposes only.

Penicillamine is another medication available for investigation only. Reports of its clinical use from Germany, Austria, France, and the United Kingdom as well as the United States demonstrate a marked degree of remission in 80 percent of the patients who are able to tolerate it. There is a high incidence of toxicity in almost all who receive it. It has been stated that for those who can tolerate it, a degree of disease control greater than that heretofore experienced with any other agent may often be achieved.

NITROGEN MUSTARD

Despite the initial enthusiasm which accompanied the first trials of nitrogen mustard, results have been generally disappointing. One of the greatest difficulties is that even when injected intraarticularly, systemic symptoms, including nausea, vomiting, and changes in white blood-cell count, may occur.

NONSPECIFIC THERAPY

The injection of foreign proteins, such as typhoid vaccine, or the mechanical production of high body temperatures is still recommended by some in the treatment of arthritis, but is of little or no value. Such measures are possibly no more than indirect ways of stimulating the beneficial secretion of endogenous ACTH and cortisone by nonspecific stress.

Intelligently planned analgesia coupled with constant, well-supervised *active* motion of all affected joints, except those most acutely inflamed, remains the cheapest and at the same time the most effective conventional management of rheumatoid arthritis. It is obvious that in all except the most severe cases such treatment can be given regularly at home or at a specialized outpatient department. As long as the patient is able to help himself there is no need for expensive hospitalization.

PHYSICAL THERAPY

Physical therapy is probably the most neglected, single effective therapeutic agent in the management of rheumatoid arthritis. Its aim is not the arrest of the inflammatory process, which it could not hope to accomplish, but rather the maintenance of the greatest possible mobility of involved joints for the longest possible period of time, the prevention of immobilizing muscular atrophy from disuse, and the retardation of the irreversible connective-tissue changes that result in contractures, deformities, and ankylosis. The modern concept of physical therapy in the management of rheumatoid arthritis is that of control of pain, prevention of immobilization, maintenance of function, and rehabilitation, rather than the old-fashioned concept of providing only heat and maintaining an adequate blood flow through massage and infrared and high-frequency electric waves.

Although whirlpool baths (as one form of moist heat) are indeed helpful, they are not indispensable. The bathtub can be effectively used in underwater exercises in order to increase blood circulation through the muscle mass. Simple homemade apparatus may be employed for the exercise of fingers, shoulder muscles, and leg muscles. These installations consist of a set of steps of varying height, a wooden "ladder" for finger exercises, bouncing putty for the same purpose, a simple wheel with an adjustable radius attached to the wall, wall bars, and simple pulley systems enabling patients to exercise against their own strength, and a bicycle stand with a graded resistance brake.

Exercises must be instituted progressively under a physician's direction, starting with a session that will neither hurt nor fatigue the patient, but which is designed to make clear to him the reasons for undertaking the quasi-religious course of exercises he is to make his daily habit. The extent of effort that is compatible with each patient's state of health must be carefully determined. It is often amazing how much more exertion a patient may take without ill effect than is estimated at the beginning of therapy. While the extent of effort in each session is individually determined and increased regularly, the schedule should, if possible, be a daily one without breaks, except when there is a contraindication, such as extreme inflammation of a joint or intercurrent disabling disease. These exercises to preserve joint range of motion are active in nature and avoid resistance unless an increase in muscle strength is a goal. Such resistive exercises should be undertaken only with strict professional guidance.

The patient can often be trusted to conduct his own exercise sessions at home, but a check should be made and new exercises added at least once a week. The Rheumatism and Arthritis Foundation has recognized this need and in some cities provides visiting physical therapists to conduct and supervise such therapy in patients' homes.

In order to apply these techniques effectively and safely, the supervision of a trained physical therapist is necessary, and the physician should be thoroughly familiar with the scope and limitations of the technique. However, where these prerequisites are not available, it is still worthwhile for the practitioner to attempt to give the patient the benefit of the simpler forms of exercises. Should resistive exercises be indicated, the principles have been recorded briefly by Watkins and may be summarized as follows:

It is well known by empirical observation, for example in the case of professional weight lifters, that muscle strength can be increased if muscles are exercised progressively against a near-maximal resistance. If this is done regularly, against increasing resistance that calls for a near-maximal voluntary effort, the effect of such exercises may be just as dramatic and significant in a patient whose muscle strength is impaired as it is in the normal person whose muscles are being subjected to such training with the aim of increasing strength over and above that initially present. Experience has shown that such exercises must be repeated not more often than 30 times in sequence and daily with one rest day each week. At the outset it is determined what load can be lifted by any given muscle 10 times and not more. This is called the *10-repetition maximum* and is used as the baseline for these exercises.

Exercise is begun with 50 percent of the 10-repetition maximum. This is used 10 times, and then, after a brief rest period, the load is increased to 75 percent of the 10-repetition maximum. This load is lifted 10 times and then the full 10-repetition maximum load is lifted 10 times. It has been found that, if the exercises are repeated 50 to 100 times, their effectiveness is reduced rather than increased, since the average patient cannot produce maximum muscle contractions under the conditions of this exercise more often than about 30 times in succession.

The rest day each week is set aside to determine a new 10-repetition maximum upon which to base the exercises of the following week. At first there may be a rapid increase of strength, which is due in part to the fact that the patient has acquired skill for some particular type of exercise, but thereafter one may expect a steady and progressive increase in the 10-repetition maximum.

The technique is easiest to apply where the range of motion of a joint is relatively normal, but it becomes more complicated when it is necessary to exercise muscles that cannot freely move a segment of the extremity. This is best accomplished under the guidance of a competent physical therapist.

In the presence of subacute inflammation, resistance exercises must be used with caution, and they should not be used when acute inflammation is present. Except for these limitations, all affected joints should be exercised regularly. But in addition, special attention should be given to strengthening those muscles that will be most necessary later on to increase the patient's independence in daily needs, even though the joints in their vicinity may not be involved in the disease process. The technique is most useful for strengthening the quadriceps muscle in the case of knee involvement. It is extremely helpful to train a patient with multiple joint involvement, one who is still able to walk, to develop strong arm musculature that will make it easier for him to use crutches if the disease continues to develop. It is likewise desirable to develop a degree of ambidexterity, if involvement of either hand is likely to become incapacitating, and not to wait until this has come about. A great degree of tact and psychological acumen is required to achieve these preventive goals without unduly frightening the patient about what may be ahead for him.

PRINCIPLES OF JOINT PROTECTION

At the proper time, one should introduce the patient to preventive and protective measures related to his involved joints.

1. *Exercise.* The majority of the exercises in any arthritic program should be active in nature

and devoid of stress. Passive exercises, in many instances, may evoke involuntary protective muscle spasms which prevent satisfactory ranging. The patient is much less apprehensive when he can control his own activity. Sling suspension lends itself well to exercising arthritic joints. By neutralizing gravity and eliminating friction, it allows the patient to exercise specific joints of an extremity suspended in air quite freely.

2. *Positions of deformity.* In performing routine daily activities, patients frequently use certain joint positions which tend to foster deformity. For instance, many people, upon getting out of bed, push up with their fingers flexed into a fist, thus putting great stress on the knuckles. The open palm should be used. Opening jars and using manual can openers puts stress on the collateral ligaments of the fingers. Mechanical devices should be installed.

3. *Joint strength.* One should always use the strongest joint for the job. Instead of lifting a roasting pan out of the oven by using fingers and thumbs on the handles, put insulated mits on and place hands under the pan, thus taking the weight on wrists and elbows. Carry a heavy purse or shopping bag on the forearm, near the elbow instead of by the fingers.

4. *Joint stability.* Each joint should be used in its most stable, anatomical, and functional plane. One should learn to rise straight up from a chair instead of leaning to one side and pulling up over a table. This habit can place great rotational and lateral forces on the knee. Available quadriceps power should be used more advantageously. Push up using the arms of the chair, increase the height of the chair seat or install grab bars at appropriate places.

5. *Patterns of movement.* Incorrect patterns of movement caused by muscle imbalance or habit may lead to eventual deformity. When rising from a chair, hip and knee extension should occur concurrently, not sequentially, and the patient should straighten up completely before moving away. One should sit slowly and gently rather than flopping through the last few inches. It is important to maintain good posture at all times.

6. *Joint stasis.* It is good practice not to hold a joint or muscle in one position for an undue length of time. Muscles have a tendency to tire quickly during static holding. Not only is circulation hindered, but different parts of articular surfaces contact each other in different segments of the joint range, and holding in one position adds to the wear and tear at that point. Any activity taking longer than ten minutes should be done seated, but the patient should probably not remain seated for more than twenty minutes at a time.

7. *Endurance.* One should never attempt an activity that cannot be stopped immediately if it turns out to be beyond one's power to complete. If one uses a sliding board to transfer from chair to bed, one cannot get hung up in the middle of the transfer because of sudden collapse.

8. *Pain.* At all times pain must be respected. If an activity causes frank pain—stop it. One must learn to differentiate pain from discomfort. The latter usually recedes during a rest period and should be expected.

9. *Weight.* Excessive weight should be avoided. This includes not only the patient's own obesity, but wearing heavy coats, carrying heavy loads, etc. Household equipment should be put on wheels or a simple wheeled utility cart can be used to convey heavy objects.

In general, one should eliminate a regular, productive activity only as a last resort. Work toward work simplification by analyzing the task to be done, eliminating unnecessary steps, or combining operations. In other words, one must evaluate the possibility of making changes in either the method, equipment, order of work, or the finished product.

HOT AND COLD MODALITIES

Most arthritics experience significant relief from moist heat treatments. These may be provided by whirlpool baths for the extremities, the Hubbard tank for full body immersion, and by hot packs. At home, a bathtub may substitute for the whirlpool and hot (hydrocollator) packs may be purchased for home use. They are kept in a deep pot of water and heated as needed. They must be well wrapped in heavy toweling to prevent burns.

Paraffin provides an excellent medium to supply heat to the hands. One needs blocks of paraffin, such as those used in home canning, mineral oil, and a double boiler. Place six parts of paraffin to one part of mineral oil in a total quantity sufficient to cover the hands in the top of the double boiler. Heat until the mixture reaches 120° to 128° F. Test with a thermometer. At that point, remove from the heat and let it cool until a thin film begins to form on the top. Dip one hand at a time into this cooling mixture and remove immediately, allowing a thin film to remain on the hand. Repeat this until the hand is covered with enough layers to simulate a thick glove. Wrap the treated hand in wax paper and then a heavy towel. After 30 minutes, the fingers can be wriggled, thus loosening the paraffin, which can then be returned to the double boiler for reuse.

In some instances, soaking a painful joint alternately in hot and cold water helps to relieve discomfort. This is called a *contrast bath*. For this treatment, one needs two containers large enough to immerse the affected joints. A double sink or two oval plastic buckets might be ideal. Fill one container with hot water at 105° to 110° F and the other with cold water at 50° to 65° F. Test with a thermometer for accuracy. First, immerse the painful joint in the hot water for ten minutes and immediately transfer it to the cold water for one minute. Reduce the time in the hot water to four minutes followed by one minute in the cold. Repeat this sequence for 25 to 30 minutes, with the last immersion always being in the hot water.

There are occasional patients who claim to feel worse with heat and sometimes benefit from ice-pack applications.

In many cases, ankyloses will develop in some joints in spite of all therapeutic efforts. These should never be allowed to cripple the patient without thorough exploration by competent orthopedists for the possibilities that restorative joint surgery might have to offer. The use of surgery in a medical condition is nearly always an admission of defeat by the internist. It should be stated, however, that this is one situation in which surgery can be extremely helpful to the internist, assisting him to prevent by mechanical means some of the deformities that are apt to occur and to correct others when they have occurred.

Among surgical procedures that may be helpful are the following:

Hip: arthroplasty to relieve pain in a patient who must continue to work. This may be a cup arthroplasty, a Moore prosthesis, or the recently developed total hip replacement.

Knee: synovectomy, arthrodesis, surgical osteotomy, femoral stem replacement, or tibial metallic implants of the McKeever and MacIntosh design.

Hand: synovectomy, joint debridement, arthrodesis, arthroplasty, sometimes in combination with relocation of tendons, tenectomy, and tenodisis.

Spine and neck: fusion of C-1 to C-2 when x-rays show distinct subluxation.

Foot: removal of the head of the metatarsal and proximal portion of the first phalanx to provide substantial relief from dropped metatarsal heads.

Of these surgical procedures, the one under active discussion is synovectomy. In the past, most surgeons waited until the patient's joints had undergone extensive destruction before advising this procedure. Recently, the pendulum has swung the other way. Particularly for the knee, wrist, and hand, when there has been marked synovial thickening, early synovectomy is now considered important in preserving joint function. It is no longer considered necessary to wait until the disease is inactive before operating.

In the hand, synovectomy might be combined with relocation of the extensor tendons to the fingers, which may have slipped down into the intermetacarpal spaces. If there has been destruction of the interphalangeal joints, arthrodesis might be performed to restore the function of grasp.

Correction of hand deformity has a tremendous value to the patient psychologically as well as physically. The hand, like the face, is constantly exposed to social interaction.

OSTEOARTHRITIS

Osteoarthritis is a degenerative joint disease that is also designated as *hypertrophic arthritis, degenerative arthritis, arthritis deformans,* and *senescent arthritis.* The pathological changes found in affected joints consist of degeneration of the hyaline articular cartilage, which increases friction as the joint surfaces move against each other. Weight bearing by the unprotected joint surfaces results in abnormalities in the subchondral bone, with the most pronounced lesions and bone condensation in those areas bearing the greatest weight. The resulting mechanical stresses produce hypertrophy and marginal proliferation.

The etiology of osteoarthritis is not well understood except perhaps for the fact that all joints undergo some degree of degeneration with advancing age. It is quite unexplained, however, why degenerative joint disease is present in most joints at advanced age but causes symptoms and distress only in some patients and not in others with equally severe joint changes of wear and tear. Irritation resulting from disturbed joint mechanics, aseptic necrosis, metabolic disorders, as in gout or hemophilia, vascular disorders, endocrine disturbances, and hereditary factors, has been considered as possibly being of importance in the etiology of symptomatic degenerative joint disease, but only rarely can any one or a combination of these factors explain its presence.

Regardless of which joints are affected, the symptomatology is quite uniformly the same and consists of pain aggravated by temperature or humidity changes and by weight bearing, stiffness after rest and tenderness to palpation, crepitus on motion, and often enlargement of the joint (by marginal osteohypertrophy), usually without synovial exudate.

The onset is usually insidious and occurs after the age of 40, except in cases of trauma or artificial menopause. There are no definitive abnormal laboratory findings. Roentgenographic examination of affected joints reveals thinning of the articular spaces due to loss of the cartilaginous joint surface, lipping of marginal bone, and varying degrees of damage in the subchondral bone. Table 3 lists the most frequent special forms of hypertrophic arthritis according to the joints most frequently involved.

CONVENTIONAL TREATMENT

The time-honored treatment for degenerative joint disease is salicylates, rest, and physical therapy. Rest includes the avoidance of imposing undue mechanical stress upon joint surfaces. This includes the use of orthopedic devices intended to minimize weight bearing by affected joints. Such measures include posture-correcting devices, arch supports, and supports for pendulous abdomens and breasts. In obese persons reduction of weight is indicated and certainly will reduce the strain placed upon weight-bearing joints.

In osteoarthritis of the cervical spine, intermittent traction exerted by means of a cervical traction apparatus may be helpful. A portable apparatus which may be hung over a door is available for home use. A plastic bag can be filled with water to certain levels which represent so many pounds. Symptoms of pain and paresthesias can often be ameliorated with faithful usage. Intermittent periods of rest during the day are beneficial in most cases of this disease.

Symptomatic relief is sometimes obtained by physical therapy. Analgesics, especially salicylates, are often indicated and are very useful in the treatment of this form of arthritis. A number of

Table 3. Forms of Hypertrophic Arthritis

Site	Remarks
Terminal interphalangeal joints (Heberden's nodes) and other finger joints	More frequent in women than men, usually appearing after 40
Knee joints	Often of traumatic origin; even severe hypertrophic changes may be asymptomatic
Spinal articulation	Especially in lumbar spine, hypertrophic changes occur with age and are often asymptomatic
Sacroiliac joint	Also often affected without causing any clinical difficulties
Hip joints (malum coxae senilis; morbus coxae senilis)	Mostly in males; can be extremely incapacitating in advanced stages because of pain through degeneration of cartilage and exostoses; often preceded by congenital anomalies of hip joint, trauma, or vascular necrosis of head of femur
Rib joints	Each of the 44 rib joints (costovertebral and costotransverse) can be the site of degenerative disease and cause pain referred to chest or abdomen

drug, vitamin, and hormone treatments have been recommended, but with the exception of those discussed below, they are useless. All authorities agree that the removal of foci of infections has no value whatsoever in the treatment of osteoarthritis.

Modern Methods of Treatment

Some of the features of conventional therapy—control of obesity to reduce the patient's weight and relief of affected joints by orthopedic measures designed to reduce weight carrying—are still useful in the modern management of degenerative joint disease. Modern rehabilitation methods aimed at muscle education may sometimes aid in relieving the strain of weight bearing in degenerating joints; this is particularly true in osteoarthritis of the spine and of the knees. These educational exercises to increase joint mobility may be facilitated by intraarticular corticoid injections, which seem to be quite successful in degenerative joint disease in most locations, least perhaps in malum coxae senilis. Systemic treatment with ACTH or cortisone is usually not helpful in osteoarthritis. Whenever degenerative joint disease is associated with osteoporosis, as it often is, the use of estrogens (in women), androgens (in men), or a combination (in women and men) is indicated, and gratifying results can often be obtained.

Since hormonal therapy and systematic muscle exercises have been introduced into the management of degenerative joint disease, the indications are that the rational use of these newer measures yields better palliative results in the treatment of osteoarthritis.

Finally, orthopedic surgery has made technical advances in the reconstruction of some of the most frequently affected joints.

GOUT

Gout may quite appropriately be discussed under the general heading of arthritis for two reasons: first, the most dramatic and painful lesion of this disease entity is arthritic in nature, and second, much like that of rheumatoid arthritis, the therapy of gout has been radically changed by modern developments. Gout is a fairly widely distributed, insidious, and chronic disease, about which there is much misinformation, and the diagnosis of which is often missed.

The diagnostic difficulty is understandable, since the disease is the result of an error in metabolism of purine bodies causing a persistent accumulation of uric acid in the organism, and since there is often no sign or symptom preceding the acute attack of articular pain. In later stages of the disease, uric acid may be deposited in joints and in soft tissues, resulting in gouty arthritis or tophi formation.

The mechanism whereby the accumulation of uric acid is brought about is not clear. Some have postulated an inability of the kidneys in patients with gout to excrete uric acid at a normal rate; others have suggested an excessive rate of formation of uric acid as the factor responsible for gout. Be that as it may, modern methods, using isotope tracer techniques in man, have clearly demonstrated that the "miscible pool" of uric acid (the portion of the substance which is dissolved throughout the organism and participates in metabolic processes at any given time) is 944 to 1,238 mg. in normal subjects and ranges from 1,909 to 3,667 mg. in patients with gout. The rate of turnover of this metabolic pool was found to be 53 to 96 percent of the pool per day in normal subjects and only 35 to 50 percent of the pool per day in patients with gout. This anomalous behavior of the metabolically active uric acid is often, but not always, reflected in an abnormally high concentration of uric acid in the serum of patients with gout, even during the attack-free, asymptomatic period.

Gout, or a clinical syndrome like gout, can be produced by injecting urate microcrystals into the joint. The deposition or presence of sodium urate crystals within the synovial fluid with concomitant reaction to them is actually a cause, if not the cause, of a gouty attack.

One current theory describes the cyclic nature of the disease process. With hyperuricemia, the tissues become supersaturated, and the urate crystals are extruded into the synovial cavity. They are then ingested by the leukocytes or white blood cells, a process accompanied by an increase in anaerobic metabolism. With this anaerobic metabolism and development of lactic acid, the pH drops within the synovial cavity. This causes more white blood cells to pour out and ingest even more crystals, with redness, heat, and swelling of the joint occurring as manifestations of the battle. It is even hypothesized that colchicine works by stopping the ingestion of the crystals by the leukocytes.

The lower limit of uric acid in serum of most gouty males is 6 mg. per 100 ml. Once the serum uric acid is elevated in a patient with gout, it will remain abnormally high except after the use of uricosuric agents. There is definite evidence that gout is a familial disorder and in many instances some blood relatives of gouty patients will be found to have serum uric acid levels which are abnormally high, even though they themselves have no symptoms of the disease. These people actually suffer from the inborn metabolic error and are clearly candidates for later clinical attacks of gout. There would be ample reason, and it would reflect good preventive medical judgment, to treat such hyperuricemic persons as gouty patients in the attack-free stage.

One should never rely on only one test to make the diagnosis. At least two determinations by a competent, reliable laboratory should be made.

DIFFERENTIAL DIAGNOSIS AND SPONTANEOUS COURSE

Once gout has been suspected, the diagnosis is easy and confirmation may be obtained by therapeutic trial. When a patient is observed during an acute attack, gout may readily come to mind, but it is often overlooked when patients complain about relatively vague and sometimes multiarticular pains. In such cases the typical tophi are usually absent, and the correct diagnosis has to rest on suspicion, elevated serum uric acid, and therapeutic trial with colchicine. Study of the family history may reveal gouty relatives or ancestors. In men, particularly in the endomorphic male, gout is much more probable than in women, since less than 5 percent of those affected are women.

There are other clinical phenomena that should call attention to the possibility of gout. One of them is idiopathic renal lithiasis. Any renal stone or gravel passed should be examined chemically, and if urates are present in large amounts, the serum uric acid should be measured. Albuminuria without azotemia is another entity that sometimes precedes or accompanies gout.

The acute attack, which suddenly and severely involves one (classically the metatarsophalangeal joint of the large toe) or several peripheral joints of the extremities, has to be differentiated from other acute arthritides. This is not always easy, since systemic symptoms, such as fever and elevated sedimentation rate, are also often found in gout. Rheumatoid arthritis and osteoarthritis are quite readily distinguishable from gout. The possibility of gout, however, should never be dismissed until a positive diagnosis has been finally established. It is fortunate that there is a specific medicament, colchicine, for the acute pain of the gout attack. This enables the physician to conduct a therapeutic test in suspicious cases, which, if positive, definitely establishes the diagnosis. A positive diagnosis can sometimes be made by tissue biopsy of synovial membrane or of subcutaneous nodules. The tissue is fixed in alcohol and stained by the DeGalantha method for urates. Birefringence of urate crystals can be demonstrated by means of polarized light* and helps in identifying urate crystals under the microscope.

X-ray films of the affected joint cannot be relied upon for early diagnosis, since typical findings of osseous tophi and articular destruction may occur only in the late stages of disease.

The course of untreated gout varies a great deal, so that classifications into various phases of the disease, as proposed by some textbooks, have little significance. The disease may remain latent for long intervals between acute attacks, and gouty arthritis with bone and joint destruction may not develop for many years after the first attack. On the other hand, attacks may recur with greater frequency, and gouty arthritis may develop relatively early. In part these differences reflect varying severities of the disorder, and in part they are caused by extraneous factors. Thus, the age at which the first attack occurs seems to be of some importance. The earlier in

life the first attack, the more severe the course of the disease.

A great many predisposing and provoking factors may accelerate the course of the disease and cause acute attacks. Most important among these are dietary excesses and surgical operations, as well as microtraumas (which may be incurred in various sports), and extreme changes of weather. Certain medicinal agents, such as liver extract, Salyrgan, ergotamine tartrate (Gynrgen), chlorothiazide (Diuril), vitamin B, and insulin; transfusions, bleeding, and purging also can induce acute attacks.

CONVENTIONAL THERAPY

The conventional therapy of gout is entirely empirical, and no doubt some of the present measures will appear somewhat inept once more becomes known of the disease mechanisms. Some aspects of conventional therapy, however, are still of more than historical interest, since the modern advances described in the next section have not as yet provided an entirely adequate rational plan of management for the gouty patient.

DRUGS

The old-fashioned prophylactic treatment included the taking of a purge (about 20 gm. of magnesium sulfate, for example) and repeated doses of 1.0 mg. of colchicine every 2 or 3 hours at the slightest premonition of an acute attack, until either the symptoms subsided or gastrointestinal distress appeared. Colchicine is still being used in this manner but purges are no longer prescribed.

If an acute attack occurs, the patient under conventional therapy should be put to rest, and the administration of colchicine should be initiated. Colchicine is available in tablets or granules of 0.53 or 0.65 mg. Two of these should be taken by mouth immediately at the onset of the attack, and subsequently one every 2 to 3 hours until pain is relieved, or until gastrointestinal symptoms appear. The response of the acute attack to colchicine is usually rapid, and addi-

---

* The American Optical Co., Rochester, New York, provides polarizing filters free of charge.

tional analgesics or narcotics are rarely indicated. If necessary, however, codeine, 0.032 to 0.065 gm., may be used every 4 hours. Salicylates, with codeine or alone, may also be helpful.

The uricosuric agents conventionally used are salicylates and cinchophen. The latter is dangerous, the former quite effective but outdated by recent developments. Salicylates have been used in doses of from 3 to 5 gm. per day, alone or in combination with sodium bicarbonate or aminoacetic acid (Glycine).

It is believed by many that the continued use of colchicine in the attack-free interval alleviates the severity of the disease and renders acute attacks less frequent. For this purpose, one tablet of 0.5 mg. of colchicine daily is recommended or, in mild cases, on 3 to 4 days of each week.

DIET

In the interval between acute attacks, as well as during an acute attack, it is believed that certain measures can modify and attenuate the course of gout. Foremost among these is diet. A purine-free diet that is low in fat, high in carbohydrates, and high in protein (low-purine proteins) is usually assumed to be indicated in an acute attack, and traditionally alcohol is forbidden. Modern thinking on the therapy of gout, however, has liberalized the dietary measures and no longer prohibits alcohol.

It is still believed by many that a low-purine diet prevents the accumulation of urates, and that the gouty subject should be placed on a diet containing 100 to 150 mg. of purines, compared to a normal purine diet of 600 to 1,000 mg. Foods that contain from 150 to 1,000 mg. of purine bodies per 100 gm. and are to be avoided completely are sweetbreads, anchovies, sardines, liver, kidney, brains, meat extracts, and gravies.

The following items contain 75 to 100 gm. of purine bodies, and one of them may be taken once a week: bacon, beef, calves' tongue, carp, chicken soup, codfish, duck, goose, halibut, lentils, liver sausage, meat soup, partridge, perch, pheasant, pigeon, pike, plaice, pork, quail, rab-

bit, sheep, shellfish, squab, trout, turkey, veal, venison.

The following items contain less than 75 mg. of purine bodies per 100 gm., and one item from this list may be allowed on four days of the week: asparagus, bluefish, bouillon, cauliflower, chicken, crab, eel, finnan haddie, ham, herring, kidney beans, lima beans, lobster, mushrooms, mutton, navy beans, oatmeal, oysters, peas, salmon, shad, spinach, tripe, tuna fish, whitefish, various oatmeal and rye breads and crackers, whole-wheat bread, whole-grain cereals, bran cereals.

Most other foods, including the following, are low in purine content and should form the basis of the diet: most beverages, butter, breads (except those listed above), corn products, cereals (except those listed above), spaghetti, macaroni, noodles, cheeses, eggs, fruit, gelatin, milk, nuts, peanut butter, pies, sugar and sweets, and vegetables not listed above.

It is generally believed that a patient with gout should acquire the habit of drinking large amounts of water to increase urine flow and to prevent formation of urate gravel and calculi.

MODERN TREATMENT

Quantitative clinical research carried out by means of isotope techniques, modern clinical experience, and the discovery of new uricosuric agents have done much to render the management of the patient with gout more rational and more effective. Since it has been shown recently that such simple substances as carbon dioxide, formic acid, lactate, acetate, glycine, and serine may be precursors of uric acid, it seems hardly justifiable to hope to achieve much by limiting purine intake, since these simple precursors may also derive from carbohydrates, fat, and protein. The rational diet for a gouty subject is therefore a well-balanced one, fairly rich in proteins and with reasonable amounts of fat and carbohydrates, but with avoidance of a few food items of particularly high purine content (see above). A large amount (from 1 to 4 quarts) of plain drinking water or alkaline table water should be taken daily.

There is no evidence that alcohol per se aggravates metabolic dysfunction, and therefore it is not justifiable to forbid alcohol because of the presence of gout. The occasional gouty patient in whom a given alcoholic beverage may be a provoking agent will sooner or later recognize its deleterious effect and can then avoid it.

Colchicine, in the conventional treatment of the acute gout attack, is still the most potent weapon for this phase of the disease despite our total ignorance of its mechanism of action. Its value during the attack-free interval is not proved.

ACTH has been recommended for the treatment of the acute attack, but it is questionable whether it offers more relief than colchicine. The same is true for cortisone and its derivatives, which are less effective than ACTH. Intraarticular Prednisolone injections are at times quite effective in arresting pain and inflammation in acute attacks of gout.

Phenylbutazone (Butazolidin) is yet another agent that has been acclaimed in the treatment of acute gout. About 800 mg. per day is given by mouth in four doses. There is a considerable incidence of toxic side effects, and the beneficial effects are not always as striking as those of colchicine. Butazolidin, like ACTH, may be used as a secondary agent in colchicine-resistant cases, as it is particularly helpful in terminating stubborn attacks or in breaking the chain of acute attacks recurring within a few days, and it has the advantage of being effective by mouth. Dosage is 200 to 400 mg. by mouth, followed by 100 mg. two to four times daily for 2 or 3 days only. This is followed by 1 to 2 mg. of colchicine daily for 1 to 2 weeks.

The discovery of probenecid (Benemid-p [di-n-propylsulfamyl-benzoic acid]) represented a significant advance in the management of gout since the discovery of colchicine. Probenecid is of no use in the treatment of the acute attack, but if taken continuously in doses of 1 to 2 gm. per day, it decreases the miscible pool of uric acid by inhibiting tubular reabsorption, thereby increasing urinary excretion of uric acid. Many patients have taken probenecid continuously for many years with no important toxicity being observed. When continuous probenecid therapy is used no other dietary measures are necessary, since uric acid is readily excreted. There is no evidence that the metabolic deficiency is corrected, but renal excretion is increased sufficiently to prevent the accumulation of uric acid and the gouty state is thereby masked. Acute attacks, which may occur early during probenecid therapy, even though serum uric acid levels have become normal, become infrequent or no longer occur, and elevated serum uric acid levels return to normal.

The large amounts of uric acid excreted during probenecid therapy, especially at the beginning, make it necessary to ensure a large daily fluid intake (2 to 4 liters), and in the presence of a strongly acid urine it may be desirable to give some sodium bicarbonate. Salicylate counteracts the effect of probenecid and must not be given while probenecid is being used. The treatment indicated for an acute attack occurring during probenecid therapy is the same as that adopted in the absence of probenecid administration—namely, colchicine. Some patients (5 to 10 percent) are intolerant toward probenecid and some (up to 27 percent) fail to respond.

The newest approved drug for the prophylactic management of gout is Zyloprim (4-hydroxypyrazole [3,4-d] pyrimidine) or Allopurinal. This is a xanthine-oxidase inhibitor which has been under investigation since 1962. This compound is effective in altering uric-acid metabolism without disrupting the biosynthesis of essential purines. Clinical studies have amply confirmed its desirable effect on uric-acid metabolism as well as its value in the management of gouty arthritis. Zyloprim is endowed with no antiinflammatory properties, so no alleviation of acute gouty attacks may be expected.

The effectiveness of Zyloprim may be regulated by the daily dosage. Approximately one week may be required for the full effect of the drug on the serum uric-acid concentration to be manifest. Conversely, three or four days may elapse following discontinuation of the drug before the serum uric-acid concentration returns to pretreatment levels.

Undesirable side effects from the daily ingestion of Zyloprim have been reported clinically in small numbers of patients. The drug is well tolerated by most patients when taken by mouth in from two to four divided daily doses. Minimal distress from gastrointestinal irritability has been reported, as well as a pruritic maculopapular rash and a slight leukopenia, in a small percentage of patients.

The recommended dose of Zyloprim varies from 200 to 600 mg. a day. Patients with mild gout respond to quantities not greater than 400 mg. a day. After the drug has been continued for several months, the effective dose may be decreased.

NONARTICULAR CAUSES OF JOINT PAIN

During the past ten years, the author has seen many patients referred to his clinic for physical therapy who came with the diagnosis of arthritis. Some had even been told, after x-rays had been taken, that these had confirmed the diagnosis. Subsequent review of these x-rays often revealed normality. In all instances, investigation of these cases demonstrated the pain to be in soft tissues adjacent to or in the vicinity of joints. They fell into fairly set syndromes relating to specific joints.

SHOULDER

There are three common areas of involvement around the shoulder joint. The middle area of the upper border of the trapezius muscle is a very common site for pain. The patient will usually complain of shoulder discomfort, and also aggravation of this discomfort by movements of the head and neck, particularly in the direction of the involved area. Examination reveals an exquisitely tender area to pressure, and it is usually firm and nodular. In many instances, it follows trauma, but at times the etiology is obscure.

A second area is anterior to the shoulder at the site of the biceps-muscle origin. This usually creates pain to internal and external rotation of the shoulder as well as abduction.

The third area is quite well known by even most patients, and this is the subdeltoid bursa.

ELBOW

The usual syndrome seen around the elbow is also fairly well defined and is commonly known as *tennis elbow*. This creates symptoms in flexion and supination, and tenderness is present to pressure over the radial head.

HIP

A trochanteric bursitis is quite commonly seen at the hip joint. While this does give symptoms during joint activity and ambulation, the patient also has symptoms when lying in bed on the affected side.

A second problem relates to pressure on the sciatic-nerve root with radiation of pain into the buttock, which many patients interpret to be hip pain. Since the treatment of this condition is quite different from that of the other situations now being discussed, an awareness of this possibility and accurate diagnosis is essential.

KNEE

The knee joint is probably the most common offender. Most people know of the prepatella bursitis or housemaid's knee. Syndromes involving, in particular, the medial ligament and, to a lesser extent, the lateral ligament do not seem to be as widely recognized. The pain experienced by the patient is often more severe and protracted than arthritic pain. The patient complains of pain even at rest in bed at night, and most will state that the pain is worse descending stairs as opposed to ascending stairs. Definite swelling is at times visible.

ANKLE

The medial and lateral ligaments of the ankle are also involved in pain around the joint. It most commonly follows trauma to the ankle, such as a sprain, and is usually symptomatic upon weight bearing.

DIAGNOSIS OF ABOVE SYNDROMES

In all the above situations except for the sciatic-root pressure, the diagnosis may be made three ways.

1. An adequate history, taken by asking the appropriate questions, will suggest the precise syndrome, if one is aware of its possibilities.

2. In all instances, direct palpation over the area will produce the pain experienced by the patient.

3. Two cc. of 2 percent procaine, or other local anesthetic, placed directly into the area of discomfort will almost immediately obliterate the tenderness caused by palpation and will also significantly decrease or eliminate the pain when the patient reproduces the active motions which have consistently created the discomfort.

TREATMENT

There are three levels of treatment which may be pursued, depending upon the patient's time and financial status. A trial at-home treatment may be given, which would include moist heat, active exercises, and a course of Butazolidin or Butazolidin Alka in doses of 100 mg. 4id, for about 2 weeks. Most other medications do not help in what can be very stubborn processes. Butazolidin works in only 40 to 50 percent of the cases.

A second level of management would include daily physical therapy. A program which has given significant relief to 80 to 85 percent of the patients includes hot packs, ultra sound, massage, active exercises, and ace bandaging of the areas, if these are around weight-bearing joints.

The third level of treatment involves injecting a steroid such as prednisolone tertiary butyl acetate in 1-cc. doses following local anesthesia directly into the site of discomfort. In all these areas, except the upper border of the trapezius, the needle point should actually touch bone and the medication should be injected at that spot. This is done every other day for three to five injections; it completely relieves the symptoms in about 96 percent of the patients. Immediate diagnosis and adequate treatment can prevent weeks to months of severe disability in these patients and also shield them from many unsatisfactory and unnecessary surgical procedures, which many have undergone before discovering the correct solution.

REFERENCES

ARTHRITIS AND OSTEOARTHRITIS

ABRAMS, N. R. In Hollander, J. L. (Ed.). *Comroe's Arthritis and Allied Conditions* (6th ed.). Philadelphia: Lea & Febiger, 1960.

BAILEY, R. W., BONNER, C. D., BROOKS, ROY W., GAUNT, W. D., JACOBSON, W. E., KAYE, R. L., MALONEY, J. M., and MINNO, A. M. The subtleties of diagnosing joint pain. *Patient Care* 2:68, March, 1968.

BAILEY, R. W., BONNER, C. D., BROOKS, ROY W., GAUNT, W. D., JACOBSON, W. E., KAYE, R. L., MALONEY, J. M., and MINNO, A. M. Treating rheumatoid arthritis: Plenty of alternatives, but no magic. *Patient Care* 2:18, April, 1968.

BAILEY, R. W., BONNER, C. D., BROOKS, ROY W., GAUNT, W. D., JACOBSON, W. E., KAYE, R. L.,

MALONEY, J. M., and MINNO, A. M. Long-term management of patients with gout, osteoarthritis, ankylosing spondylitis. *Patient Care* 2:70, June, 1968.

BARTON, E. M. Abnormal serum proteins as aids in diagnosis of rheumatoid arthritis and systemic lupus erythematosus. *Med. Clin. N. Amer.* 43:607, 1959.

BONNER, C. D. Effectiveness of multiple short-interval intraarticular injections of hydrocortisone acetate in rheumatoid and osteoarthritis. *Arch. Int. Rheumatology* 2:3, 1959.

BONNER, C. D. Intraarticular injections for osteoarthritis. *Rheumatism* 16:84, 1959.

CALKINS, E., COHEN, A. S., and SHORT, C. L. Long term chloroquine therapy in rheumatoid arthritis. *Med. Clin. N. Amer.* 45:1219, 1961.

CORDERY, J. C.   Joint protection—A responsibility of the occupational therapist. *Am. J. Occup. Ther.* 19:285, 1965.

DeLORME, T. L.   Restoration of muscle power by heavy-resistance exercises. *J. Bone Joint Surg.* 27:645, 1945.

DeLORME, T. L., and WATKINS, A. L.   *Progressive Resistance Exercise: Technique and Medical Application.* New York: Appleton-Century-Crofts, 1951.

GERBER, D. S.   Histidine found effective in relieving R.A. symptoms. *Clin. Trends Rheumatology* 2:3, 1971.

GOODMAN, L., and GILMAN, A.   *The Pharmacological Basis of Therapeutics.* (4th ed.). New York: Macmillan, 1970.

HARTFELL, S. J., GARLAND, J. G., and GOLDIE, W.   Gold treatment of arthritis. *Lancet* 2:784, 834, 1937.

HENCH, P. S., KENDALL, E. C., SLOCUMB, C. H., and POLLEY, H. F.   The effect of a hormone of the adrenal cortex (17-hydroxy-11-dehydrocorticosterone: Compound E) and of pituitary adrenocorticotropic hormone on rheumatoid arthritis. *Proc. Mayo Clin.* 24:181, 1949.

HENCH, P. S., et al.   Ninth rheumatism review. *Ann. Intern. Med.* 28:66, 1948.

HOLLANDER, J. L.   In Hollander, J. L. (Ed.). *Comroe's Arthritis and Allied Conditions* (6th ed.). Philadelphia: Lea & Febiger, 1960.

KUZELL, W. C., SCHAFFARZICK, R. W., BROWN, B., and MANKLE, E. A.   Phenylbutazone (Butazolidin) in rheumatoid arthritis and gout. *JAMA* 149:729–734, 1952.

MONTGOMERY, M., PICZ, C. G., and ARONSON, A. R.   Early diagnosis of arthritis and allied disorders. *Med. Clin. N. Amer.* 44:29–48, 1960.

RUDD, Y. L.   Better method for cervical traction in the aged orthopedic patient. *J. Amer. Geriat. Soc.* 11:283–286, 1963.

SELYE, HANS.   *Textbook of Endocrinology.* Montreal, Canada: Acta Endocrinologica, 1947.

SHORT, C. L., and BAUER, W.   The treatment of rheumatoid arthritis. *New Eng. J. Med.* 227:442–450, 1942.

SHORT, C. L., and BAUER, W.   The course of rheumatoid arthritis in patients receiving simple medical and orthopedic measures. *New Eng. J. Med.* 238:142–148, 1948.

SOKOLOFF, L.   Biopsy as a diagnostic procedure in rheumatic disease. *Bull. Rheumat. Dis.* 7 (Suppl.): 55 (Oct.) 1956.

STEINBROCKER, E., BERKOWITZ, S., EHRLICH, M., ELKIND, M., and CARP, S.   Phenylbutazone therapy of arthritis and other painful musculoskeletal disorders. *JAMA* 150:1087–1091, 1952.

STEINBROCKER, E., TRAEGER, C. H., and BATTERMAN, R. C.   Therapeutic criteria in rheumatoid arthritis. *JAMA* 140:659–662, 1949.

STEPHENS, C. A. L., JR., YEOMAN, E. E., HOLBROOK, W. P., HILL, D. F., and GOODWIN, W. L.   Benefits and toxicity of phenylbutazone (Butazolidin) in rheumatoid arthritis. *JAMA* 150:1084–1086, 1952.

STILLMAN, J. S. (guest editor). Arthritis and rheumatism. *Med. Clin. N. Amer.* 45:5–45, 1961.

WAINE, H.   Current concept and management of osteoarthritis. *Med. Clin. N. Amer.* 45:1337–1348, 1961.

WATKINS, A. L.   Practical applications of progressive resistance exercises. *JAMA* 148:443–446, 1952.

GOUT

BARTELS, E. C.   Long term (six to seven years) therapy of gout. *Med. Clin. N. Amer.* 44:447–452, 1960.

BARTELS, E. C.   Available uricosuric agents. *Med. Clin. N. Amer.* 44:453–463, 1960.

GUTMAN, A. B.   Keeping the patient with gout employable. *Industr. Med. Surg.* July, 1953.

GUTMAN, A. B., and YU, T. F.   Current principles of management in gout. *Amer. J. Med.* 13:744–759, 1952.

HENCH, P. S.   In Beeson, P. B., and McDermott, Walsh (Ed.). *Cecil-Loeb Textbook of Medicine* (13th ed.). Philadelphia: Saunders, 1971.

SEEGMILLER, J. E.   The present day treatment of gout. *Med. Clin. N. Amer.* 45:1258–1272, 1961.

TALBOTT, G. H.   *Gout and Gouty Arthritis.* Modern Medical Monographs. New York: Grune & Stratton, 1953.

TALBOTT, G. H.   Gouty arthritis, diagnosis and treatment. *Calif. Med.* 79:220–226, 1953.

TALBOTT, G. H.   *Gout* (3rd ed.). New York: Grune & Stratton, 1967.

WYNGAARDEN, J. B., and JONES, O. W.   The pathogenesis of gout. *Med. Clin. N. Amer.* 45:1241–1258, 1961.

3

Stroke

The clinical syndrome which today is commonly called *stroke* has been known by many names. In fact, physicians continue to refer to stroke patients as *hemiplegics*, *hemiparetics*, and *CVA's* almost interchangeably.

Hemiplegia was originally a term derived from the Greek words *hemi-*, half, and *plegia*, strike. It describes a condition of one-sided paralysis. It is a disease of the arterial blood supply to the brain and can be caused by a variety of pathological situations.

Strokes often occur in persons in "the best of health," but a careful history usually demonstrates that many of them have preexisting hypertension or high blood pressure. A stroke is usually sudden and a very frightening event for the patients as well as their families. There is often a regrettable tendency to look with pessimism on such patients, in the belief that they are destined to lead a useless and hopeless existence and that they will most likely succumb to another stroke within the near future. This is not necessarily true. With proper care, which must begin immediately at the time of the cerebral vascular accident, many of these patients will return to useful life and their life expectancy can often be prolonged. Whether the additional years of life for such patients will be a burden to them and their families or a comfortable, useful, and often enjoyable time depends not only on the extent and course of the disease, but also, in large measure, on the quality of the treatment given and on the perseverance of the rehabilitation team.

STROKE

Stroke is the third cause of death in the nation. For those stroke victims who die, and for those who have a spontaneous recovery and function normally, there is, actually, no problem. Stroke is the first crippler in the United States, however, and leaves more than a million and a half individuals disabled to some degree every year. An increasing number are now getting proper treatment, but too many still are victims of indifference, ignorance, and neglect and may find themselves confined to a useless existence and chronic institutionalization. There is no excuse for this. It is a result of apathy and lack of knowledge on the part of practitioners combined with old-fashioned notions ingrained in the minds of laymen that a stroke is the end and that the poor patient has suffered enough and should be left alone.

In order successfully to rehabilitate a person afflicted with stroke, one must be convinced, and those around the patient must believe, that with the proper measures at least enough function can be restored to render the patient self-sufficient; and they must feel that it will be more convenient for those caring for the patient if he is rehabilitated than if he is allowed to vegetate. There are situations where widespread damage resulting from cerebral vascular disease has destroyed learning ability and efforts at rehabilitation are doomed to failure. Proper selection of candidates is therefore necessary and should be made by a physician who has experience, if not board qualifications, in physical and rehabilitation medicine. Once unfavorable cases are eliminated, there remains a vast group of patients who can be rehabilitated and for whom neglecting to try this procedure would be malpractice and unforgiveable.

TYPES OF STROKE

The term *cerebrovascular* applies to all diseases in which one or more blood vessels of the brain are primarily involved in a pathological process. An abnormality of the vascular wall, occlusion by thrombus or embolus, change in the caliber of lumen, and altered permeability to plasma and blood cells would all be grouped under this term.

The outline below is a classification of cerebrovascular diseases reported by an ad hoc committee of the Advisory Council for the National Institute of Neurological Diseases and Blindness of the Public Health Service. The basis of the classification is pathology, except in those disease categories in which only clinical features are known.

  I. Cerebral infarction (pale, red, hemorrhagic, and mixed types)
    A. Thrombosis with atherosclerosis
    B. Cerebral embolism
      1. Of cardiac origin
        a. Atrial fibrillation and other arrhythmias (with rheumatic, arteriosclerotic, hypertensive, congenital heart disease)
        b. Myocardial infarction with mural thrombus
        c. Acute and subacute bacterial endocarditis
        d. Heart disease without arrhythmia or mural thrombus
        e. Complications of cardiac surgery
        f. Nonbacterial thrombotic (marantic) endocardial vegetations
        g. Paradoxical embolism with congenital heart disease
      2. Of noncardiac origin
        a. Atherosclerosis of aorta and carotid arteries (mural thrombus, atheromatous material)
        b. From sites of cerebral artery thrombosis

        c. Thrombus in pulmonary veins
        d. Fat
        e. Tumor
        f. Air
        g. Complications of neck and thoracic surgery
        h. Miscellaneous: rare types
        i. Of undetermined origin
    C. Other conditions causing cerebral infarction
      1. Cerebral venous thrombosis
      2. Systemic hypotension
      3. Complications of arteriography
      4. Arteritis (see VI)
      5. Hematologic disorders (polycythemia, sickle-cell disease, thrombotic thrombopenia, etc.)
      6. Dissecting aortic aneurysm
      7. Trauma to carotid
      8. Anoxia
      9. Radioactive or x-ray radiation
     10. With tentorial, foramen magnum, and subfalcial herniations
     11. Miscellaneous: rare types
    D. Cerebral infarctions of undetermined cause
  II. Transient cerebral ischemia without infarction
    A. Recurrent focal cerebral ischemic attacks (previously called *vasospasm*) usually associated with thrombosis and atherosclerosis
    B. Systemic hypotension (simple faint, acute blood loss, myocardial infarction, Stokes-Adams syndrome, traumatic and surgical shock, sensitive carotid sinus, severe postural hypotension)
      1. With focal neurological deficit
      2. With syncope
    C. Migraine
  III. Intracranial hemorrhage (including intracerebral, subarachnoid, ventricular, rarely, subdural)
    A. Hypertensive intracerebral hemorrhage
    B. Ruptured saccular aneurysm (if unruptured, see IV A)
    C. Angioma (if unruptured, see IV B)
    D. Trauma
    E. Hemorrhagic disorders (leukemia, aplastic anemia, thrombopenic purpura, liver disease, complication of anticoagulant therapy, etc.)
    F. Of undetermined cause (normal blood pressure and no angioma)
    G. Hemorrhage into primary and secondary brain tumors

H. Septic embolism, mycotic aneurysm
I. With hemorrhagic infarction, arterial or venous (see under I and VII)
J. Secondary brainstem hemorrhage (temporal-lobe herniation)
K. Hypertensive encephalopathy
L. Idiopathic brain purpura
M. With inflammatory disease of arteries and veins (see under VI, VII)
N. Miscellaneous: rare types

IV. Vascular malformations and developmental abnormalities
    A. Aneurysm—saccular, fusiform, globular, diffuse (if ruptured, see III B)
    B. Angioma (including familial telangiectasis, trigeminal encephaloangiomatosis—Sturge-Weber-Dimitri disease, retinal-pontine hemangiomas) (if ruptured, see III C)
    C. Absence, hypoplasia, or other abnormality of vessels (including variations in pattern of circle of Willis)

V. Inflammatory diseases of arteries
    A. Infections and infestations
        1. Meningovascular syphilis
        2. Septic embolism
        3. Arteritis secondary to pyogenic and tuberculous meningitis
        4. Rare types (typhus, schistosomiasis mansoni, malaria, trichinosis, etc.)
    B. Diseases of undetermined origin
        1. Lupus erythematosus
        2. Rheumatic arteritis
        3. Polyarteritis nodosa (necrotizing and granulomatous forms)
        4. Cranial arteritis (temporal)
        5. Idiopathic granulomatous arteritis of aorta and its major branches

VI. Vascular diseases without changes in the brain
    A. Atherosclerosis
    B. Hypertension arterio- and arteriolosclerosis
    C. Hyaline arterio- and arteriolosclerosis
    D. Calcification and ferruginization of vessels
    E. Capillary sclerosis, etc.

VII. Hypertensive encephalopathy
    A. Malignant hypertension (essential, chronic renal disease, pheochromocytoma, etc.)
    B. Acute glomerulonephritis
    C. Eclampsia

VIII. Dural sinus and cerebral venous thrombosis
    A. Secondary to infection of ear, paranasal sinus, face, or other cranial structures
    B. With meningitis and subdural empyema
    C. Debilitating states (marantic)
    D. Postpartum
    E. Postoperative
    F. Hematologic disease (polycythemia, sickle-cell disease)
    G. Cardiac failure and congestive heart disease
    H. Miscellaneous: rare types
    I. Of undetermined cause

IX. Strokes of undetermined origin

Of the nine groupings above, the first three include the types of stroke seen most frequently. Focal arterial disease of the brain can also be classified into three stages by the clinical status of the patient.

These three stages are defined as *impending* or *incipient stroke, progressing stroke,* and *completed stroke.* In the first stage, brief, transient episodes of neurological dysfunction take place, but the status of the patient returns to normality in between. During the second stage, the neurologic deficit continues to progress or gets worse while still in the early phase of symptomatology. The completed stroke has reached its maximum neurological deficit, has been stable for hours or days, and then may begin to show improvement.

The most common type of cerebral vascular accident is caused by a thrombosis of one of the arterial systems involved in supplying blood to the cerebral hemispheres. At one time such strokes were thought to occur only in the cerebral arteries themselves. With modern techniques, however, it has been possible to demonstrate that thromboses take place not only in these arteries, but also in the basilar-vertebral arterial system, the circle of Willis, within the carotid artery near its bifurcation and in its immediate branches. The thrombotic phenomenon may be represented by extensive arterial involvement whereby long segments of arteries are occluded with calcific and fatty deposits or by one plaque strategically placed at a narrow point of passage.

Disease of the cerebral vessels themselves is usually heralded by a singular episode which may be slow in onset. The patient may be left with complete or partial paralysis or may recover. Disease in the basilar-vertebral system or carotid tree, however, may create symptoms at first which are transient and minor. They are often referred to as *transient ischemic attacks* (TIA). The person may suffer a momentary loss of speech or have a weakness of one extremity. Such transient findings should serve as a warning of more serious problems to come and stimulate investigation of the cause. It is not enough to make the diagnosis of thrombosis. The specific site should be determined if possible, because some lesions of the carotid arteries lend themselves to surgical removal or bypass grafts, while others may be alleviated by anticoagulant therapy. The arrival at a correct diagnosis and the institution of appropriate corrective treatment may prevent a major neurological catastrophe with residual disability.

Obstruction in the carotid artery may be heralded by a bruit, Grade I to IV, which can be heard by stethoscope when placed over the artery. This diagnostic procedure has not received sufficient recognition within the medical profession and should be incorporated into the regular routine of all physical examinations. The presence of a bruit plus transient symptoms should stimulate immediate investigation and definitive treatment. Palpation of the carotid artery will give confirmatory information, as the thrombosed vessel will show a decreased pulsation.

Patients who suffer from strokes caused by cerebral emboli usually fall into younger age groups. Stroke is primarily secondary to heart disease with atrial fibrillation. It can also be caused by other cardiac disorders, such as bacterial endocarditis, a mural thrombus following myocardial infarction, cardiac surgery, or by fat and air. With modern methods of arrhythmia control and anticoagulation, the instance of this type of accident is diminishing. Frequently, however, the anticoagulation procedure or the attempt at rhythm conversion takes place after the embolus has occurred and initial damage has been done. There are also situations where, following anticoagulation to prevent the above,

bleeding takes place in the brain substance, also creating a stroke problem.

Subarachnoid hemorrhages can also cause strokes in a certain percentage of patients so afflicted. These are caused by aneurysms of the various arteries. The clinical sign of this condition can vary, from the patient who ruptures an aneurysm and develops no neurological deficit, suffering only a headache or stiff neck, to the patient who dies. Death happens in 50 percent of the cases. In between is the patient whose aneurysm ruptures out of the subarachnoid space and into brain substance. Correct location of the aneurysm is vital, as it may be possible to obliterate it surgically and prevent further bleeding. Many aneurysms are located in the circle of Willis, but other arteries are also commonly involved. Some patients can have more than one aneurysm present, all or any combination of which can rupture. Not all locations lend themselves to surgical intervention.

The frank intracerebral hemorrhage is usually caused by a significant elevation in blood pressure and, in 85 to 90 percent of the cases, results in death. Of those who survive, many have experienced such massive cerebral damage that they are unable to cooperate in any rehabilitation process. A small percentage of this group, however, will still have significant potential for rehabilitation, and this potential should be utilized.

The above four entities include the most frequent causes of cerebral vascular accidents. There are other processes which can damage the same areas of the brain and result in similar strokelike syndromes. Included among these are: trauma caused by automobile accidents, falls from heights, blows from blunt objects; expanding lesions both benign and malignant; vascular inflammatory disease; and hematological disorders.

Another stroke syndrome related to symptomatic vertebral-basilar artery ischemia is known as the *subclavian steal syndrome*. This occurs when there is stenosis of the subclavian artery proximal to the origin of the vertebral artery.

The arm on the side of the stenosis may be supplied by retrograde flow in the ipsilateral vertebral artery, and during exercise, blood of a sufficient quantity can be diverted from the vertebral system to the arm to cause symptoms of brainstem ischemia.

Intracerebral hematomas are also found in younger people, secondary to bleeding of undetermined etiology. Etiology of the cerebral vascular accident can be quite varied. Each requires a different type of preventive measure. The residual physical disability is similar for each, and the team approach to the rehabilitation of each individual applies.

PREVENTION

In many instances strokes can be prevented. It is well known that there are so-called risk factors which additively increase the possibility of experiencing this problem. High up on the list is hypertension, or high blood pressure. This is almost causative in frank cerebral hemorrhages, but it is also a very contributory ingredient toward cerebral thrombosis. It is interesting to note that high blood pressure seems to have a predilection for certain ethnic groups and individuals in poverty areas. In most instances, the people in poverty areas belong to the minority ethnic groups. Hypertension among the blacks is almost twice as prevalent as among the whites. It happens at a much earlier age, is much more severe, and frequently leads to cerebral hemorrhage and death. It is said that 80 percent of hypertension under age 65 is found in blacks. They rarely have lesions which are accessible for surgery or correction and rarely have transient ischemic attacks. A high percentage of hypertension has also been found in the Chicano population.

There are many excellent treatment modalities for hypertension in this day and age, and if the disease process is conscientiously ferreted out among the high-risk populations, it can be controlled in most instances. Many of these individuals also have poor dietary control. There is a tendency to eat saturated fats, egg yolks, and various dairy products, all of which contribute toward arteriosclerosis which, in turn, is another contributing factor toward cerebral thrombosis. People should also try to keep their weight at a normal level, because individuals who are obese also have a tendency to increase their blood pressure, if they are hypertension prone, and this produces one additive risk factor.

Cigarette smoking has been incriminated as also has diabetes; the former should be stopped if possible and the latter kept under strict control. Uric-acid levels should also be evaluated in the blood and appropriate measures instituted to keep them at normal levels. Unfortunately, most individuals in the United States engage in very little physical exercise. To keep in the best of health, one should see to it that at least 3 to 4 days a week some type of physical activity is done, such as walking, bicycling, swimming, ice or roller skating, calisthenics, etc. The popular fad of jogging is not necessarily a good practice for all individuals.

PHYSICAL SIGNS

Much emphasis has always been focused upon the motor disability by all individuals concerned in the stroke situation. This is probably because the inability to lift an arm or a leg or use it for any functional purpose is quite a shocking and visible experience. Most people are also concerned about mobility and ambulation; hence the inability to walk because of muscular weakness and dysfunction receives major attention. It is, of course, true that motor deficits are almost always part of a stroke patient's disability.

In the typical situation, the patient usually will have some return of motor power in the lower extremity, while the upper extremity may remain useless; however, all types of combinations may be seen, from the patient who has a completely flaccid paralytic upper and lower extremity to the patient who may get full return in the upper extremity and have a residual paralysis of the lower. There are all shades of muscle weakness and ability in between. Usually, initially, these extremities are flaccid, and if motion is to return, they begin to develop the spastic element. This is of great importance, because if there is too much spasticity (usually seen in the upper extremity), it may be, again, impossible to use this extremity for any functional purpose.

Many patients and families focus on the upper extremity to the point that they would be willing to wait forever for an improbable return of function or ability rather than learn how to work around this deficit. Therefore, it is important for the physician to be very frank with the patient at the outset so that he does not sit and wait for something that may not happen at all.

There are many excellent techniques (to be described later) which make the person with only one functional extremity a very competent individual. It can usually be predicted that the patient who does have some return of hip flexion, if he is educable, can probably learn to ambulate with appropriate supporting mechanisms.

Less commonly seen is a sensory deficit on the affected side of the body. However, knowledge, on the part of physician and nurse, of the presence of this deficit is most important for a number of reasons. If heat modalities are to be utilized, one must be sure that the patient is not burned by a too hot pack. Also, if the patient may be exposed to open radiators, pipes, smoking, or matches, sensory information is vital information to have. Sensory deficit in the upper extremity may create additional problems. Even when motor return takes place, if a patient is unable to feel objects, such as pencils, cups, etc., in the affected hand, it may be a significant handicap, depending upon what his job may be.

Homonymous hemianopsia is seen in a certain percentage of cases. The presence of this deficit has many implications. It should be considered in the proper placing of the patient in a nursing unit, so that his available vision is directed toward the overall center of activity. Bedside table, water pitcher, food tray, etc., all should be placed on the side of the patient's active vision. Those who take care of the patient must be aware of the problem and approach him from this same direction, if they expect him to work up to his best potential.

Incoordination is a less common finding, but its presence is important in the overall prognosis. In the affected upper extremity, if motor power is restored, incoordination interferes with fine dexterity, and there may be difficulties in manipulating things such as buttons and cuff links in dressing techniques.

Patients who have a lesion in the dominant hemisphere on the left may have speech problems or aphasia. For the patient, this may be the most frustrating area of his disability. All members of the rehabilitation team must have a complete understanding of this deficit. They must realize, too, that the lesion creates more than just speech difficulties. It embraces the whole area of language and can involve reading, writing, recognition of objects, and ability in arithmetic. See Chapter 13.

Individuals who have a lesion on the right, nondominant hemisphere may be subject to perceptual and cognitive problems which may interfere with the final total product. These individuals will have deficits in the area of dressing, because they will not be able to interpret the shapes and forms of what to others are familiar objects; they may have difficulty in geographical situations, such as finding their way around, even in familiar surroundings; they may have difficulty in copying structural problems, such as duplicating three blocks in a certain arrangement; and they may have difficulty in recognizing facial characteristics. They may have a tendency toward denying the left side and may neglect bringing it into useful activities.

TREATMENT

There are probably three basic stages in the treatment of the stroke patient.

The first phase takes place immediately at the time of the stroke. It must be remembered that rehabilitation starts at the time of the cerebrovascular insult. All patients should be seen by a physician, and an accurate diagnosis must be made. In order to guarantee appropriate interest and treatment, stroke units have been recommended for general hospitals. The stroke committee of the Massachusetts Heart Association Inc. developed the following as a possible model for a stroke unit:

Definition: A *stroke unit* may be: (A) a team of specialists knowledgeable about the care of the stroke patient, who consult throughout a hospital wherever the patient may be; or (B) a special area of the hospital providing beds for stroke patients who are again cared for by a team of specialists. As an alternative, the above could be incorporated as an integral part of an existing rehabilitation service.

Purpose: To save lives; to make accurate diagnoses; to prevent complications, such as contractures, deformities, bedsores, and incontinence; to start mobilization and ADL [activities of daily living]; to institute proper referral for achievement of maximum potential.

Necessary Components: For A and B: An enlightened administrator who is able to see that early and comprehensive treatment of the stroke patient is financially sound, results in better bed utilization by more rapid discharge, improves hospital mortality statistics and also its image in the community. This concept of treatment has been accepted in other areas of physical disability.

A cooperative and interested medical staff that is willing to refer its stroke patients to the care of the special unit while still maintaining medical supervision of its patients.

A potential for continuing education of staff members—both medical and allied health—concerning the comprehensive care of the stroke patient.

Built-in designs where possible and feasible for research at all levels.

A team composed of the following:

1. A physician with sincere interest in and knowledge of the problems of stroke patients. He must have had experience or accept training in evaluating physical disability, setting goals, prescribing physical restorative techniques, and assessing progress. He must be knowledgeable about bracing and splinting and aware of psychosocial consequences. He must be willing and able to lead the team.

2. A registered nurse who has training in the principles of rehabilitation nursing and procedures necessary for the activities of daily living (ADL).

3. A registered physical therapist.

4. A social worker.

5. A consulting neurologist to provide definitive diagnosis if required to recommend further investigation if needed.

Depending upon the length of patient stay:

6. The services of a consulting physiatrist.

7. A registered occupational therapist.

8. A certified speech pathologist.

This team must be prepared to work closely with one another and to meet at least weekly for problem solving, progress reports, and constructive discussion. It must be able to provide:

1. Early and sustaining medical treatment.

2. Measures to prevent contractures, such as range of motion and proper positioning of weak or paralyzed extremities.

3. Measures to prevent loss of bladder and bowel integrity.

4. Measures to prevent bedsores and dehydration.

5. Early mobilization.

6. Initial competency in ADL.

If the services of a consulting occupational therapist and speech pathologist are available, the following should be provided:

7. Mental stimulation and assessment of learning deficits and potential abilities.

8. Assessment and stimulation of communication.

For A: If a special area cannot be set up, the team must be prepared to work throughout the hospital. This requires a great deal of education for all ward personnel, because the nurse trained in rehabilitation cannot be on all patient care units at all times. The rehabilitation nursing will depend upon the attitude of the other nurses and the competition for their attention by what they may consider "more interesting patients." This type of rehabilitation knowledge by all nurses should be the ultimate goal.

For B: A special patient-care-unit area, consisting of a specific number of beds under the supervision of a nurse trained in rehabilitation specialties, should be set up with adequate space for wheelchairs, properly equipped bathing and toileting facilities, wardrobe closets and dressers, so that the patient may wear his own clothes, and rules which keep the patient out of bed when medically cleared.

The rehabilitation process should be designed in order that the patient will achieve his maximum potential. This may be done by means of the hospital's own restorative program, if it has been set up for long-term care, or by referral to a comprehensive rehabilitation center, an extended-care facility, or a home program. Referral should be made on the basis of the restorative, personal adjustment, and *long-term-care* needs of the patient and not for the convenience of the hospital in accepting the first available discharge plan in order to free a bed.

The above describes the type of situation not available in many hospitals. This should not discourage these hospitals from using their available staff.

Hospitals where similar units have been established have demonstrated decreased mortality while providing better functional abilities. The use of oxygen, intravenous therapy, antibiotics for pulmonary infections, etc., must be given priority during the initial cataclysmic period.

Once the patient has been stabilized, the second phase of treatment, which may be called *preventive rehabilitation measures,* should begin. There are several complicating problems that can happen at this stage, if an attempt to prevent them is not made. (These are covered in greater detail in Chapter 8.) It is important to prevent contractures of affected extremities. Those seen most commonly are of the shoulder, fingers, knee, and ankle. Once firmly established, they are painful and difficult to reverse. Prevention can be accomplished by training nurses or aides to perform passive range of motion exercises.

I. Definition of passive range of motion (PROM): Extent of movement within a given joint achieved by an outside force, without the assistance or resistance of the patient. (It should be noted that ROM is one of the most important therapeutic routines that can be performed for the patient. Permanent or long-term partial disability can be prevented.)

II. Purpose of PROM:
   A. Prevention of:
      1. joint contractures
      2. pain in affected extremities
   B. Maintenance of:
      1. circulation
      2. joint motion

III. General principles:
   A. Good body mechanics through the procedure:
      1. position the patient flat in bed with his involved side as close to you as possible.
      2. bed or exercise table should be at the level of the nurse's waist.
      3. use a wide foot-base of support while keeping back straight.

   B. Keep movements within a pain-free range —watch the patient's facial expressions.
   C. Do each full motion 5 to 6 times—smoothly and slowly—coming to a complete stop after each motion is completed.
   D. Do not exceed the patient's existing range of motion. Do not use force.
   E. Support the extremity at the joint. For an arthritic patient or any patient with a painful joint, the extremity should be supported in the muscle area.

IV. Specific procedures:
   A. Neck (flexion, extension, rotation)
      Support back of patient's head with palms of hands, and, placing thumbs in front of each ear, flex his head forward to chest. Extend to chest. Extend by returning to original position. Rotate by turning head to side, flexing head forward, and returning to original position with face in opposite direction.
   B. Shoulder (flexion, extension, abduction, adduction, internal and external rotation):
      Flex and extend by supporting the patient's arm by the wrist and elbow joints and raising the patient's arm straight up over his head. (Do not allow it to come out to the side.) (If shoulder is flail or subluxed, do not go beyond 100°.) Abduct by supporting the shoulder with one hand. Cradle the patient's lower arm with your other hand, then, while keeping the patient's arm at bed level, move it away from his side until it reaches 90°. To rotate, abduct the patient's arm, flex the elbow at 90°, bring the forearm toward the bed, palm down. Then, bring the forearm toward the top of the bed, palm up.
   C. Elbow (flexion, extension, supination, pronation):
      Support the patient's wrist and elbow joint, keeping the upper arm stationary on the bed. Flex the elbow, taking patient's wrist toward his shoulder. For extension, reverse the procedure. Supination and pronation are achieved by slightly flexing the elbow. Grasp the patient's hand as though you were shaking hands with him and turn the palm upward, then downward.
   D. Wrist (flexion, extension):
      Flex the elbow. Hold the forearm. With your other hand, flex the wrist forward (palm down) and backward (palm up).
   E. Fingers (flexion, extension, abduction, adduction):

Flex the elbow, cup your hand over the back of the patient's hand so that your fingers extend slightly beyond his. Curl the patient's fingers down beginning with the fingertips until they form a fist. To extend them, reverse the procedure until they are completely straight. To abduct, place the patient's hand on the bed, fingers straight. Move one finger sideways away from the adjacent one and then move it back. Do this to each finger.

F. Thumb (opposition):
Flex the elbow. Keeping the fingers straight, move the thumb away from the hand. Move the tip of the thumb to the base of the adjacent finger, then back to its original position. Continue this motion with every finger base.

G. Hip (extension, flexion, abduction, adduction, internal and external rotation):
To flex, support the heel and knee. Lift the lower leg, keeping it parallel to the bed. Do not allow the patient's leg to be abducted or rotated. Slowly, move his knee toward his chest. Take your hand out from under his knee, place it on top, and continue guiding the knee toward his chest. To extend, reverse the movement. Be sure to replace your hand under the knee as you return the leg to the bed. To abduct, support the leg by the heel and knee. Keeping the leg flat, move it out to the side. Do not allow the leg to roll outward. To rotate, place your hand above the patient's knee and the other over his ankle; roll the thigh in; roll the thigh out. The hand over the knee should perform most of the movement.

H. Knee (The knee joint is flexed and extended in the hip flexion and extension exercises.)

I. Ankle (dorsiflexion, plantar flexion):
With the patient's leg lying flat on the bed, put the heel of your hand on the ball of his foot and extend your fingers along the lateral and medial sides to stabilize it. Keep your other hand over his knee to keep it straight. Bring his foot upward, keeping it straight, then move the foot downward by bringing the heel back and up (plantar flexion).

J. Toes (flexion, extension):
Stabilize the leg by placing one hand over the ankle. Place fingers over the patient's toes and curl them down, then bring them up.

As soon as the patient is able, it is worthwhile to instruct him in doing his own ranging exercises. This is particularly important, if the arm has a residual amount of paralysis, even at discharge. A home-exercise program can be followed.

I. Purpose of self-ranging:
A. To keep the affected extremities free from deformity and from becoming stiff and painful by maintaining as much ROM as possible per joint.
B. To make putting on and removing clothing and maintaining hygiene easier.

II. General procedures:
A. All exercises should be done four sessions per day.
B. Each exercise should be repeated ten times or as tolerated.
C. Precautions!
1. Some of the exercises may be painful for the patient, and these should be performed only within his pain tolerance.
2. Some patients tend to overdo when exercising and can produce pain in their extremities from this. These should be supervised so that they do not exceed the specified ranges on the ten repetitions per exercise.

III. Specific procedures:
A. Shoulder flexion: forward upward motion of the arm, from side to shoulder height.
1. Hold affected arm as if cradling a baby, grasping arm at the elbow.
2. Lift arms to shoulder height.
B. Shoulder abduction: upward motion of the arm away from the side of the body. Cradle affected arm on top of stronger arm.
1. Assume cradle position.
2. Move arms from side to side. Swing through as though rocking a baby.
C. External rotation—in wheelchairs or chairs with armrests:
1. Position elbow of affected arm inside wheelchair armrest.
2. With other hand, grasp forearm of the affected extremity and push forearm away from body, being careful that arm remains stabilized against wheelchair.
D. Elbow flexion and extension:
1. Grasp affected extremity at the wrist and bend arm to touch each shoulder alternately.
2. Still grasping arm at wrist, pull arm down between legs to straighten it out.
E. Forearm pronation and supination:
1. Grasp affected arm just above the wrist,

holding it on lap. Turn so that the palm of the hand is facing up.

2. Turn in opposite direction so that the palm faces down.

F. Wrist flexion and extension:
1. Grasp involved hand at palm.
2. Bend wrist up and down.

G. Wrist—ulnar and radial deviation:
1. Grasp involved hand at palm.
2. Move hand from side to side without moving forearm.

H. Finger flexion and extension:
1. Place involved hand on lap or table, palm up.
2. Straighten involved fingers and then bend them into a fist.

I. Thumb abduction:
1. Place involved hand on lap in neutral position, palm up.
2. Place thumb and index finger of uninvolved hand between the thumb web of the involved hand at base of thumb and below index finger.

3. Spread thumb and index finger of uninvolved hand so that thumb web of involved hand is spread open. Precaution: Do not exert pressure at ends of fingers and thumb, thus hyperextending joints.

J. Thumb opposition:
1. Place involved hand on lap, palm up.
2. Grasp base of thumb of involved hand and move it out from palm, making a bridge toward the tip of the little finger.

K. Shoulder-girdle exercise:
1. Sit with shoulders level.
2. Shrug right shoulder and relax, then shrug left shoulder and relax.
3. Now bring your shoulders "to attention," as it is done in the military. Try to touch your shoulder blades together. Then relax.

The second way that contractures are prevented is by positioning the patient and his extremities properly, whether he be in bed, in a chair, or in an upright position.

BED POSITIONING AND MOBILITY

Nursing Responsibilities	*Prime Objectives*

Equipment necessary:
1. Condition of bed requirements:
  a) Bed—flat
  b) Surface—firm:
    (1) Mattress—firm
      or
    (2) Bedboard—solid
      or hinged (portable)
  c) Footboard—solid
	To maintain body in good postural alignment.
	
	To promote good physiological function of all body systems.
	
	To assist in preventing foot drop, support correct anatomical position.
	To prevent weight of covers.
	To use as exercise board.

Supine. (*See* Fig. 1.)
1. Body position desired:
  a) Body—straight line
  b) Head and neck extension
  c) Shoulders level
  d) Hips level
  e) Feet at ease against footboard—toes up, right angle to leg.
Caution: if spasticity is present, modify above as necessary.
	Make certain body is in good alignment.
	Teach, explain, maintain good alignment.

2. Method to attain body position:
  a) Move nonaffected side near edge of bed. Teach patient to:
    (1) Grasp affected arm at wrist and place across abdomen.
	Teach patient to assist in moving nonaffected side near edge of bed to allow space for positioning of affected arm.

(2) Place nonaffected foot under weak knee, slide toward ankle and bend knees.

(3) Lift affected leg, keeping feet crossed.

Encourage patient to perform independently to extent of his capability.

(4) Grasp mattress edge or rail with non-affected hand at same time.

(5) Dig nonaffected heel and elbow into mattress, raise hips, move to edge of bed.

(6) Keep same hand grasp, dig nonaffected elbow into mattress, raise head and shoulders, move to edge of bed.

(7) Realign trunk and extremities.

3. Move patient down in bed. Teach patient to:

Teach patient to assist in moving down in bed.

a) Grasp affected arm at wrist, place across abdomen.

b) Grasp edge of mattress or side rail with nonaffected hand.

c) Bend nonaffected knee, keeping foot firm on bed.

d) Dig nonaffected heel and elbow into mattress and slide down in bed. (Support affected leg.) Repeat until feet touch footboard.

Teach importance of footboard.

4. Hip:

a) Preferably provide trochanter roll, otherwise, padded sandbags. Trochanter roll should be placed from iliac crest to just above the knee.

Avoid external rotation and flexion.

b) No sandbags necessary with trochanter roll.

c) Double trochanter roll—fold bath blanket into thirds.

Teach, explain, maintain position of extension.

d) Teach patient to help you when applying trochanter roll.

(1) Grasp affected arm at wrist—place across abdomen.

Teach patient turning.

(2) Grasp rail or mattress edge with non-affected hand.

(3) Bend nonaffected knee, dig heel and elbow into mattress and roll.

(4) Place bath blanket from iliac crest across to about one inch above knee.

(5) Roll patient back and pull blanket out to edge of bed and anchor it.

5. Knee:

No pillow or roll under knee.

Avoid knee flexion.
Teach, explain, maintain position.
Note: knee flexion contracture of more than 20° leads to inability to learn to walk; transfer from bed to chair or chair to toilet.

Caution: re spasticity.

6. Feet:

a) At ease against footboard.

b) Toes up.

c) Right angle to legs.

Avoid plantar flexion.
Teach, explain, and maintain position of dorsiflexion.

Nursing Responsibilities	*Prime Objectives*

Caution: re spasticity.

    7. Heels:

        a) Elevate—use pad under Achilles tendon just large enough to raise heel from mattress. — Avoid pressure.

        b) Rest over space between mattress and footboard. — Teach, explain, maintain position of elevation.

    8. Head:

        a) Support with small or flat pillow

        b) No pillow optional — Avoid forward flexion contracture. Teach, explain, and maintain head extension. Prevent rounded shoulders, chest cramping, obstructed air way.

Upper Extremities

    9. Shoulder:

        a) Move affected arm away from body. — Prevent frozen or tight shoulder.

        b) Support arm with large pillow. — Teach, explain, maintain shoulder abduction.

        c) Tuck pillow well up in axilla.

    10. Elbow:

    Place on pillow extended or slightly flexed. — Avoid flexion contracture. Teach, explain, maintain flexion.

    11. Wrist and Fingers:

        a) Support affected hand on pillow in line with forearm. — Prevent wrist flexion (wrist drop). Teach, explain, maintain extension position (functional position).

        b) Use "cock-up" splint or towel splint (smooth cover if spastic). *See* section on splinting.

        c) Keep fingers slightly flexed. Use hand roll or towel splint. If hand roll is used, place roll in the hand at a slant. Thumb and fingers to be around the roll with the thumb opposite the index finger. Hand size and severity of contractures determine size of roll. (*See* Fig. 2.) — Avoid extension. Prevent complete flexion. Teach, explain, maintain fingers semiflexed as much as possible.

Hand Rolls: The basic hand roll is made by using two washcloths or other material of similar size and consistency. The size of the patient's hand and the severity of contractures determine the desired circumference of the roll. (*See* Fig. 3.)

Making Hand Rolls: To make the basic roll, place one cloth on top of the other, fold in half, roll loosely and secure with masking tape. The roll should be firm but not hard.

If this basic roll will not stay in place, one of the following variations may be used:

1. Place the basic roll inside a narrow piece of stockinette and stitch the ends together. The stockinette wraps across the back of the hand. The length of stockinette needed depends upon the size of the hand. (*See* Fig. 4.) To provide firm, smooth surface, the roll may be placed in a suitably sized paper cup.

2. Use webbing with velcro sewn to each end. Roll up this strap inside the basic roll and wrap ends around wrist, fastening with the velcro. (*See* Figs. 5A & B.)

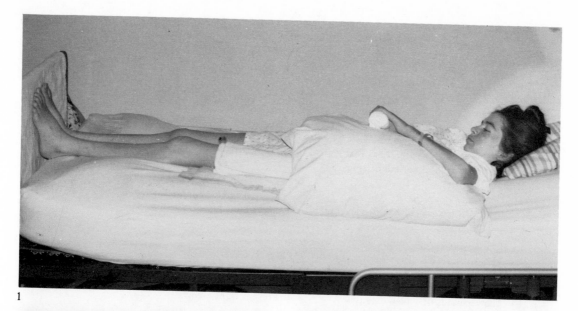

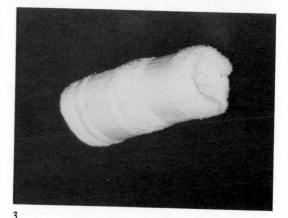

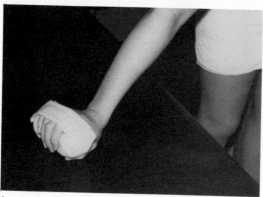

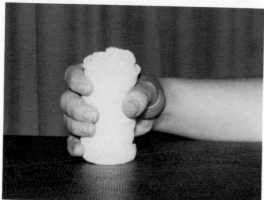

FIG. 1. Correct position for supine patient.

FIG. 2. Correct placement of hand roll in a paralyzed upper extremity.

FIG. 3. Basic hand roll, usually made by rolling up washcloths.

FIG. 4. Basic hand roll held securely on hand by placing roll in stockinette material and wrapping it across the back of the hand.

Nursing Responsibilities   *Prime Objectives*

3. Use a small blanket or bath towel. Roll material under to desired thickness, slide thumb under roll and fold sides of material over the forearm. Secure at the wrist with a pin. (*See* Fig. 6.)

Alternate Positions: *See* Figures 7A, B, & C. Alternate arm positions for back-lying. That in Figure 7C should be used only for short periods of time.

Allow alternating positions of involved arm to provide comfort and to prevent joint stiffness.

12. Arm:
    a) Use pillow doubled.
        (1) Affected arm at shoulder level on bed.
        (2) Rotate shoulder outward.
        (3) Elbow at right angle.
        (4) Palm facing upward.
        (5) Wrist extended.
        (6) Hand roll in palm.

Prevent tight shoulder

    b) Allow periods of elbow extension.
        (1) Affected arm abducted as much as width of bed allows.
        (2) Elbow fully extended, palm facing ceiling. Hand roll in palm.

Prevent tight elbow.

Side Lying (*See* Fig. 8.)
Turn on unaffected side starting with affected side near you. Position to be maintained no longer than two hours.
Caution: know when to turn more frequently.

Change of position prevents complications other than contractures.

Teach patient the need for turning and how to maintain correct position.

Essential steps:
    1. Move affected side to edge of bed.
      Teach patient to:
      a) Grasp affected arm at wrist and place across abdomen.
      b) Place nonaffected foot under affected knee and slide toward ankle and bend knees.
      c) Lift affected leg and move toward affected side.
      d) Keeping feet crossed, dig nonaffected heel and elbow into mattress, raise hips, and move to edge of bed.
      e) Keeping same hand grasp, dig nonaffected elbow into mattress, raise head and shoulders, and move to edge of bed.
      f) Repeat same as necessary to reach side of bed.
    2. To turn onto unaffected side
      Teach patient to:
      a) Keep affected arm on abdomen and feet crossed.
      b) Grasp mattress edge or rail with nonaffected hand.
      c) At the same time, dig nonaffected heel and elbow into mattress; raise hips and roll onto nonaffected side.

Teach self-care.
Nurse instructs and assists where needed.

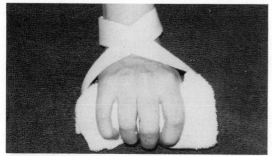

5A

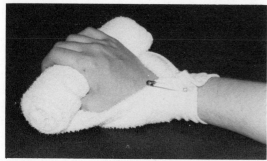

5B

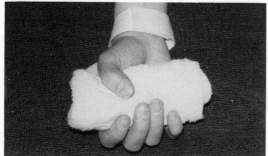

6

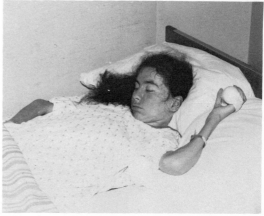

7A

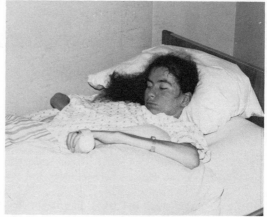

7B

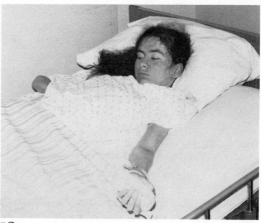

7C

FIG. 5. Basic hand roll secured to hand by velcro straps.

FIG. 6. Adequate hand splint formed from a towel and fastened at the wrist.

FIGS. 7A, B, C. Alternate positions for upper extremity of supine patient.

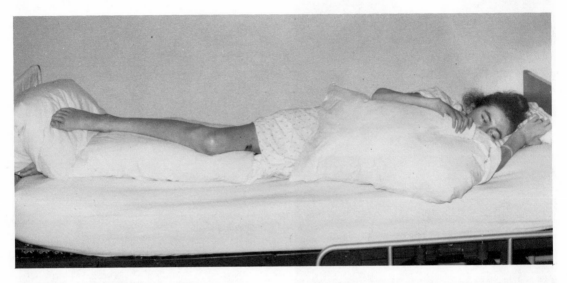

FIG. 8. Correct position for side-lying patient.

Nursing Responsibilities	*Prime Objectives*

3. Upper extremities
   a) Head:
      (1) Small support (size to correspond to distance between neck and tip of shoulder).

      (2) Head and trunk in straight line (same as in good standing position).

   Avoid forward flexion contracture.
   Avoid obstructed airway.
   Teach, explain, maintain neutral position.
   Prevent backstrain.

   b) Arm: (affected)
      (1) Away from body at shoulder level.
         (a) Support on pillows to give anatomical alignment.
         (b) Place pillows in front of patient and away from face.

   Avoid obstructed airway.
   Teach, explain, maintain position of abduction.

      (2) Elbow: slightly flexed
      (3) Hand: maintain same position as when supine.

   See Supine position

4. Lower extremities
   a) Hips:
      (1) Push up and distribute weight evenly.
      (2) Affected hip must not drop forward.

   Prevent dislocation of hip.

      (3) Support affected leg with one, two, or three large pillows, knee flexed as necessary.

   Prevent pressure on unaffected leg.

   b) Feet:
      (1) Support affected foot on pillow.
      (2) Elevate nonaffected ankle, using ankle roll if indicated.

   Prevent pressure.
   Prevent foot drop.
   Teach, explain, maintain position of dorsiflexion.
   Prevent pressure.
   Teach, explain, maintain position of elevation.

Prone Position:

Make sure patient can medically tolerate this position; consult doctor if necessary.

Change of position.

30 minutes 2 to 3 times a day; increase as tolerated. Maintain all night if patient can tolerate with usual regular changes being done.

Prevent complication other than contractures.

Teach patient the need for turning and how to maintain correct face-lying position.

Essential Steps:

1. If side-lying, remove pillows from between knees.

   Teach patient to:

   a) Grasp rail or edge of mattress and roll onto back.

   b) Realign body position.

2. Have patient move down in bed. (*See* step #4 under Supine, except feet not to touch footboard.)

3. Move involved side to edge of bed.

4. Turn to unaffected side:

   a) Place: (nurse does this)

      (1) foam pad or small pillow beside abdomen.

      Prevent lordosis or hyperextension of lumbar spine.

      (2) small pillow beside lower leg, if no space at foot of bed.

      Permit dorsiflexion

   b) Teach patient to:

      (1) Grasp affected arm at wrist and place along side of body.

      (2) Place nonaffected foot under weak knee and slide to ankle, bend knees.

      (3) Keep feet crossed.

      (4) Grasp head of bed frame with nonaffected hand.

      (5) At the same time, dig nonaffected heel into mattress and roll onto abdomen.

      (6) Adjust entire body in straight line.

      Nurse will need to assist patient where necessary.

Upper Extremities

1. *Head:* No pillow best. May use flat pillow.

   Prevent hyperextension of lumbar spine.

2. *Shoulder:*

   a) Place pads under each shoulder.

   Prevent subluxation of head of humerus.

   b) Adjust shoulders downward (away from ears).

   Maintain shoulder external rotation.

3. *Elbow:*

   a) Flat on bed and away from body.

   Allow alternating positions.

   b) Straight or slightly flexed.

4. *Wrist:*

   a) Flat on bed and palm down.

   Teach, explain, maintain functional position. Prevent wrist drop.

   b) Place hand roll in palm.

5. *Fingers:*

   Maintain same position as explained under *Supine*.

   See Supine position.

6. Thumb:

   Maintain same position as explained under *Supine*.

   See Supine position.

Nursing Responsibilities   *Prime Objectives*

Lower Extremities
  1. *Knees:*
     Avoid knees touching each other.   Prevent pressure.
  2. *Feet:*
     a) Should hang over edge of mattress.   Avoid plantar flexion.
     b) If above not possible, support lower leg   Teach, explain, maintain position of dorsiflexion.
        with pillow and knees slightly flexed.
     Note: Check alignment of legs in relation to
        entire body.

From Prone to Supine
  1. Assist patient in moving affected side to edge   Teach turning from prone to supine position.
     of bed.
     a) Grasp head of bed frame directly over
        affected side.
     b) Raise chest and push away from bed with
        nonaffected hand, and using nonaffected
        foot, roll onto back.
     c) Realign body position.

The third way to assist in preventing contractures is the proper utilization of static splints.

INDICATIONS FOR HANDSPLINTING

A. Description of Hand: Flail hand
   Purpose of Splint:
   1. To prevent deformities.
   2. Protection—(gravity weight of hand pulls wrist into extreme flexion, overstretches extensor tendons, and can lead to permanent deformity which interferes with ease of application of clothes and is not cosmetic).
      If voluntary motion should return, hand is properly balanced to use.
   Type of Splint:
   1. Simple cock-up stabilized wrist and palmar support (fingers and thumb free).
      or
   2. Full hand splint, fingers and wrist and thumb stabilized in functional position.
   Length of time to be worn:
   As soon as possible post stroke; to be worn as night splint and majority of day in *combination with frequent* ROM periods.
   Precautions or Special Instructions:
   Watch for edema (may require wider straps for more even pressure). Check sensation. If patient lacks sensation, check very carefully for inaccuracies of fit.

B. Description of Hand:
   Partial return of voluntary motion (generalized weakness, muscles below fair). Isolated not pattern motion.

Purpose of Splint:
   1. Prevent deformities.
   2. Give means for prehension.
   3. Transfer power from one joint to another.
   4. Provide assistance for weakened muscles.
   5. Fingers cannot function with an unstable wrist; patient anxious to use fingers in normal manner: attempt to encourage muscle balance rather than substitution.
Type of Splint:
   1. Simple cock-up wrist support for stability
      or
   2. Wrist splint with action-hinged wrist joint to assist weak muscle and to prevent extreme motion in stronger muscle.
Length of time to be worn:
   During therapy for specific hand activity, or for special ADL.
Precautions or Special Instructions:
   Worn in conjunction with muscle-strengthening program. May be supplemented by night-resting splint: usually a temporary device only.

C. Description of Hand:
   Spastic finger and wrist flexors (no isolated motion).
   Purpose of Splint:
   1. To prevent further deformities.
   2. To correct deformity (only in conjunction with active stretching treatment).
   3. Cosmesis.
   Type of Splint:
   Full hand splint, fingers, wrist, thumbs stabilized in functional position below stretch reflex.

Length of time to be worn:

Initially worn for one-hour intervals to build up tolerance. Eventually worn majority of day and night with self-ranging periods in between.

Precautions or Special Instructions:

As soon as any spasticity is noted in the affected hand, a splint should be constructed before contractures begin. If spasticity is severe, initial splint will need to conform to flexed position to prevent further tightening. Emphasis would be on a stretching process with splint to hold.

Note: This splint is the most difficult for the patient to tolerate; and a compromise in design as well as continual refitting is essential.

METHOD FOR APPLYING HANDSPLINTS

1. Acquaint yourself with purpose of the splint so that the patient's needs for this special attention are understood.
2. Do range of motion exercises to all joints— hand and wrist. (time: 2 to 3 minutes).

   If hand is spastic:

   1. Grasp base of thumb and gradually pull out of palm into a position of extension.
   2. Grasp four fingers and, with patient's wrist in a neutral or flexed position, gradually pull fingers into extension and hold until tension relaxes.
   3. With thumb and fingers held in extension, gradually pull wrist out of flexion into a neutral position and hold again until tension is reduced.

3. Place handsplint on relaxed hand, aligning patient's wrist to wrist area of splint and fasten with wrist strap.
4. Adjust position of fingers so that they lie along surface of splint and do not pull away; carefully strap just above middle joint of fingers.
5. Adjust position of thumb.
6. Fasten strap on forearm.
7. Refasten all straps, making sure they are snug but still loose enough that a finger can be easily slipped between the strap and patient. Precaution: if too tight, circulation would be hindered.
8. If upon wearing splint, the hand appears to get out of position:

   1. Remove splint and do more thorough ROM exercises.
   2. Observe if straps are inaccurately placed.
   3. Do not have patient continue wearing

splint if he is adopting a worse position through inaccurate fit.

   4. Notify therapist to reevaluate.

9. Upon removal of handsplint, do range of motion exercises to reduce stiffening caused by splint; and check for reddened areas which are still obvious *one half* hour after removal. Immediately after removal it is common to see some marks, but these should disappear in one half hour.

   If reddened areas remain, check with therapist:

   1. Splint may require adjustments.
   2. Patient may require frequent short applications of splint to build up tolerance.

10. If any rash appears, remove splint and notify therapist. Some patients appear allergic to certain types of splinting materials.
11. Determine length of time splint should be worn with therapist or doctor. Within long periods of wearing, *remove splint every several hours for range of motion* and reapply.
12. Where possible encourage patient to apply splint or assist in the application.

TYPES OF SPLINTING MATERIALS

ORTHOPLAST-ISOPRENE

(Johnson & Johnson)

Description: Thermoplastic

Sizes: $\frac{1}{8}$"x12"x20"—plain
       $\frac{1}{8}$"x18"x24"—perforated

Malleable at 170° F (any heat source). Dry heat preferable for self-bonding—no glue necessary; surface must be clean, however, so use nonflammable household cleaner.

Warm material can be applied directly to patient. Sets in 8 to 10 minutes.

Suitability: Easily malleable and strong; does not stretch. Best for large splints, cock-up or full hand. Needs minimal reinforcement.

Time for Construction: Cutting, heating, and molding: 15 to 20 minutes. Finishing: 30 minutes.

Special Considerations: Appears nonallergenic.

Approximate Cost: $5.50—full hand splint.

PRENYL

(Ortho-Industries)

Description: Thermoplastic

3 thicknesses, $\frac{1}{16}$", $\frac{1}{8}$", $\frac{3}{16}$"

Size: 13"x22"

Malleable at 140° F. May be bonded (using

Prenyl cement). Can be molded directly on the patient (sets in 20 minutes).

Suitability: Especially good for small splints with compound curves. Material can be stretched and fit can be precise. Larger splints, i.e., full hand splint needs a rib reinforcement for added stability.

Time for Construction: Cutting, heating, and molding: 15 to 20 minutes. Finishing: 20 to 30 minutes.

Special Considerations: Some patients have developed a skin reaction to Prenyl.

Approximate Cost: $5.50—full hand splint.

It should be strongly stated that the prevention of contractures does not depend upon the use of only one of the three described situations above, but by the use of all three at appropriate intervals during the day. Without a hand splint, for instance, the fingers develop flexion contractures. If one uses the hand splint all the time, then extensor contractures will form. Either of these is disabling. Therefore, the proper alternation of range of motion exercises, proper positioning, and proper splinting should be utilized. Contractures of the shoulder may make it impossible for the person to dress himself with one arm. A flexion contracture of the knee or a contracture of the Achilles tendon may make it impossible for the patient to ambulate.

Another major problem is the occurrence of decubitus ulcers. Many of these may be prevented by ensuring the proper mobility of the patient as early as possible. Any stroke patient, uncomplicated by coma or other serious medical problems, should be mobilized out of bed within 48 hours. This includes those with cerebral thrombi and emboli. More caution must be utilized for patients with hemorrhagic disease because they usually require a period of 3 weeks in bed. During that time, attention to above details of proper positioning and range of motion should take place. Patients can develop pressure areas not only from lying in bed in one position too long, but also from sitting in a chair too long. Whenever possible, patients should be taught how to change position in bed and in wheelchairs fre-

quently. In addition to seeing that these patients are kept dry and well powdered, it is important to see that their nutrition is adequately maintained and that their blood status is within normal limits; one should avoid movements of the patient which create shearing forces which injure the small blood vessels supplying the skin.

There are a number of pieces of equipment that assist in the prevention of bedsores. One should be familiar with the use of alternating pressure mattresses, Stryker frames, and water mattresses. In lieu of the very expensive commercial type of water mattress available, an inexpensive air mattress can be bought at a store such as Sears & Roebuck and half filled with water. This provides a very effective, inexpensive water mattress for these patients. The nurses find it much easier to manipulate the patients on these than on the commercial variety.

For the wheelchair many types of cushions may be used, such as foam rubber, Stryker gel, or bio-float cushions, some of which utilize water and air mixtures. The traditional donut should be avoided.

Bedsores occur, usually, over bony prominences, such as the greater trochanter, the sacrum, the malleoli at the ankles, and the heel. These are the areas that should be protected. Bunny boots are helpful for the heels. It must be remembered that once the decubitus takes place, it may take months for it to heal, and this may be the final reason for a long-term institutionalization that could have been prevented in the first place.

Integrity of the urinary bladder is most important. There is too great a tendency to catheterize many patients and leave the catheter in for an inordinate length of time, utilizing the justification that this will keep the patient dry and prevent bedsores. It must be remembered that the bladder is basically a muscle and if it is kept empty from catheter drainage for long periods of time, it can contract and decrease the bladder capacity. These patients must void frequently and often cannot make the john in time. Thus they develop iatrogenic incontinence. If, during the acute illness, the catheter is necessary, it should be a closed setup with the loop of tubing from the catheter positioned at least 6 inches above the pubis, so that the bladder can expand and push the urine over this loop. This device maintains some bladder tone. As soon as possible, the catheter should be removed, and the patient should be taken to the toilet with privacy at set intervals to start a functional bladder program.

Attention should also be paid to the bowels. All too frequently, these patients are victims of severe impactions and must go through the uncomfortable and undignified process of digital disimpaction. Again, with proper attention to mild laxatives as necessary, proper fluid intake, and (most important of all) being placed on the toilet at the appropriate time each day and given the necessary privacy, a routine of defecation can be reestablished.

Another frequent complication is that of dehydration, mainly because the nursing staff does not have time to see that patients actually take in the water which is placed on their bedside tables. This type of patient presents a very apathetic, seemingly unmotivated affect and may be considered an unlikely rehabilitation candidate. When adequate water has been provided, however, and when he has been hydrated, he becomes quite alert, cooperative, motivated, and an excellent candidate. Proper attention to all these matters makes the stage-three part of the treatment much simpler, much shorter, and less expensive.

Stage three provides the amount of physical restoration or rehabilitation that the patient needs. In some instances, if treatment outlined above has been adequately performed, the patient may be able to go home from the general hospital already at a functional level; or it may be possible to send him home and have the visiting nurse or homemaker come in and carry out the rest of the restorative process. In many instances, however, the residual deficits are too

great and too complicated; they require the knowledge of a team of experts to accomplish a satisfactory rehabilitation process.

It is no longer sufficient to consider that all strokes respond to the same old routines of treatment which were used in yesteryear. Intense study has brought into focus and clarified several puzzling aspects of stroke behavior and treatment. It has made it possible for each team member to contribute a bit more skill, culminating in a better understanding of the problems, and providing newer avenues of therapy.

NURSING

In a rehabilitation facility, the rehabilitation nurse plays a major role. In essence, she and her fellow staff members are involved with the patient 24 hours a day, 7 days a week. Their support of, and contribution to, the overall program is felt in many areas.

At the time the patient is admitted, an initial evaluation is made. The nurse's critical judgment will play a major part in the attainment of patient goals. These depend heavily on her abilities to *assist* the patient in what he is doing for himself. This reverses her old traditional role of *doing* for him. The nurse's major responsibility at this point is to continue questioning and evaluating. An attempt is also made to make the patient feel at home. He is dressed in his own clothes and is allowed to bring personal belongings which will help make his stay more enjoyable. See Figure 9.

Activities of daily living (ADL) provide a means by which the entire nursing staff can remain dynamic. One might call it a concise check list that provides vital individual information. Training the patient to dress, bathe, go to the toilet, etc., is striking directly at the basics of disability. Inadequacy of performance in these areas will often end in chronic institutionalization. See Figure 10.

A matter of considerable importance is the patient's adjustment to his own body. It is a difficult task, requiring a great deal of patience from the nurse. The ability to do independent transfers is a large step toward independence. The method of transfer must employ safe, good body mechanics, and be consistently practiced by all members of the staff. See Figure 11.

The initial instruction related to ambulation and the use of assistive devices is begun by the physical-therapy department. The nurse then becomes the reinforcing tool by assisting the patient with ambulation on weekends, teaching the family safety factors, and guiding patient expectations. There are many assistive devices available. Those chosen will depend upon the severity of gait and mobility impairment, but the nurse is a definite aid in reemphasizing the most functional and aesthetic gait possible. See Figure 12.

Certain patients have a visual-field defect of one half of the eye on the affected side. This is called *homonymous hemianopsia*. The nurse's function with this problem becomes mainly a teaching one. She must help the patient compensate for this loss by placing his food tray within his field of vision, communicating with him from that side, and explaining to family members what this impairment entails. See Figure 13.

The nurse, as an integral part of the team, has endeavored to care for, teach, and help the patient regain most of what previously created his independence. She has made a concrete contribution toward that day when he can leave the rehabilitation unit as a person who has not had to relinquish his dignity, his sense of self, or his participation as an important, functioning member of society.

PHYSICAL THERAPY

Physical therapists base their treatment of the stroke patient on principles grouped into four techniques: those of Dr. and Mrs. Karl Bobath, Signe Brunnstrom, Margaret Rood, and Dr. Herman Kabat. The latter's techniques are more commonly known as *proprioceptive neuromuscular facilitation* (PNF) and are also connected with Dorothy Voss and Margaret Knott.

All these schools of thought share a basic concept: there are two primary motor functions developed in sequence, which are called *stability* and *mobility*. The patient must have proximal stability in order to have functional distal mobility.

A combination of these four approaches may be used. The primary goal is maximal functional ability. This may include wheelchair mobility, transfers, use of affected arm in activities of daily living, and ambulation. To reach these goals, it is necessary first to focus on trunk balance or trunk stability. Rolling, done passively and actively, promotes awareness of movements of the upper and lower trunk and activates dynamic control. This is also translated into a necessary functional activity enabling the patient to turn in bed and come to a sitting position. Resistance is added at the shoulders and/or hips to recruit and strengthen musculature. See Figure 14.

The on-elbows position is used to develop stability of the shoulder girdle. As the patient shifts weight onto his affected side, he is causing joint approximation. This stimulates joint receptors which, in turn, facilitate contraction of the shoulder musculature, thus increasing shoulder stability. This is the beginning step leading to a nonweight-bearing shoulder movement and is part of the basic philosophy in the Bobath approach. These same principles are followed as the patient progresses in the developmental sequence from on-elbows to all-fours and to upright kneeling. See Figure 15.

In the kneeling position, resistance can be given at the shoulders and at the hips to strengthen shoulder, trunk, and hip stability. The type of resistance given, reciprocal resistance or rhythmical stabilization (PNF) is designed to help the patient establish control of postural muscles in an antigravity position. See Figure 16.

In conjunction with stabilizing activities, the therapist also uses special stimuli and reflexes to facilitate the function of particular muscle groups. Some of the stimuli that facilitate, inhibit, or activate response are associated reactions, icing

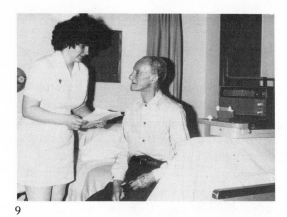

9

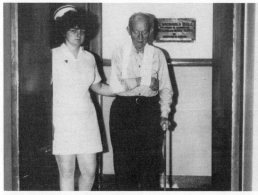

12

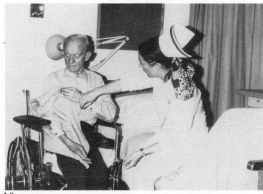

10

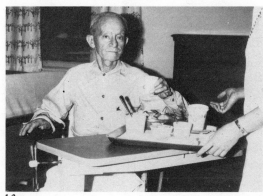

13

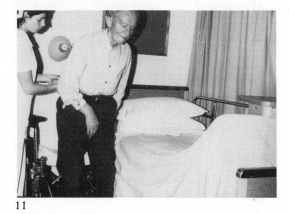

11

FIG. 9. The nurse attempts to make the patient feel at home; she encourages his dignity by allowing him to wear his own clothes or keep personal comfort items such as radio, watch, electric shaver, or even television set.

FIG. 10. The nurse instructs the patient on how to dress with one hand.

FIG. 11. The nurse instructs the patient on how to transfer properly from bed to wheelchair. Note that she functions from patient's affected side.

FIG. 12. The nurse augments and reinforces safety in walking on the ward, once it has been reached in physical therapy. Note arm sling for flaccid upper extremity of standing patient.

FIG. 13. Food tray should be presented to patient with homonymous hemianopsia and placed within his remaining field of vision.

stimulus, and quick stretch, such as Marie-Foix. See Figures 18 and 19. Associated reactions can be defined as the movement or increased muscle tone of the affected limb in response to voluntary or reflex activity in the opposite limb. One of many associated reactions is reciprocal flexion and extension of the lower extremities. Studies undertaken by Signe Brunnstrom demonstrated that flexion of the unaffected lower extremity facilitates extension of the affected extremity. See Figure 17.

In addition to associated reactions, a procedure used to elicit a mass flexion response is passive plantar flexion of the toes (quick stretch) which is referred to as the *Marie-Foix reflex* or *Bechterev's reflex*. See again Figure 18. While reflex contractions and/or associated reactions are being evoked, the patient is asked to superimpose voluntary motion in conjunction with the reflex contraction. As more voluntary control is gained, the therapist relies less on the use of reflex excitation. The patient is asked to attempt to initiate the movement completely voluntarily.

As the patient gains gross voluntary control in musculature, other stimuli are used to facilitate isolated and more coordinated movements. Figure 19 shows a quick icing stimulus to wrist extensors. Quick application of ice tends to evoke reciprocal action of superficial mobilizing muscles, as these areas are heavily supplied by A-size sensory fibers. Once a response is elicited, resistance is applied to prolong and strengthen the agonist response.

Response, whether it be stabilizing or mobilizing, is the primary purpose of treatment. The role of the physical therapist is that of the activator of response. By combining the various procedures of these four schools of thought, one possesses a greater selection of skills which help the stroke patient to gain his maximal functional abilities.

OCCUPATIONAL THERAPY

Perceptual-motor problems dealing with spatial relations are a common complication in the re-

habilitation of the stroke patient and are seen most commonly in parietal disease.

Symptoms manifested may often be attributed by staff to lack of motivation, inattention, or senility. Once diagnosed, however, and assimilated into the treatment plan, management of the patient becomes easier.

Figure 20 shows a completed drawing of a person by a patient which demonstrates internal spatial disorientation. Unilateral neglect of one side of the body, usually the left, is commonly observed in dressing. See Figure 21. The patient may consistently fail to incorporate that side in other motor activities, such as wheeling the chair. Unilateral neglect is often seen in the absence of, as well as in the presence of, homonymous hemianopsia.

The range-of-motion class not only provides the patient with self-ranging techniques but also provides sensory stimulation to the neglected side of the body. Group support and the laying-on-of-own-hands make this modality enjoyable and effective. See Figure 22.

Hemianopsia and/or unilateral neglect make mealtime particularly difficult for the patient and nurse. The nearly full plate appears to indicate poor appetite or disinterest. Actually the patient may not see the food on one half of the plate, let alone his napkin, fork, or any items to one side of the midline. See Figure 23A and B. The plate and items on the plate must be consistently positioned to the unneglected side of the body if the patient is to eat alone; otherwise, he must be continually reminded to turn his head in order to see.

Another common mealtime difficulty is abnormal judgment of perspective and depth, seen in the pouring of liquids. The patient needs to be trained to put the bottle neck or the spout against the lip of the glass. See Figure 24A and B.

Frequently, objects made of the same material and having the same color become confusing, even though their areas of use are very different, such as a water jug and a urinal. A front view of the objects may suggest over-

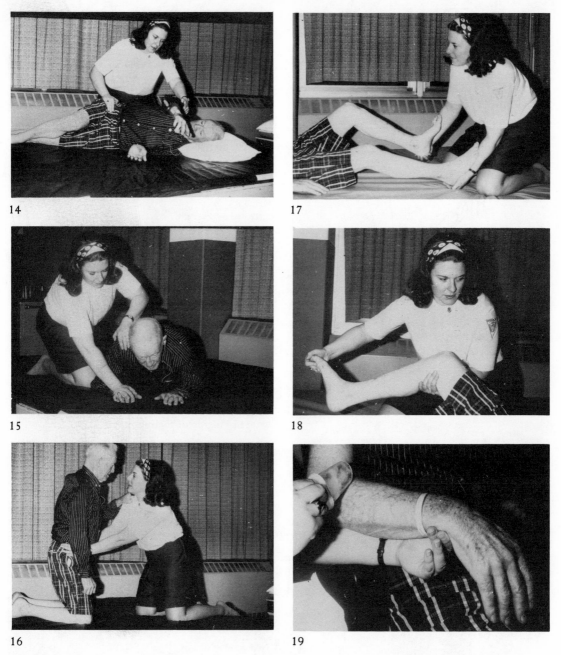

14

17

15

18

16

19

FIG. 14. PNF technique of resisted rolling. Resistance is applied at shoulders, hips, or both.

FIG. 15. Bobath technique using developmental sequence and joint compressing. Patient is in on-elbows position and approximation is applied through the shoulder.

FIG. 16. PNF technique. Rhythmical stabilization is applied at hips.

FIG. 17. Brunnstrom technique using associated reactions (lower-extremity synkinetic movements) with resistance.

FIG. 18. Brunnstrom technique using Marie-Foix or Bechterev's reflex to facilitate lower-extremity flexion.

FIG. 19. Rood technique using quick icing to stimulate wrist extensors.

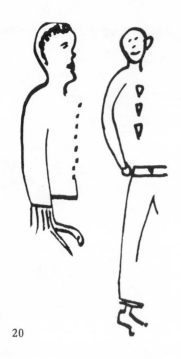

20

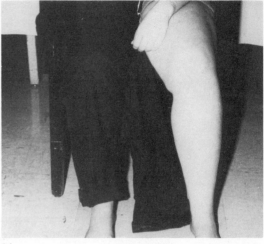

21

FIG. 20. Drawing of human figure leaves out half of body, demonstrating the perceptual motor problem, internal spatial disorientation.

FIG. 21. Unilateral neglect in dressing. Patients feels completely dressed, while in reality he has totally ignored one lower extremity.

FIG. 22. Group engaging in self–range-of-motion activities becomes more aware of their affected sides by the laying-on of their own hands.

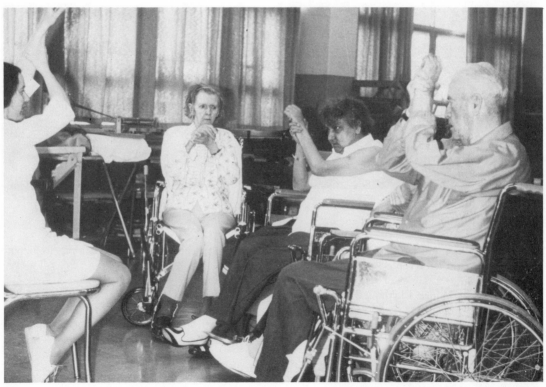

22

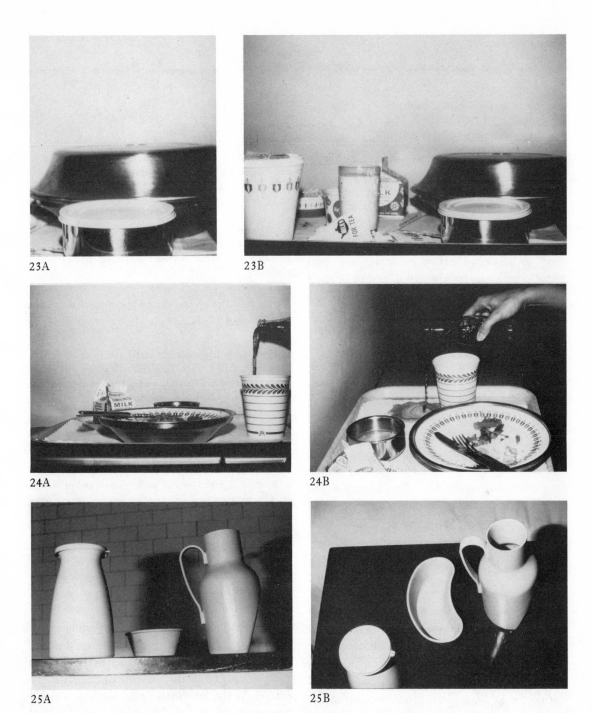

23A   23B

24A   24B

25A   25B

FIGS. 23 A & B. A. Hemianopsic patient may thus perceive his meal tray and wonder why it contains no fluids. B. Adequate fluids are present but may be missed by the patient if not called to his attention.

FIGS. 24 A & B. A. Patient seems to be pouring liquid into cup. B. Patient is really pouring liquid onto tray because of a defect in his depth perception.

FIGS. 25 A & B. A. Similarly colored and unfamiliar objects on the bedside table seem crowded to patient with space-perception problems. B. Objects actually are not crowded.

crowding of the bedside table, when in reality, the objects are placed at different spatial depths and there is plenty of room on the table for manipulation. See Figure 25A and B.

Evaluation of observational information, analysis of physiological and cognitive demands of tasks, and evaluation of the psychological need to perform are necessary before any retraining can be started.

Other questions which need to be answered are: What are the clues to which the patient needs to be alerted? How important are opto-spatial perceptions for this task—or can intellect and verbal reasoning also bring about the desired function? What minimal, general abilities must the patient have for the task to be successful? Can the task be learned subcortically rather than cortically? Does the task demand the understanding of an abstract concept, or is it composed of more easily learned concrete steps?

The therapist must answer many questions and know, not only the approach, but the quality of response expected in the teaching of any task requiring a new type of integration so that the patient may utilize his fullest capacities and potentials with some genuine satisfaction and dignity.

LANGUAGE THERAPY

The use of language, or the ability to devise, use, and manipulate a system of symbols for effective communication, is a distinctly human activity. Without language man is unable to organize his experiences in a way meaningful to himself and to others. Without language, man is at the mercy of a chaotic internal and external world. As William James said in one of his lectures in the mid to late 1800s:

We have no organ or faculty to appreciate the simply given order. The real world as it is given objectively at this moment is the sum total of all its being and events now. But can we think of such a sum? Can we realize for an instant what a cross-section of all existence at a definite point of time would be? While I talk, and the flies buzz, a sea gull catches a fish at the mouth of the Amazon, a tree falls in the Adirondack wilderness, a man sneezes in Germany, a horse dies in Tartary, and twins are born in France. What does that mean? Does the contemporaneity of these events with one another, and with a million others as disjointed, form a rational bond between them and unite them into anything that means for us a world? Yet, just such a collateral contemporaneity, and nothing else, is the real order of the world. It is an order with which we have nothing to do but get away from as fast as possible. As I said, we break it; we break it into histories, and we break it into arts, and we break it into sciences; and then, we begin to feel at home. We make ten thousand separate serial orders of it, and on any one of these, we react as though the others did not exist.

A. N. Whitehead, in two speeches delivered in 1915 and 1916, said:

It is not true that we are directly aware of a smooth-running world, which in our speculations we are to conceive as given. In my view, the creation of the world is the first unconscious act of speculative thought; and the first task of a self-conscious philosophy is to explain how it has been done . . .

I emphasize the point that our only exact data as to the physical world are our sensible perceptions. We must not slip into the fallacy of assuming that we are comparing a given world with given perceptions of it. The physical world is, in some general sense of the term, a deduced concept.

Our problem is, in fact, to fit the world to our perceptions, and not our perceptions to the world.

Without language then, man is unable to shut out experiences irrelevant to the task at hand. Without language, man is unable to stabilize and internalize his outer world that he may, with some confidence, make decisions and act upon them. He is often unable to reconstruct the past, organize the present, or plan for the future. As the human skeleton provides a stable framework against which muscles may act and interact, language creates the inner certainty without which man cannot intelligently act.

One aspect of language utilization comes through the visual sense. Unlike concrete objects, a symbol's meaning is affected by its orientation in space and its relationship to other symbols and their orientation in space. A stroke patient with impaired visual perception may exhibit symptoms of right-left, and up-down confusion, which result in number and letter inversions and reversals, defective recognition of words, and impaired scanning abilities.

The letter W turned upside down becomes an M. The number 9 turned upside down becomes 6. The small letter d turned around becomes the letter b. The juxtaposition of the letters in the word on changes the word to no.

Language retraining with the visually impaired patient involves helping him to become conscious of direction, to become cognizant of the left-right orientation that is necessary for reading, and to learn left-handed writing when indicated. This last visual-motor task trains the left hand to move horizontally from abduction to adduction instead of the accustomed adduction to abduction from the body's midline. This is a totally new task and is often difficult to master. However, multisensory feedback to the brain often aids in reinforcing the total visual-verbal picture.

Leslie A. White said: "Today we are beginning to realize and to appreciate that the symbol is the basic unit of all human behavior and civilization. It was the exercise of the symbolic faculty that brought culture into existence, and it is the use of symbols that makes the perpetuation of culture possible. Without the symbol, there would be no culture, and man would be merely an animal, not a human being."

SOCIAL SERVICE

The social worker, in conjunction with other members of the rehabilitation team, is vitally interested in restoring the stroke patient to his highest level of function. A prime social-work goal is to bring about improvement in total social functioning within the limitations of the patient's physical disability and his social situation.

At the time of his admission to Youville Hospital, the patient and his family are interviewed by the social worker. It is important to assess, as soon as possible, the patient's social situation, his role in the family in the past, and his role to be in the future. By being aware of this, the social worker can aid the family in adjusting to changes brought about by the stroke.

Group therapy led by a social worker (MSW) can be quite beneficial. Briefly, the group meets weekly to permit discussion of thoughts and concerns, anxieties and fears, regarding disability. Because the members of the group are all stroke victims, many of their problems and concerns are similar. Discussing these issues can lead to a better understanding of their condition and can also be supportive and reassuring.

When the patient has reached his maximum functioning, discharge plans are discussed with him and his family. If he will be returning home, the team will visit his home prior to his discharge. The patient accompanies the team. This is a good opportunity to observe how the patient and family members carry over skills learned in therapy to the home situation. It is also an opportunity to determine if the patient needs special equipment or adaptive devices in order to continue to function maximally. Patients often state that they find this visit reassuring, and it increases their self-confidence. See Figure 26 and Chapter 19.

There are some special techniques and equipment aids which should be described. One of the basics of a good rehabilitation program is efficiency in activities of daily living. For the patient who is left with a nonfunctional upper extremity, there are a number of little aids and pieces of equipment that can be used to make life simpler and more complete.

There are also many ways to become functional in household and kitchen activities, using the one good arm. Figure 27 demonstrates the use of a special rolling pin to prepare dough for baking. Figure 28 shows a stirrer which can be used in pots on the stove. Note the pot handle placement—between two suction-based uprights so the pot will remain stable. A towel placed alongside a cup and saucer will soak up any spillage. See Figure 29. Glasses may be washed utilizing a brush attached to suction cups as seen in Figure 30. Nails sticking up appropriately

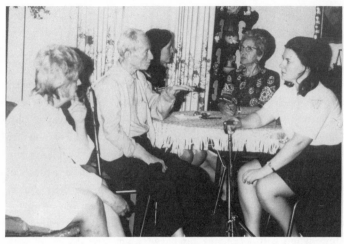

FIG. 26. Home evaluations by the team are essential in many instances to ensure the patient's functioning to maximum capacity. Following initial evaluation of patient's capacity to function, physical therapist, occupational therapist, and social worker make recommendations to patient and his wife.

ADL AIDS AND EQUIPMENT

Dressing

Equipment	Purpose
Buttonhook	Assist patient with limited ROM and muscle weakness to dress independently.
Elastic thread	To eliminate need to button and unbutton cuff on unaffected side.
Velcro	To make fastenings on clothing easier to handle for patients who lack fine finger dexterity or lack finger musculature.
Tongs—wooden and metal	Assist with LF's dressing, for reaching, picking things up off the floor.
Long shoehorn	To assist with shoes.
Heel assist	Holds heel of shoe firmly so foot can slip in more easily.
One-handed tying	*First Preference*—Independent shoe tying.
Zipper lacing	*Second Preference*—Independent shoe tying when patient is unable to learn one-handed tying.
Elastic lacing	Independent shoe tying.

Hygiene

Equipment	Purpose
Suction-cup handbrush	To clean nonaffected hands and nails.
Long-handled bath sponge	To wash back independently.
Soap mitten	Independent washing.

Emery board clamped to table	Method for one-handed person to file fingernails.
Slip-X strips	To prevent slipping in bathtub or shower.

Eating

Rocking knife	To cut meat independently.
Plate guard	Independent eating.
Wet paper towel	To keep plate from sliding on table when eating.

Miscellaneous

Wheelchair bag Walker bag Shoulder bag	To carry personal items.
Nonskid disc	To prevent patient from slipping from wheelchair. Also used with dishes.
Clip-on ash trays	For wheelchair patient who smokes.
Left-handed scissors	For patients who must use left hand for cutting.
Electric scissors	To cut material more easily.
Card holder	For patient who is unable to hold playing cards.

from a board, as in Figure 31, make it possible to slice and peel apples, potatoes, or onions impinged thereon. The same board with a right-angled elevated border makes it possible to butter bread by stroking toward oneself. See Figure 32. A one-handed electric can opener is also available. See Figure 33. Figure 34 demonstrates how silverware may be cleaned using a suction brush. A one-handed mincer is commercially available. See Figure 35. Once the work is

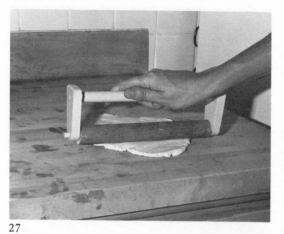

27

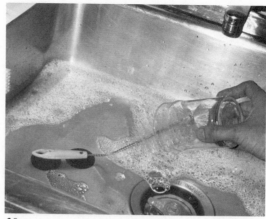

30

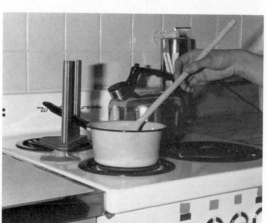

28

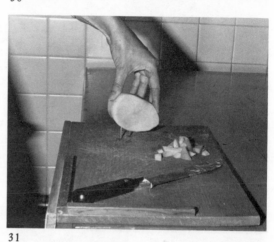

31

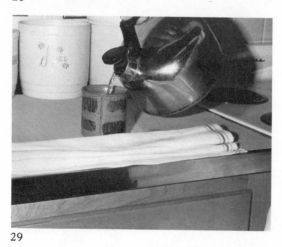

29

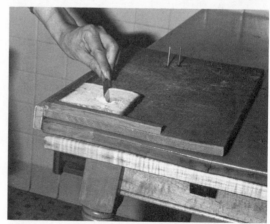

32

FIG. 27. Rolling pin for the one-handed.

FIG. 28. Stirring a pot whose handle is stabilized by suction-cupped gadget with two vertical prongs.

FIG. 29. A severe burn from hot liquids may be prevented by placing folded towel beside cup to absorb spillage.

FIG. 30. Suction cup brush to wash the insides of glasses.

FIG. 31. Foods which need to be peeled may first be impaled on nails sticking through board.

FIG. 32. By applying an elevated right-angled border to the board in Figure 31, patient can butter bread with one hand by stroking knife toward himself.

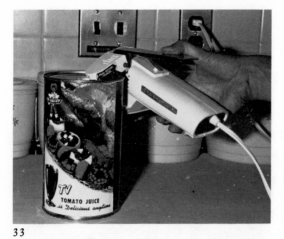

33

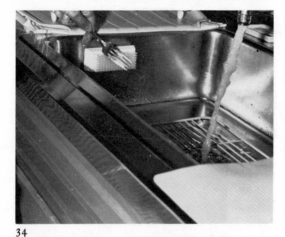

34

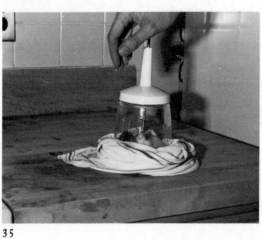

35

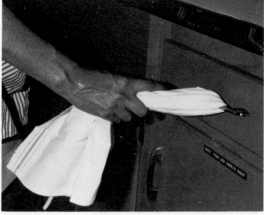

36

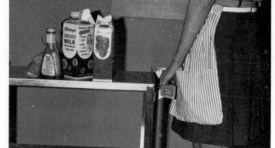

37

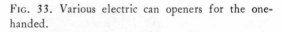

FIG. 33. Various electric can openers for the one-handed.

FIG. 34. Small suction-cupped brush to clean silverware.

FIG. 35. Mincer for the one-handed.

FIG. 36. Patient can dry wet functional hand securing the towel on a drawer handle.

FIG. 37. Clip-on apron and utility cart.

done and the hand is washed, it can be dried on a towel pulled through a drawer handle. See Figure 36. Cleanliness and transportation for small objects are provided by a clip-on apron and utility cart, as in Figure 37.

The ability to dress oneself with one functional upper extremity is always a challenge. Many patients are licked before they start and are satisfied to have someone else do the job. For those individuals who really want to be independent, however, there are techniques which may be learned and can provide a great deal of satisfaction once they have been mastered.

ONE-HANDED DRESSING TECHNIQUES

PULLOVER SHIRT

1. Place shirt on lap with label facing down (back of shirt will be up) and neck away from you.
2. Using unaffected hand, gather up the back of the shirt to open armhole. Push it up to above the elbow.
3. Gather back of shirt up to collar and work shirt sleeves up higher on both arms. Hold tight to gathered shirt—duck head, and pull shirt over.
4. Pull shirt down in back (by leaning forward slightly) and straighten front.

Removing pullover shirt:
1. With unaffected hand, gather shirt up to collar in back.
2. Duck head and pull shirt over.
3. Take shirt off unaffected arm.
4. Then off affected arm.

BRA

Style I:
1. With unaffected hand, slide bra around back at waist level and fasten hooks in front.
2. Turn bra around.
3. Put affected arm through shoulder strap and work it up to shoulder.
4. Put unaffected arm in other shoulder strap, work up to shoulder and adjust bra. (It may be helpful to add elastic inserts to straps for more give.)

Removing Bra:
1. Work strap down affected arm and take arm out.
2. Same for unaffected arm.
3. Turn bra around and unhook it.

Style II: (can be used for stretch bra)
1. Hook bra first.

2. Put on same as a pullover shirt: (1) put affected arm through shoulder strap; work strap to above elbow; (2) put unaffected arm through shoulder strap to above elbow; (3) gather back of bra, duck head, and pull over; (4) adjust bra.
3. Remove same as for Style I.

Style III: (Have bra cut in front and sew velcro strips on.)
1. With unaffected hand, slide bra around back and pat velcro strips together (at waist level).
2. Put affected arm through strap and work strap up to above elbow.
3. Put unaffected arm through strap and work strap up to shoulder.
4. Adjust bra.
5. Remove same as for Style I.

BUTTON-FRONT SHIRT

Style I:
1. Pick up shirt by collar. Put on lap with label facing up—collar next to abdomen and shirttail draped over knees.
2. With unaffected hand, open sleeve for the affected arm from the armhole to cuff.
3. Pick up affected hand and put it into sleeve.
4. Pull sleeve up over elbow.
5. Put unaffected hand into armhole, then raise arm up and out to put sleeve on.
6. Gather up the back of shirt, lean forward, duck head, and put shirt over.
7. Work shirt down over shoulders, then leaning forward, reach back and pull tail of shirt down.
8. Line up shirt front; match button to correct buttonhole, and button from bottom up.

Removing Shirt:
1. Unbutton shirt.
2. Lean forward. With unaffected hand, gather shirt up in back, duck head, and bring shirt over head.
3. Take unaffected arm out of sleeve, then the affected arm.

Style II:
1. Pick up shirt by collar and put on lap with label facing up—collar next to abdomen and shirttail draped over knees.
2. With unaffected hand, open sleeve for affected arm from armhole to cuff.
3. Pick up affected hand and put it into sleeve.
4. Pull up over elbow.
5. Pick up collar at the point closest to the unaffected side.
6. Hold collar tight. Lean forward, bring shirt up over affected shoulder and around the back to the unaffected side.

7. Put unaffected hand into armhole. Raise arm up and out to put sleeve on.
8. Straighten shirt out over shoulders and pull shirttail down.
9. Line up shirt front. Match button to correct buttonhole and button from bottom up.

Removing shirt:
1. Unbutton shirt.
2. Using unaffected hand, take shirt off shoulders on both sides.
3. Work shirt sleeve off unaffected arm.
4. Leaning forward, and using unaffected hand, pull shirt across back to affected side.
5. Take shirt off affected arm.

PANTS
1. While sitting down, move unaffected leg across midline of body toward affected leg.
2. Pick up affected leg under knee, lift, and cross over unaffected leg.
3. Pick up pants at waist (check to make sure they are opened completely) and place on lap with front facing up and pant legs hanging over legs.
4. Grasp center front of pants and bring pants down toward feet.
5. Put pant leg over affected leg and pull up to just below the knee.
6. Uncross legs.
7. Put unaffected leg into pants and pull up over knees.
8. Stand and pull pants up, then fasten zipper or button.

Removing pants:
1. Unfasten pants.
2. Stand and let pants drop.
3. Sit and cross affected leg over unaffected leg.
4. Remove pants from affected leg.
5. Uncross legs.
6. Remove pants from unaffected leg.

SOCKS
1. Sitting down, bring unaffected leg across midline of body toward affected leg.
2. Pick up affected leg under knee, lift and cross over unaffected leg.
3. Spread top of sock with thumb and fingers so it can go over toes, then pull sock over foot. Make sure heel is in correct position.
4. Pull sock up leg, making sure it is wrinkle-free.

Removing socks:
1. Slide sock down affected leg (after legs are crossed).

2. Slip sock over heel and pull off.
3. Remove from unaffected foot.

SHOES
1. Sitting down, cross affected leg over unaffected leg.
2. Pull tongue of shoe up through laces (so that it won't be pushed down into shoe as foot goes in).
3. Put shoe on, being careful to have all toes in.
4. If shoe does not go on easily, after shoe is half on, uncross legs, put shoehorn into heel of shoe, and put direct downward pressure on knee while intermittently moving shoehorn back and forth.
5. Fasten ties.

To provide the proper positioning of a paralyzed upper extremity, it may be necessary to supply various types of arm-support devices.

I. SLINGS:
A. Purpose:
1. Support for the affected arm.
2. Prevent and control edema.
3. Assist in maintenance of standing and walking balance by stabilizing arm in one place.
4. Control increase of pain from random motion of painful shoulder while walking, by generally supporting arm in shoulder joint.
B. Precautions: Slings should be worn only in conjunction with standing or walking activities, since the positions in which the arm is held in a sling (elbow flexion, pronation and internal rotation) are the positions which most often develop contractures in a spastic arm. Thus, the sling promotes deformity and immobilization if worn constantly.
C. Description:
1. Navy blue trough (commercial—DePuy Mfg.) with straps and slide buckle. This sling is designed to support weight of affected arm across back (not around neck).
a) Self-application: Version A
1. Patient places sling across lap with closed elbow section toward affected arm and straps forward. See Figure 38A.
2. He works sling onto arm as he would a sleeve, making certain that his arm passes beneath both

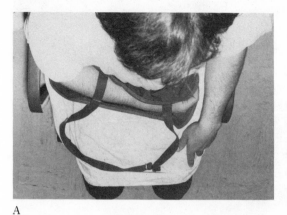

A

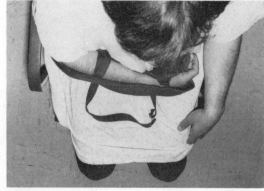

B

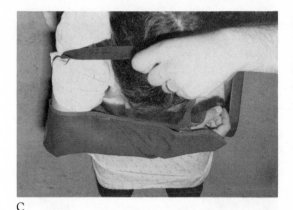

C

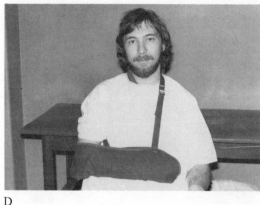

D

FIGS. 38 A through D. Self-application of a commercial sling (version A).

straps and that it is adjusted properly on elbow.

3. Both straps must then be pushed down between the patient and his affected arm. See Figure 38B.

4. The elbow strap is pulled around the elbow, up and behind the affected shoulder, and over patient's head. See Figure 38C.

5. The wrist strap is brought to the inside again. See Figure 38D. The sling can be tightened by pulling end of strap toward nonaffected shoulder until affected hand is positioned higher than elbow. Pull up and back when loosening sling, grasp buckle by both edges, tip buckle down, and pull down. Pull loosened strap over head and remove sling. (Remind the patient *not* to loosen the strap completely, otherwise it will be necessary to rethread it through the buckle.)

b) Self-application: Version B

1. Shake out sling so straps pull correctly from top of trough. Hold in front of you with elbow pocket toward affected side. See Figure 39A.

2. Drop strap loop over head. See Figure 39B.

3. With strong arm, pull affected arm totally through loop, so that strap falls behind affected shoulder and elbow.

4. Run nonaffected arm into trough under both straps, grasp affected arm, and pull into trough (as though putting on shirt sleeve). See Figure 39C.

5. Adjust so that affected elbow is supported in trough pocket. Pull end of strap at buckle to raise affected hand to proper position. See Figure 39D.

2. Rancho Sling: Webbing with wrist and elbow loops at both ends; adjustable buckle at wrist; to be worn by any hemiplegic patient whose walking or standing

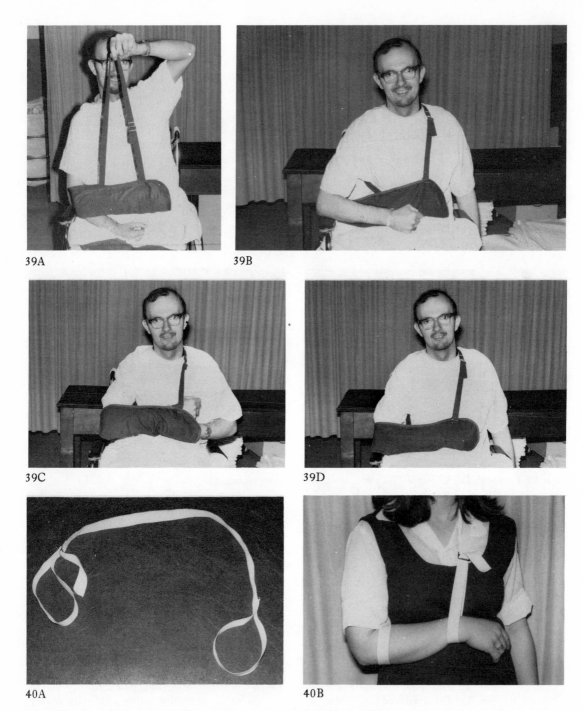

39A

39B

39C

39D

40A

40B

FIGS. 39 A through D. Self-application of a commercial sling (version B).

FIGS. 40 A & B. Rancho sling.

balance would be improved by the use of a sling. (See Fig. 40A and B.)

Application:

a) Patient slides elbow cuff into place.

b) Passes strap between elbow and self.

c) Around neck.

d) Over unaffected shoulder.

e) And onto affected wrist.

3. Webbing Sling—Type A (Fig. 41A and B.)

  a) Two-inch webbing fitted and constructed by therapist in occupational therapy to support a subluxed or painful shoulder. (Adequate mechanical leverage to totally reduce a severely subluxed shoulder is not possible to achieve by any sling yet devised, because of lack of shoulder-girdle stability on the affected side.)

  b) Construction:

    1. Preshrink webbing (shrinks approximately 2 inches).

    2. Starting at affected shoulder prominence, wind webbing behind, then in front of arm, over shoulder, behind and across back, under arm on nonaffected side of the body, and under affected wrist. Then attach with velcro in front of affected shoulder.

    3. Sew overlap of straps on shoulder prominence.

  c) Application:

    1. Patient usually needs assistance in positioning this tightly enough on shoulder.

    2. Sling should be applied directly to shoulder and elbow (not via hand-arm route).

    3. Next, sling goes under nonaffected arm, comes forward and beneath affected wrist, and is fastened with velcro on strap near affected shoulder.

4. Webbing sling—Type B (Fig. 42A and B.)

  a) Construction:

    1. Preshrink webbing (shrinks approximately 2 inches).

    2. Start by placing neck section properly to distribute weight across back (2 to 3 inches below neck).

    3. Then form cuff for affected arm by bringing webbing in front,

then behind arm, and meeting at affected shoulder prominence.

    4. Stitch securely at shoulder.

    5. With remaining webbing on nonaffected side, bring webbing in front of and under affected wrist, forming a wrist loop. Either stitch loop in position or use velcro for adjustable positioning.

  b) Application:

    1. Patient may need assistance in positioning tightly enough on shoulder.

    2. Sling should be applied directly to shoulder and elbow (not via hand-arm route).

    3. And then, wrist-loop section is brought behind neck, in front of unaffected shoulder, and slipped onto affected wrist.

  c) Modification:

    1. To prevent the affected arm from slipping out of the sling, a strap may be sewn to the mid-back portion and mid-front portion of elbow-shoulder strap and attached with velcro just above wrist.

    2. Application is similar to that of type B sling with the addition of adhering the strap with velcro just above the affected wrist. See Figure 42C and D.

II. ARMBOARDS

  A. Purpose:

    1. A general support for the affected arm while patient is seated in wheelchair.

    2. Assist in maintenance of sitting balance.

    3. Armboards should be used by any hemiplegic patient with a spastic or nonfunctional extremity, since an abducted position of the shoulder anatomically aligns humerus into glenoid fossa (shoulder joint) and should be the best position for prevention of subluxation from dependence.

    4. Theoretically, this device is preventive in nature and should be applied *early* post onset to provide optimal positioning of the affected extremity before contractures or subluxation are evident.

  B. Precautions: Referred motion, from excessive trunk motion while navigating the wheelchair, may cause shearing or scraping of affected elbow on armboard. Check pa-

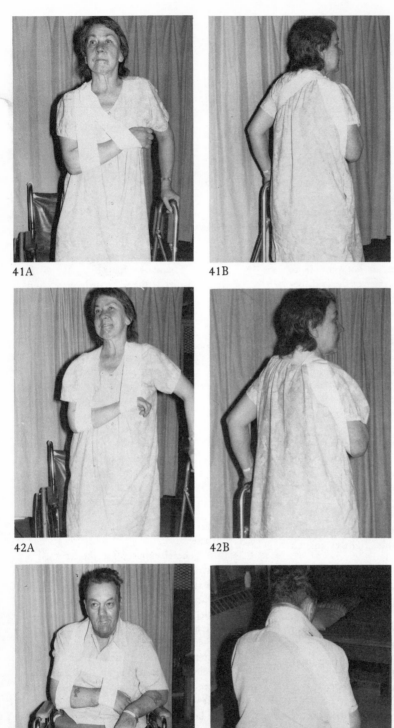

41A 41B

42A 42B

42C 42D

Figs. 41 A & B. Type A webbing sling.

Figs. 42 A & B. Type B webbing sling.

Figs. 42 C & D. Type B webbing sling modified to prevent arm from slipping out.

tient's skin regularly. Remedy or prevent this problem by properly applying synthetic sheepskin section to elbow area or armboard.

C. Description: See Figure 43.

1. A Royalite runner can be slid onto the arm of the wheelchair as the underneath attachment. It may also need velcro strap attachments for lateral stability. See Figure 44.
2. The ironing-board type cover is removable for washing.
3. Straps are attached where indicated.
4. Some may have a built-up hand area to duplicate functional position of hand: wrist neutral, palm elevated, IP joints in some flexion.

D. Application:

1. Since armboard may need to be removed to allow adequate space for transfer either in or out of wheelchair, gently slide or push runner onto arm of chair; fasten straps underneath.
2. Place patient's arm on board, apply straps, teach patient application when possible. Fingers should not extend beyond end of board unless this is preferred by therapist. Patient need not wear splint with armboard (if armboard duplicates position) unless otherwise indicated by therapist.
3. With some chair and arm combinations, the patient's elbow may protrude. This is often because chair armrests are too high. Exchange chair if possible or attach elbow guard or angle skateboard.

III. SUSPENSION SLINGS

A. Purpose:

1. A general support for the affected arm.
2. Reduction of edema.
3. Antigravity support which allows independent exercise of minimal musculature of shoulder and elbow. (Other devices, i.e. sling and armboard, prevent motion.)

B. Precautions:

1. The metal support which is attached to wheelchair may get out of alignment and become an obstacle when going through doorways.
2. The referred motion into the affected arm while navigating the wheelchair may produce shoulder pain, since the weakened musculature is not adequately stabilizing the shoulder joint.

3. The distal end of the metal support rod can be a hazard to personnel working with patient. (Foam rubber or a small red rubber ball should be attached to the end of the rod for protection.)
4. Severe spasticity may prohibit effective use of this device.

C. Description: (See Fig. 45.)

1. An inverted L-shaped rod is supported by a special bracket attached to wheelchair.
2. A spreader bar with a wrist and elbow sling is attached to rod.

D. Application:

1. Basic equipment is attached to wheelchair by occupational therapist and need not be removed, since equipment does not interfere with transfer, etc.
2. Slings are positioned with the largest one under the elbow and the smaller one supporting the wrist, with the thumb through the thumbhole.
3. The therapist will establish the correct height of each sling, and the slings should not be lengthened or shortened during application.
4. The suspension rod should be parallel to the armrest. If it gets out of position, first loosen thumb screw on bracket, then realign rod, and retighten thumb screw. *Never* just twist rod, as this will damage bracket.
5. Patient can learn to apply slings by first inserting nonaffected arm through wrist sling, then through elbow sling, and grasping affected arm and pulling through both slings (similar to putting on shirt sleeve).
6. If suspension is being used to reduce edema, make sure slings are in correct sequence, with wrist supported well above elbow level.

Frequently, ambulation, which is a major goal in most patients' minds, must be aided by some type of bracing mechanism. In a few instances, because of severe residual paralysis of the lower extremity, a long leg brace may be necessary. This long leg brace has a drop lock on the medial aspect of the upright, so that it can be controlled by the nonaffected arm. It is a major job to teach the patient to put this long leg brace on himself so that he can be independent.

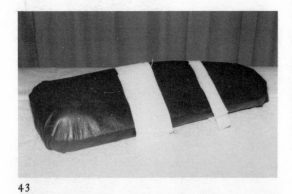

43

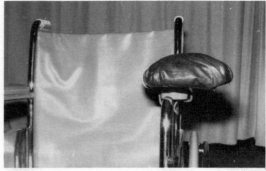

44

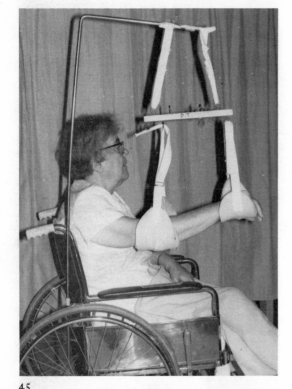

45

Fig. 43. Armboard that can be attached to wheelchair arm.

Fig. 44. Armboard secured to wheelchair by Royalite runner.

Fig. 45. Suspension sling attached to wheelchair by L-shaped rod and special bracket.

Figs. 46 A, B, C. Application of temporary elastic bandage assist.

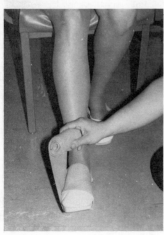

46A

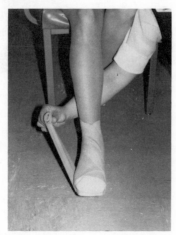

46B

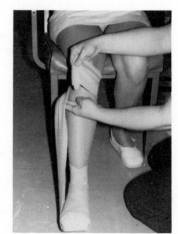

46C

APPLICATION OF A LONG LEG BRACE
BY A HEMIPLEGIC PATIENT

A. Preparations:
1. There should be a long shoehorn within reach.
2. Patient should be seated in a locked wheelchair or in a straight armchair that is stabilized so that it cannot slide, facing a mat or bed that is the same height as the chair, or nearly so, about 18 inches away from it.
3. The tongue of the shoe attached to the brace should be tucked up through the shoelace so that it will be out of the way when the foot is inserted into the shoe.
4. With the knee locked, the brace is stood on the floor beside the patient's unaffected side.

B. Instructions to the Patient:
1. Using unaffected hand, cross affected leg over unaffected leg.
2. Place brace across chair and bed on affected side, so that it forms a "bridge," with the heel of the shoe resting on the bed.
3. Lift affected leg and place it so that it rests on top of the brace.
4. Slide proximal cuff of brace under thigh.
5. Grasp affected leg close to ankle and insert foot into shoe as far as it will go.
6. Fasten proximal cuff of brace.
7. Unlock brace and by grasping medial upright, bend leg, and lower foot to floor.
8. With toes well into shoe and heel touching back of shoe, insert shoehorn into heel of shoe.
9. Work foot into shoe by alternately pressing down on knee with unaffected hand and pulling up on shoehorn.
10. Fasten shoelaces.
11. Grasp medial upright of brace just below knee and place leg back on bed. Straighten knee.
12. Lock brace and tighten knee pad. Extremity is now ready for weight-bearing. If patient is not about to walk, brace should be unlocked and foot lowered to floor or pedal of wheelchair. Otherwise, lower foot to floor with brace locked.

C. Locking and unlocking brace:
In order for the brace to be easily locked or unlocked, its proximal and distal portions must be in line with one another, so that the drop lock can slide easily over both of them, where they come together at the hinge.
1. Place the heel of the braced extremity on a raised surface, such as a bed, chair, or footstool, so that there is pressure *upward* on the *distal* portion of the brace.
2. With the heel of the hand on the medial upright just above the knee, apply pressure *downward* on the proximal portion of the brace.
3. While still maintaining the downward pressure with the heel of the hand, use the fingers of the same hand to slip the ring lock distally, to lock the brace, or proximally, to unlock it.

More commonly a short leg brace is utilized, because most patients are able to control the affected knee. If there is too much tendency to back knee, an appropriate Swedish knee cage, which prevents genu recurvatum, can be added to the short leg brace. One can get a good idea of how the patient is going to function in this short leg brace by using a temporary elastic bandage assist. Its purpose is to support the foot in a neutral position for ambulation. It should be worn only during walking practice, until such time as a brace may be obtained.

1. Patient, wearing shoes, is seated with foot to be bandaged resting flat on floor. Person applying bandage kneels on floor, facing him.

2. Start bandage at lateral aspect of dorsum of foot, bring it medially, then under the sole. See Figure 46A.

3. Make two or three circular turns around the foot, securing the free end of the bandage firmly.

4. Make several figure-eight turns around the foot and ankle, applying strong tension in the direction of dorsiflexion and eversion. Bring the last loop under the metatarsal heads. See Figure 46B.

5. With strong upward tension, pull the remaining bandage to the lateral aspect of the leg just below the knee.

6. With one hand maintain the upward tension on the portion which stretches from the

foot to the knee. With the other hand, pass the remaining bandage behind the leg and around to the front, making a circular turn. See Figure 46C.

7. Continue the circular turn *under* the portion which is being held taut and around the upper calf again.

8. Repeat the circular turns until the bandage is used up, each time maintaining, or even increasing, the tension on the vertical portion. Be sure to keep the bandage as wide and as free of wrinkles as possible, to avoid problems with circulation and innervation.

9. Pin or tuck in the free end of the bandage.

When the patient shows that he is adequately able to ambulate outside the parallel bars with a quad cane, a short leg brace may be ordered. If the patient has a great deal of spasticity in the ankle, a 90-degree stop may be necessary and sometimes, even a T-strap, to provide the stability of the ankle in the proper position. Otherwise, a Klenzak spring type of ankle may be put into the brace, thus allowing ankle mobility. Again, it becomes necessary for the patient to learn how to put the brace on independently.

1. Patient is seated in wheelchair with brakes locked or in straight chair with arms, situated so that it cannot slide.

2. Patient crosses affected leg over unaffected leg.

3. He must pull tongue of shoe through laces, so that it will not slide down into the shoe when it is being applied.

4. Holding brace at junction of inner upright and calf band, he brings it behind leg so that heel is between the two uprights.

5. Patient turns toe of shoe slightly medially and slides foot into shoe.

6. With toes well into shoe, and heel touching back of shoe, he inserts shoehorn into heel of shoe.

7. Then he grasps upright bar and swings foot to floor.

8. Patient works foot into shoe by alternately pressing down on knee with unaffected hand and pulling up on shoehorn.

9. Finally, he fastens shoelaces and strap(s) of brace.

If the end result demonstrates that the patient is unable to ambulate, he should be trained to become independent in a wheelchair. He may be taught to manipulate the wheelchair by utilizing his unaffected arm and using the leg for steering. There are various types of wheelchairs available and a prescription should be made depending upon the needs of the patient. In all instances, one of the basics is learning how to use the wheelchair locks, because this is necessary in any transferring technique. The patient is taught to transfer from bed to wheelchair, unlock the chair, go to his destination (such as the toilet), relock the chair, and transfer on. When this is the final result, it may be necessary to make certain adaptations in the home, so that wheelchair mobility is possible. This may necessitate widening certain doorways, especially the bathroom doorway, plus providing ramps for access in and out of the house if elevators are not available.

During the past decade, the stroke problem and stroke management have begun to emerge as an entity with which all workers in the health field must contend. It has been successfully demonstrated that there can be a better life for all these people if they receive the proper dynamic management. All stroke patients who are mentally alert and who can follow simple commands deserve a trial at rehabilitation therapy. The majority will have a successful experience, and if the physical restoration is not total, the general condition and health of these patients will at least be improved.

REFERENCES

Advisory Council for the National Institute of Neurological Diseases and Blindness. A classification and outline of cerebrovascular diseases. *Neurology* 8:5, 1958.

Bobath, Berta. *Abnormal Postural Reflex Activity Caused by Brain Lesions*. London: Heinemann, 1970.

Bonner, C. D. *The Team Approach to Hemiplegia*. Springfield, Ill.: Thomas, 1968.

Bonner, C. D., et al. Stroke Units in Community Hospitals: A "How-to" Guide. *Geriatrics* 28:166, April, 1973.

Brunnstrom, Signe. *Movement Therapy in Hemiplegia*. New York: Harper & Row, 1968.

Gibson, Walker. *The Limits of Language*. New York: Hill and Wang, 1962, pp. 8–9.

Hayakawa, S. I. *Language, Meaning and Maturity*. New York: Harper, 1954, pp. 252–263.

Knott, Margaret, and Voss, Dorothy E. *Proprioceptive Neuromuscular Facilitation*. 2nd ed. New York: Harper & Row, 1968.

LaQue, Katherine. Perceptual and Allied Evaluations, Prognostic Importance in Right Cerebral Hemispheric Lesions. Unpublished data, Sept., 1970.

Perry, Catherine E. Principles and techniques of the Brunnstrom approach to the treatment of hemiplegia. *Am. J. Phys. Med.* 46:789, 1967.

Policy and Procedure Manual, Cambridge, Mass.: Youville Hospital, 1972.

Semans, Sarah. The Bobath concept of treatment of neurological disorders. *Am. J. Phys. Med.* 46:732, 1967.

Stockmeyer, Shirley Ann. An interpretation of the approach of Rood to the treatment of neuromuscular dysfunction. *Am. J. Phys. Med.* 46:900, 1967.

4

Fractures

Aged persons frequently sustain all sorts of fractures because of increasing difficulties in maintaining balance and responding quickly enough to accidental changes of body position as well as because of poor eyesight, residual weakness from minor strokes, and decreased elasticity and strength of bones. Of all fractures, the most serious is the so-called "hip fracture."

There are two major types of fractures of the hip: those involving the femoral neck and those involving the trochanteric region. About 80 percent of both types occur in people over age 60 and are more common in women than in men. This is probably because women have a slightly wider pelvis with a tendency to coxa vara; they are more prone to senile osteoporosis because they are less active; and their life expectancy over age 60 is five years longer than that of the average man.

Once the fracture has taken place, however, the prognosis is entirely different. Fractures of the trochanter nearly always unite with proper reduction and fixation. A wide area of bone is involved, most of which is cancellous, and both fragments are well supplied with blood. Late complications are rare.

On the other hand, fractures of the femoral neck involve a constrictive area with comparatively little cancellous bone; the periosteum is thin, and the cambium layer is absent. The blood supply to the distal fragment is usually adequate, but the blood supply to the proximal fragment may be impaired or entirely lacking. This can give rise to avascular necrosis and late degenerative changes of the femoral head which can contribute to a nonunion.

Mortality figures indicate that the trochanteric fracture is a serious injury. The death rate in the first three months is reported to be 16.7 percent, more than twice that for central fractures of the femoral neck. This is thought to be because the average patient is about four and one-half years older, more severe trauma is required to produce the fracture, and the operative procedure to correct it is considerably more extensive.

Many hip fractures, as well as others, could be prevented by eliminating from the environment of the aged such hazards as high steps on stairs, icy sidewalks and stairs, narrow staircases (sometimes without banisters), poor illumination, defective household implements, such as decrepit furniture, rough flooring, and loose scatter rugs. Night lights should be placed in bathrooms and in halls that have to be traversed to reach the toilet at night. In an editorial in *Geriatrics* (April, 1963), Dr. Alvarez said:

The important point to be remembered by an aging person is that he had better keep thinking of the setups for accidents. He must avoid these setups and must remember that the old man who starts to fall cannot, with his slow reflexes, weak muscles, and poor vision, recover his balance in an instant as a young and athletic man can do. I often marvel as I see a professional football star tackled about the ankles. He jumps out of the tackler's arms and goes on running. An old lady who just slips on a polished floor goes down like a ton of bricks and smashes a hip.

In years past, the patient with a hip fracture, the surgical counterpart to the victim of a cerebral vascular accident, was routinely put to bed in the surgical ward and placed in traction. Here he remained for 4 to 6 months, during which time his body muscles gradually deteriorated for the simple reason that no therapy whatever was given to maintain muscle tone. As a result of this omission, patients who survived the accident more often than not became permanently crippled and had to be sent to nursing homes, where they stayed for the rest of their lives. This resulted in the high mortality statistics which paralleled the omission of suitable therapeutic measures.

Modern, aggressive management has as its goal the patients' restoration to fullest functional capacity at the earliest possible date. Obviously, patients must be admitted to a hospital, and an x-ray examination must be made to determine the location of the fracture and the extent of its severity. In all but a few cases, early surgical repair will be recommended. Thanks to the availability of modern hospitals and advanced surgical techniques, such as early mobilization, there are few patients, even among the aged population, who are unable successfully to undergo active surgical repair. Therefore, if such a procedure should be vetoed, the reasons for such a decision must be questioned, making sure that the operation actually is a greater risk than its omission. At the same time, it should be remembered that reliance on the old methods, i.e., bed rest and traction, subjects the patient to a higher rate of mortality, a greater chance of nonunion, and a greater likelihood of permanent disability at the end of hospitalization.

The type of repair to be effected, obviously the responsibility of the physician and surgeon in charge of the case, depends on a number of specific criteria not pertinent to this book. Suffice it to say that most hip fractures are repaired by fixation of the fracture site, with any of several types of nails designed for this purpose. The nail may be driven into place during open surgery, or it may be inserted by means of a closed method, its position being checked by x-ray examination. In some cases, when there is very little of the femoral head left, or if the patient is in the age group over 75, a surgeon

may decide to remove the head, replacing it with one of several types of prostheses that are available.

The following series of illustrations demonstrate successful operative procedures for these fractures. Figure 47 shows a Smith Peterson nail in good position fixing a fracture of the femoral neck. The same type of nail is seen in Figure 48, this time, used in the repair of a trochanteric fracture. In certain situations, a nail and plate mechanism is used and Figure 49 demonstrates a Jewett nail fixing a trochanteric fracture. Figure 50 shows a Smith Peterson nail and plate also correcting a trochanteric fracture. In Figure 51 a Smith Peterson nail and plate, plus a screw, repairs a complicated comminuted sub- and intertrochanteric fracture. At times, the operation of choice may be a prosthetic replacement rather than a nail. Figure 52 shows an Austin Moore prosthesis in good position.

Unfortunately, all repairs do not go as smoothly as these, and many types of complications can be seen. Figure 53 shows a fracture of the base of the neck and adjacent trochanteric areas which was not surgically treated. Poor healing is the result. Figure 54 shows an ununited fracture. The nail and plate have been removed, as evidenced by the still visible holes in the shaft made by the screws. Reabsorption of the femoral head is taking place. Absence of the femoral head, broadening of the acetabulum, and subeburnation of the roof laterally is seen in Figure 55. An atrocious surgical result is seen in Figure 56, which demonstrates an ununited fracture of the femoral neck. An attempt at repair with a Smith Peterson nail was made, but the nail did not even bridge the fracture or enter the head. It protruded through the neck into the pelvic bone. Figure 57 shows the same fracture once the hardware had been removed. Could this result have been checked by x-ray? Fortunately, most of these patients, once the pain subsides and the local area adjusts, can still be taught to ambulate with adequate physical therapy. Figure 58 shows a trochanteric fracture

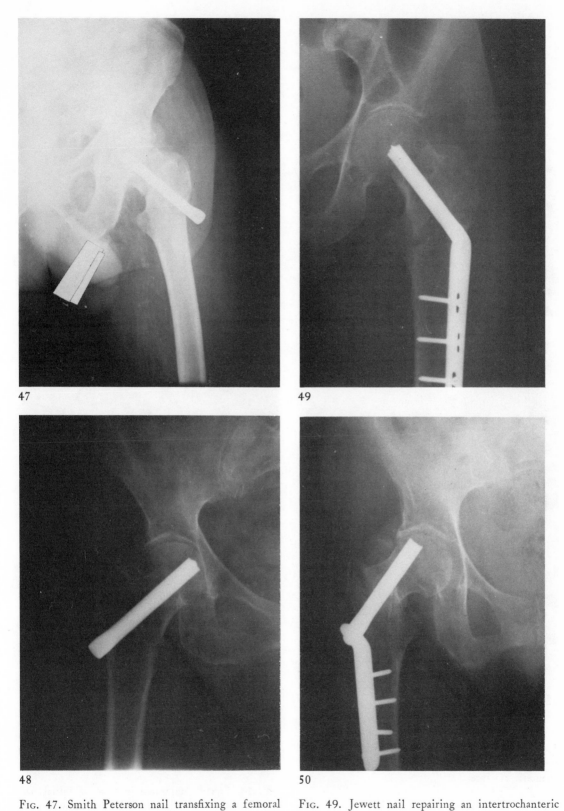

47

49

48

50

Fig. 47. Smith Peterson nail transfixing a femoral neck fracture.

Fig. 48. Smith Peterson nail used in an intertrochanteric fracture.

Fig. 49. Jewett nail repairing an intertrochanteric fracture.

Fig. 50. Smith Peterson nail and plate fixing an intertrochanteric fracture.

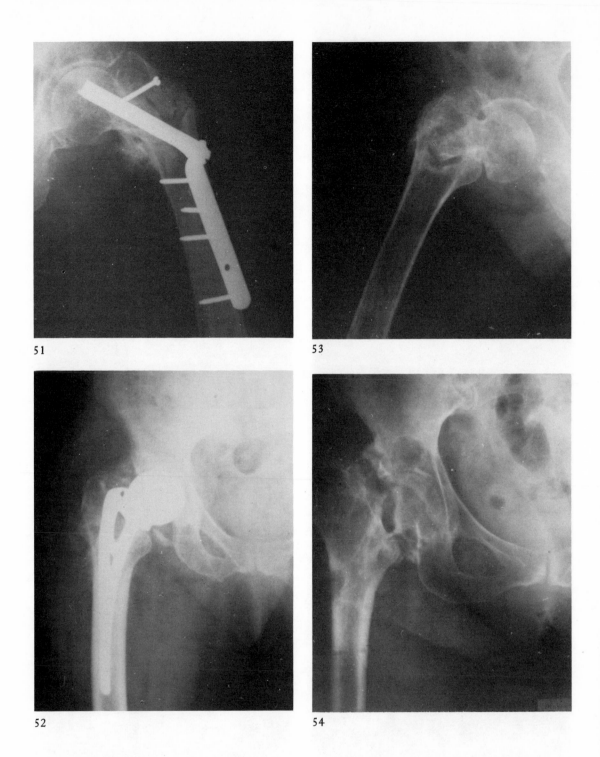

51

53

52

54

FIG. 51. Screw with Smith Peterson nail and plate repairing a comminuted subtrochanteric and intertrochanteric fracture.

FIG. 52. Austin Moore hip prosthesis.

FIG. 53. Poorly healing fracture which was not treated surgically.

FIG. 54. Fracture ununited in spite of initial nail and plate which subsequently had to be removed.

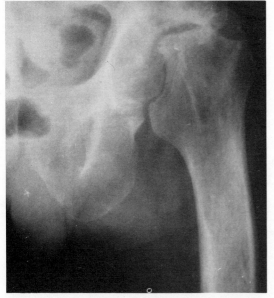

55

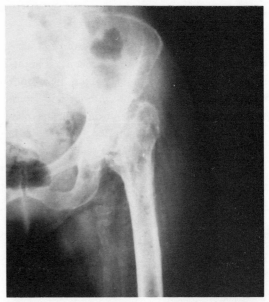

57

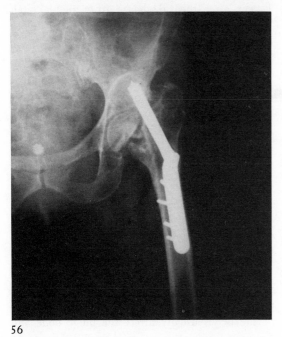

56

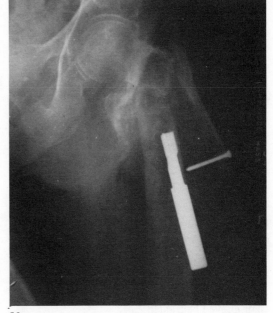

58

FIG. 55. Note absence of femoral head, broadening of the acetabulum, and subeburnation of the roof.

FIG. 56. Poor surgical result in an ununited femoral neck fracture. Note that nail failed to bridge fracture site but protruded into pelvic bone.

FIG. 57. Same hip as in Figure 56 after removal of hardware.

FIG. 58. Intertrochanteric fracture with marked separation between lesser and greater trochanters and shortening of the bone. Note nail in soft tissue posterior to upper third of femur.

with marked separation of the greater and lesser trochanter and shortening of the bone. The nail is in the soft tissue posterior to the upper third of the femur. The screw is anterior and lateral to the femur. A Smith Peterson nail and plate unsuccessfully treat an ununited fracture of the femoral neck in Figure 59. The nail protrudes from the neck into the pelvic bone. Figure 60 shows a Jewett nail causing the same difficulty. A Smith Peterson nail and screw miss a femoral neck fracture, which is ununited, and erode the pelvic bone in Figure 61. An Austin Moore prosthesis is shown in a posteriorly dislocated position in Figure 62.

The above results should clarify the fact that reparative hip surgery is not always successful, and prevention is the best thing.

Regardless of the reparative method used, the primary goal is early mobilization of the patient. This means that instead of lying at home or in a nursing home waiting for the fracture to heal, he should graduate from bed to wheelchair as soon as possible. Meanwhile, an active rehabilitation program, calculated to maintain strength in the uninvolved extremities, especially the arms, should be inaugurated. The latter consideration is especially important because good strong arms will be needed for ambulation with crutches or a walker. Great strength and stamina must be acquired before crutches can be used successfully. As a matter of fact, many people who are given crutches with no preparative therapy find that they are unable to use them at all; consequently, they continue to be tied to the chair or even bedridden.

The good leg should receive active and progressive resistance exercises for maintaining strength, because during the initial ambulatory period it must bear the brunt of the body's weight.

The affected leg requires several types of therapy: quadriceps-setting exercises to strengthen the thigh muscle; passive exercises to preserve the range of motion of the knee and ankle; and active exercises for the lower part of the leg. The end result of this program will then be a body well prepared to start on a partial weight-bearing program in which the patient uses crutches or a walker until the hip is completely healed, then gradually works up to using a cane and, finally, walks with no mechanical aids whatever, agility and general physical conditioning permitting.

In the years since early operative fixation, early mobilization and rehabilitation techniques have come into their own; statistics concerning the longevity and mortality of hip-fracture victims have more or less reversed themselves in that life expectancy has increased and deaths have shown a sharp drop. As a matter of fact, today, of those patients who could receive treatment considered adequate, 90 percent were still active 1 year after their discharge from the hospital. Furthermore, those deaths that had taken place were due to the usual diseases attendant upon old age rather than to fracture complications. These and many supporting figures of a similar nature indicate that the new techniques are here to stay because they have proved themselves. Thus, it should hardly be necessary to say that the recommendations made in this chapter, faithfully followed in behalf of any hip-fracture patients, will help immeasurably in returning them to their rightful place in society—a far happier fate than their regression to the shadowy world of the semi-invalid or total invalid, unneeded, unhappy, dependent on others for every want and need.

There are other fractures which are seen with some frequency among the elderly. Fractures of the pelvis usually affect the pubic bone and can most frequently be treated by closed methods. A satisfactory reduction can usually be made, even with such extensive injuries as separation of the symphysis pubis with fracture of the ilium.

Fractures of the shoulder may affect the surgical neck of the humerus or the head. In the former, they may be divided into two major groups: impacted and unimpacted. The impacted type occurs almost exclusively in older individuals. These people have more tendency to develop periarthritis of this area; therefore

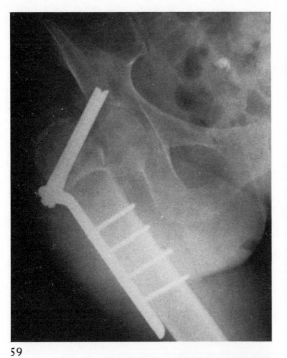

59

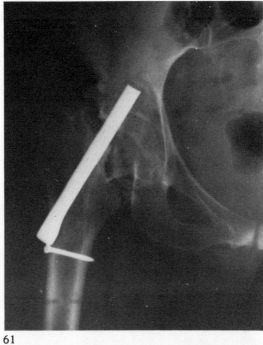

61

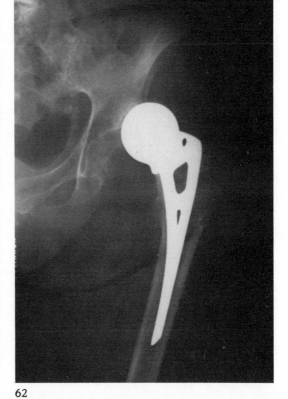

60

62

FIG. 59. Smith Peterson nail protruding from femoral neck into pelvic bone.

FIG. 60. Jewett nail protruding into pelvic bone.

FIG. 61. Smith Peterson nail and screw missing an ununited femoral neck fracture and eroding pelvic bone.

FIG. 62. Austin Moore prosthesis dislocated posteriorly.

early motion and early restoration of function are indicated. Rarely should they be manipulated to improve position, because this would require a longer period of immobilization, and restoration of function would become difficult.

Unimpacted fractures may be abduction in type. They are usually caused by a fall on the outstretched and abducted arm. Fractures that are adduction in type are caused by a fall with the arms at one's side.

Fractures of the head may be comminuted or fracture dislocations. These were rarely treated surgically in elderly people until the past three decades. When the head has fractured into several pieces and the tuberosities are avulsed, restoration to normal is almost impossible. In the elderly, conservative management in a splint for 7 to 10 days followed by exercise is justifiable. If the patient's age is less than 60, an attempt should be made to reassemble the fragments.

Colles fracture at the wrist and a bimalleolar fracture at the ankle also occur, and, as has been indicated above, may be more conservatively managed in the elderly with emphasis on less immobilization and earlier exercise. Whirlpool treatments, massage, and exercise may be indicated as physical therapeutic measures.

REFERENCES

ALVAREZ, WALTER C. Harvard Study of Accidents and the Aged. *Geriatrics*, Vol. 18:257, April, 1963. (Minneapolis, Minn.)

CRENSHAW, A. H. *Campbell's Operative Orthopedics*. St. Louis: Mosby, 1971.

5
Osteoporosis

Osteoporosis is one of the major problems of an inactive geriatric society. Current thinking best defines it as a condition in which bone density is low; in other words, there is too little bone matter within the anatomic bone volume. Although deficient in quantity, the osteoporotic bone is normal microscopically, chemically, and crystallographically. A number of newer densitometric techniques allow for reproducible measurements of bone density.

Recent intensive research by new techniques of kinetic analysis of bone turnover suggests new concepts concerning the mechanism of osteoporosis. They suggest that the primary process is increased bone resorption rather than the lack of bone formation. If true, the age-old concept of Albright's, that the primary mechanism of osteoporosis was deficient anabolic activity due to estrogen lack, may be challenged.

While awaiting the results of more definitive research, the following classification of possible causes may be helpful:

  I. Defect in osteoblasts
     A. Loss of stress and strain
     B. Lack of estrogen
        1. Postmenopausal state
        2. Ovarian agenesis—congenital
     C. Congenital osteoblastic defect—osteogenesis imperfecta
 II. Defect in matrix
     A. Loss of androgen
        1. Eunuchoidism
        2. Senile osteoporosis
     B. Invasion
        1. Gaucher's disease
        2. Malignancy

     C. Loss of protein
        1. Malnutrition
        2. Hypovitaminosis D
           a. Rickets
           b. Osteomalacia
        3. Hypovitaminosis C
        4. Cushing's syndrome
        5. Corticoid administration
        6. Hyperthyroidism
        7. Uncontrolled diabetes
III. Defect in calcium metabolism
     A. Renal rickets
     B. Hyperparathyroidism
 IV. Defect unknown
     A. Acromegaly
     B. Idiopathic osteoporosis.

Although there are many causes for the clinical syndrome of osteoporosis, the one most commonly seen in patients admitted to a chronic-disease hospital or rehabilitation center is that caused by loss of stress and strain on the bones normally created by physical activity and muscular contraction. This phenomenon occurs in isolated bones after immobilization for fracture with plaster or after paralysis of an extremity. Many patients among the older age group, however, have generalized osteoporosis because of enforced general physical inactivity. This especially involves the vertebral column and the long bones. Frequently, osteoporosis from disuse may give rise to compression fractures of the spine and fractures of the hip, which may lead to incapacity and, eventually, death.

These fractures at times occur following minimal injuries. Hip fractures have been reported in individuals who have bent over to switch the channel on a television set. Compression fractures of the spine may occur when stepping down off a high curb or when sitting down too hard in a chair which is too low. One patient was a woman who sneezed while in bed and compressed five dorsal vertebrae.

Osteoporosis is a chronic disease that often passes unrecognized and has caused more pain than many other chronic diseases; yet, in certain instances, it is more amenable to simple therapeutic measures than many other such diseases. It probably holds a record among chronic diseases for having led to false diagnoses. Anything from neurasthenia or psychoneurosis to bone metastasis of malignant disease has been diagnosed, when osteoporosis was the true offender.

In surveying the x-ray films of patients in the average chronic-disease hospital, one may encounter a large percentage that show a relatively poor density of bones, usually referred to by the radiologist as *minimal* or *mild osteoporosis*. It must be remembered that *at least* 30 percent of the calcium contained in bone must be lost before x-ray examination reveals any degree of loss of calcification. These "mild" or "minimal" cases of osteoporosis are therefore patients who have already lost *more* than 30 percent of the calcium from their skeletons. Yet customarily the finding of "mild" or "minimal" osteoporosis will be brushed aside as irrelevant in considering the problems of such patients.

In a survey made in a home for the aged (patients ranging from 65 to 90 years of age) 30 percent of the women and 20 percent of the men were found to have profound vertebral osteoporosis with one or more silent compression fractures.

If compression fractures are absent and, at the same time, x-ray studies show some spurs of hypertrophic arthritis, or some degenerative changes of the intervertebral discs, the present tendency is to disregard the decalcification and to accept the localized anatomical lesions, with their quite incurable consequences, as the source of the patient's back pain or cervical discomfort. This tendency of the physician to grasp at the localized and striking lesion, brushing aside the

systemic disease, has deprived many a patient of appropriate treatment for an illness that can be controlled. Worse than that, the mistaken diagnosis often leads to measures of immobilization which in turn aggravate the unrecognized osteoporosis that was the original source of the trouble, since perhaps the most common cause of osteoporosis is *disuse*. Regardless of the patient's age and condition previous to immobilization, the absence of the daily mechanical stresses and strains that normal activity imposes on bone rapidly leads to decalcification. The osteoclastic activity in the bone continues, whereas the osteoblasts become dormant. Consequently the matrix is decalcified rapidly; so rapidly, in fact, that marked hypercalciuria develops, leading sometimes to the formation of kidney stones. This complication is particularly to be dreaded in aged persons, who already have a tendency to senile osteoporosis and more often than not have preexisting urinary-tract infections favoring the development of kidney stones. Complete immobilization is particularly undesirable in aged people.

It is well known that fractures of the femur and of the ribs, as well as compression fractures of vertebrae, occur more frequently in aged subjects than in the young. These fracture patients usually have osteoporosis; but if they do not have it at the time of the accident, they will almost certainly get it from disuse during their enforced immobilization.

OSTEOPOROSIS AS VIEWED TRADITIONALLY

While there is a definite relationship between the gonads and bone calcification in women, this relationship is not so clear in men. Nevertheless, the condition of the bones in men who have undergone orchiectomy for cancer of the prostate should be closely watched. Estrogens may be indicated in the treatment of some of these patients, in spite of satisfactory control of bone metastasis from prostatic cancer, for the purpose of avoiding excessive loss of calcium from bone.

Bone calcification is subject to other controlling factors, such as the adrenal hormones. One of the prominent features of Cushing's disease (hyperfunction of the adrenal cortex) is osteoporosis, a condition reproduced occasionally during the prolonged administration of adrenocortical or adrenocorticotropic hormones (i.e., cortisone or ACTH). The decalcifying action of hormones, such as ACTH and cortisone or its derivatives, must be kept in mind and its effects forestalled by the proper, specific corrective measures whenever such hormones are being used for extended periods of time.

Any condition that tends to create a protein deficiency or retards the formation of connective tissue, such as malnutrition from any cause or vitamin C deficiency, may favor the development of osteoporosis. Thus osteoporosis is a disease that is to be expected in the aged or chronically ill, as many of these people suffer simultaneously from general debilitation, senility, malnutrition, hypogonadism, and vitamin deficiencies and are frequently immobilized.

The actual incidence of osteoporosis in this group is much higher than is generally realized. Physicians tend to dismiss lightly their complaints of bone aches, insecurity in walking, loss of vibration sense, easy fatigability, postural pains, shortening of stature, and changes of posture as inevitable accompaniments of physiological aging.

Bone is formed by the development of osteoid tissue through the activity of the osteoblasts, or bone matrix, which is calcified by the deposition of calcium phosphate as soon as the matrix has been formed. This is a continuous process, and the normal mass of bone is maintained by the dynamic equilibrium of osteoblasts, which form bone matrix, and osteoclasts, which continuously destroy bone.

Osteoporosis is a systemic disease usually based on a defect in the synthesis of bone matrix. Since there is lowered production of the osteoid substance, no calcification can occur. The osteoporotic patient needs, above all, adequate supplies of protein in the diet, plus the factors necessary for connective-tissue synthesis, such as Vitamin C, plus chemical factors stimulating the deficient osteoblastic activity to normal levels or beyond. Calcium and vitamin D must, of course, be present in sufficient amounts to permit calcification, which will occur when the other necessary factors are available. The optimal amounts have been found in balance studies to be around 1.5 gm. of calcium and 50,000 units of vitamin D per day. Larger doses of these substances are probably quite useless and may be deleterious.

In addition, the mechanical stresses of normal physical activity stimulate the osteoblasts to their physiological activity. Metabolic balance studies have shown that if these normal stresses are suspended by complete immobilization of otherwise healthy young adults, there immediately occurs a serious depletion of calcium in the bone, accompanied by increased excretion of phosphorus and nitrogen in the proportions in which these elements occur in bone. This takes place regardless of intake and can be corrected by resumption of the patient's normal activity, or by such artificial measures as an oscillating bed.

It has been shown by the same methods of metabolic-balance studies in man that estrogens cause an increased retention of calcium and phosphorus in the proportions in which they occur in bone. This same effect is found when androgens are given, and with the latter substances there occurs also an increased retention of nitrogen. The combination of estrogens with androgens causes an even more marked retention of phosphorus and calcium than when these hormones are given separately. Amounts of dietary calcium exceeding the recommended daily ration of 1.5 gm., even when accompanied by vitamin D, are not utilized by the osteoporotic subject and are excreted in urine and feces.

Osteoporotic patients have normal serum values for calcium, phosphorus, and phosphatase. They have aching pains, particularly in the back, anywhere from the cervical spine down to the sacroiliac region, with or without x-ray evidence of mild or minimal osteoporosis, and often flaccid, dry, atrophic skin. Characteristically, a favorable response will follow one of the therapeutic programs outlined below. Fatigue, depression, a feeling of insecurity in walking, and headaches, cervical or frontal, may often complicate the picture and should not mislead the physician into a diagnosis of psychoneurosis.

The differential diagnosis must be made against conditions with somewhat similar symptomatology, such as multiple myeloma, metastatic carcinoma, osteomalacia, hyperparathyroidism, and Paget's disease. This is sometimes difficult and can be facilitated by Table 4, modified from that in Anderson's review article.

TREATMENT

In the first place, it is imperative that a reasonable degree of physical activity be maintained in order to subject the osteoblasts to the physiological, mechanical stimulus of stress, to which they readily respond. Every surgeon knows the rapid loss of calcium that occurs in an immobilized fractured limb, to a degree where x-ray density is markedly reduced. It is well known that the fractured limb, once mobilized, quickly

recovers its normal x-ray appearance. This natural phenomenon of acute orthopedic surgery should not be forgotten when chronic problems of the osteoporotic debilitated subject are considered. The patient who has a painful spine, even with collapsed vertebrae, should not be immobilized if this can possibly be avoided. A well-constructed corset-type support can alleviate some of the immediate distress and still safely permit some activity for mechanical stimulation of the osteoporotic bone.

As the situation improves with the other therapeutic measures, simple but skillfully planned active exercises should be instituted to strengthen not only the bone but also the musculature, which may have become atrophic from prolonged disuse and consequently no longer helps to carry its share of the patient's weight. If an oscillating bed is available, it can be used with benefit for peripheral vascular tone, muscular tone, and bone salt storage.

Next in simplicity and importance are dietary measures. A calcium intake of 1.5 gm. per day is indicated, and 50,000 units of vitamin D should be given daily. To give supplementary

TABLE 4. TABULATIONS OF LABORATORY DATA WHICH MAY AID IN THE DIFFERENTIAL DIAGNOSIS OF OSTEOPOROSIS[a]

Disease	Blood Chemistry					Sternal Puncture	Bone Biopsy
	Calcium	Phosphorus	Alkaline Phosphatase	Protein	Calcium Balance		
Osteoporosis	N	N	N	N	N or −	N	N (?)
Metastatic cancer	N or +	N	N or +	N	N	N	N or +
Hyperparathyroidism	+	−	N or +	N	−	N	Osteitis fibrosa
Multiple myeloma	N	N	N	+	N or −	+	N or +
Paget's disease	N	N	+	N	N	N	N or +
Osteoporosis with sprue	N	−	+	N	−	N	Osteomalacia

N means normal, (?) indicates "of questionable value," − less, + more or "positive."
[a] As modified from Anderson, *Quart. J. Med.* 19:67–96, 1950.

calcium beyond 1.5 gm. per day might indeed do harm, since in the absence of sufficient bone matrix the calcium is not utilized and some of it will be excreted and precipitated in the urine in the form of insoluble salts, leading to kidney stones. This complication should be guarded against by maintaining an adequate urine flow, at least 1500 ml. per day, and by keeping the calcium intake at a reasonable level. A diet rich in protein, such as the osteoporotic patient should receive, contains appreciable amounts of calcium, which can be brought to 1.5 gm. per day by the use of milk (containing more than 1 gm. per quart) and calcium lactate tablets. In elderly, sedentary patients even less than 1.5 gm. of calcium may be sufficient, and smaller amounts of vitamin D should be given.

Shorr and his group have shown that strontium, a rare earth metal that is closely related to calcium, may be retained by bone equally as well as calcium, or perhaps even more readily. With strontium there is no danger of renal lithiasis, and as much as 6 to 9 gm. of this substance (expressed as strontium lactate) has been given daily for many months and years to some patients with osteoporosis and resulted in satisfactory strontification of bone without complication.

The most important part of the therapeutic regimen is the administration of androgens or estrogens, or both. Since androgens and estrogens combined are most effective, as shown in balance studies, the combinations of both are perhaps the most effective therapy. When doses are used that mutually neutralize the purely sexual effects of these hormones, such undesirable side effects as impotence and gynecomastia in men, and breast engorgement and uterine hemorrhages that sometimes accompany estrogen medication in women, may be avoided. The same is true of the possible stimulation of preexisting microscopic cancer of the prostate in man, and of virilization in women, which may occur with the administration of androgens alone. A number of oral and injectable mixtures of androgens and estrogens are at present on the market, and

the neutralizing ratios of androgen to estrogen are usually 50 mg. of testosterone propionate to 1 mg. of estradiol benzoate.* This proportion, however, may vary from patient to patient and may have to be adjusted individually, depending on any untoward side effects of estrogens or androgens that may occur.

There is some question about the wisdom of administering methyltestosterone by mouth, since cases of hepatocellular jaundice have been reported in the literature with the use of this drug. Most estrogens can safely be given by mouth, and the frequent injection of androgens can be avoided by using pellets instead, which can be inserted at intervals of as much as 3 months (75 mg. of testosterone in pellet form will, for example, suffice to neutralize 3.75 mg. of Premarin taken orally every day). In women with postmenopausal osteoporosis it is necessary to avoid excessive estrogenic stimulation of the breasts or uterus, which may occur in spite of combined estrogenic and androgenic therapy. This can be done by interrupting hormone therapy every 3 weeks for 1 week. Withdrawal bleeding from the uterus may occur whenever therapy is discontinued, and the patient should be warned beforehand of that possibility. At no other time during therapy should there be any vaginal bleeding. If it occurs at times other than upon withdrawal of medication, it must be considered as suspicious a symptom of cancer of the cervix as it would be if found in a woman receiving no hormone therapy.

Another form of treatment has been suggested whereby estrogenic therapy may be given

---

* This neutralizing ratio is expressed here in terms of a commonly used crystalline androgen and estrogen, respectively. Androgenic activity is commonly expressed in terms of milligrams of testosterone propionate, rather than in "units." In the case of estrogens extracted from urine or placenta, the estrogenic activity is expressed in international units, 1 I.U. being equivalent to 0.1 microgram (0.0001 mg.) of crystalline estrone. Occasionally the older Allen-Doisy "rat unit" is still used, and this may be from three to twenty times as potent as the international unit. This should be kept in mind when determining the actual estrogenic potency of commercial preparations.

without interruption, and overstimulation of breasts and uterus may be avoided. This is by the use of orally administered progesterone (an-hydrohydroxyprogesterone), which is given in 100-mg. daily doses for 5 days every 4 weeks, while estrogen treatment continues. In the presence of a uterine mucosa this produces a "menstrual" flow that ceases upon withdrawal of Progesterone. Again, no bleeding should occur at any other time during therapy. This form of therapy is the most physiological one in women and probably also the most effective regimen yet devised.

The optimal dosage of estrogenic hormone has not been determined. There is no evidence that large doses are more effective than smaller ones, but the most effective dose is probably somewhere around 3.75 mg. of Premarin per day or its equivalent in natural or synthetic estrogens. It is quite certain that doses below 1.25 mg. of Premarin are ineffective.

Relief is often perceptible after a few days or weeks of treatment and can progress rapidly to the point of complete disappearance of symptoms. Although the x-ray picture may not change for many months or years, since it is a poor index of those slight changes in bone density which are sufficient to alleviate symptoms, bone pain, fatigue, and insecurity in walking are greatly decreased. The patient's psychological difficulties—depression, pessimism, or irritability—also tend to disappear, and the skin takes on its normal turgescence.

Upon the cessation of therapy, symptoms promptly recur. It must be remembered that this is a substitution treatment that has to be continued indefinitely. However, gradual reduction of dosages is often possible, while the benefits of therapy are maintained. The complications of hormone therapy are few if it is managed as outlined above. Rarely, edema may occur and can usually be controlled by restricted salt intake, or, if necessary, by chlorothiazide or mercurial diuretics given at suitable intervals.

Failure of the treatment to show effect after at least a month's trial should arouse suspicion that the diagnosis of osteoporosis was mistaken, or that complicating factors exist. The differential diagnoses to be considered include, besides other systemic bone diseases, multiple myeloma and bone metastases of tumors of undetermined primary origin. When the diagnosis of osteoporosis is correct, the effects of hormone therapy (estrogens, estrogens plus androgens, or anabolic steroids) can be remarkable. However, for best results, a program designed to promote adequate physical activity must be an integral part of therapy.

CURRENT THINKING

Since Albright's original concept has come under scrutiny, the mechanism of osteoporosis has become the subject of renewed intensive research. For instance, experimental animals fed a calcium deficient diet will develop osteoporosis. If these animals are parathyroidectomized at the onset of the study, osteoporosis does not develop with this diet nor with immobilization. Therefore, can osteoporosis be due to faulty parathyroid hormone or calcitonin excretion?

A new approach has been to study the role of the skeleton as a systemic reservoir of alkali. Many experimental and clinical observations show bone involvement in the buffering of excess acid, ingested or endogenously generated. Actual increased resorption of bone in the process of buffering excess acid has been demonstrated.

Applying this observation to humans showed that high-protein diets, which are high in acid content, could greatly influence calciuria and might contribute significantly to a negative calcium balance. Therefore, the traditional concept that a high-protein diet is good for an osteoporotic patient needs to be reexamined and minutely explored.

It has also been found that potassium bicarbonate not only stimulated bone formation but prevented the development of osteoporosis in normal animals given a low-calcium diet. Preliminary studies in humans reveal that potassium-containing alkali salts lower urinary and stool calcium excretion even in experimental immobilization.

Many observers feel that the older regimes utilizing estrogenlike substances, anabolic hormones, calcium supplements, and high doses of vitamin D have shown little evidence of clinical value. It is the author's contention that many patients will respond—even dramatically at times —and that the vast majority of patients with this problem are not treated at all. Certainly, many more are salvageable while one awaits a better treatment program, and the physician should help those who are amenable in greater numbers.

REFERENCES

ALBRIGHT, F., and REIFENSTEIN, E. C., JR. *Parathyroid Glands and Metabolic Bone Disease: Selected Studies*. Baltimore: Williams & Wilkins, 1949.

ANDERSON, I. A. Postmenopausal osteoporosis: clinical manifestations and the treatment with estrogens. *Quart. J. Med.* 19:67–96, 1950.

BANGHART, H. E. A clinical evaluation of methyl androstenediol in the treatment of osteoporosis. *Amer. Pract. Digest Treat.* 5:964, 1954.

BANGHART, H. E. Osteoporosis treatment with nandrolone phenpropionate. *Penn. Med. J.* 64:984–986, 1961.

BARZEL, U. S. (ed.) *Osteoporosis*. New York: Grune & Stratton, 1970.

BONNER, C. D., and HOMBURGER, F. Jaundice of hepatocellular type during methyl testosterone therapy. *Bull. New Eng. Med. Center* 14:87–89, 1952.

CHUR, L. S. W., and ABRAMSON, D. I. Diagnosis and treatment of osteoporosis. *Geriatrics* 18:679–692, 1963.

GERSHON-COHEN, J., RECHTMAN, A. M., SCHRAER, H., and BLUMBERG, N. Asymptomatic fractures in osteoporotic spines of the aged. *JAMA* 153:625–627, 1953.

GOODMAN, L., and GILMAN, A. *The Pharmacological Basis of Therapeutics* (4th ed.). New York: Macmillan, 1970.

HART, G. M. Postmenopausal osteoporosis of the spine. *Geriatrics* 5:321–330, 1950.

HOMBURGER, F., DART, R. M., BONNER, C. D., BRANCHE, G., KASDON, S. C., and FISHMAN, W. H. Some metabolic and biochemical effects of methylandrostenediol. *J. Clin. Endocr.* 13:704–711, 1953.

KUZELL, W. C., GLOVER, R. P., BRUNS, D. L., and GIBBS, T. O. Methandrostenolone in rheumatic diseases and osteoporosis. *Geriatrics* 17:428–441, 1962.

REIFENSTEIN, E. C., JR., and ALBRIGHT, F. The metabolic effects of steroid hormones in osteoporosis. *J. Clin. Invest.* 26:24–56, 1947.

RICCITELLI, M. L. The management of osteoporosis in the aged and infirm. *J. Am. Geriat. Soc.* 10:498–504, 1962.

SELYE, H. *Textbook of Endocrinology* (2nd ed.). Montreal: Acta Endocrinologica, Inc., 1949. List of commercially available hormone preparations, pp. 34–38.

SHORR, E., and CARTER, A. C. Studies on the effects of estrogens, androgens and vitamin D_2 on the calcium and strontium metabolism. Conference on Metabolic Aspects of Convalescence, 15th meeting, Josiah Macy, Jr. Foundation, New York, March, 1947.

SHORR, E., and CARTER, A. C. The usefulness of strontium as an adjuvant to calcium in the remineralization of the skeleton in man. *Bull. Hosp. Joint Dis.* 13:59–66, 1952.

SHORR, E., PAPANICOLAOU, G. N., and STIMMER, B. S. Neutralization of ovarian follicular hormones in women by simultaneous administration of male sex hormone. *Proc. Soc. Exp. Biol. Med.* 38:759–762, 1938.

Symposium on Anabolic Therapy, held by Michigan and Wayne County Academies of General Practice, Detroit, Michigan, March 21, 1962. (Sponsored by Organon, Inc., West Orange, N. J.)

TILLIS, H. H. Clinical effects of methandrostenolone in osteoporosis. *Clin. Med.* 8:274–276, 1961.

WHEDON, G. D., DEITRICK, J. E., and SHORR, E. Modification of effects of immobolization upon metabolic and physiologic function of normal men by use of oscillating bed. *Am. J. Med.* 6:684–711, 1949.

6

Lower-Extremity Amputations

Ischemic or occlusive vascular disease is a common underlying pathological process affecting three basic areas of the body. Cerebral vascular disease or stroke has been discussed in Chapter 3. Coronary artery disease with occlusion and myocardial infarction is well known as a serious problem and is not covered in this publication. The third area of major consideration is the lower extremity; the loss of one or both legs is causing disability in increasingly larger numbers of the elderly population. During war time, a significant number of amputations done on the lower extremities are traumatic in nature. There are also a number of amputations each year caused by industrial, farm, automobile, and motorcycle accidents. These usually occur in younger age groups. In the geriatric groups, incident studies show that per 100,000 population, the number of elderly patients with gangrene, which necessitates surgical removal of a lower extremity, increases each year. Survival studies reveal that patients who now survive the operative procedure live longer than similar patients have in the past. Therefore, every effort at rehabilitation must be applied. The fact must also be faced, however, that a patient who has survived amputation surgery for as long as five years has the real possibility of losing the remaining extremity.

With the realization that the number of geriatric amputees is increasing from year to year, there has been, fortunately, a change in philosophy on the part of many surgeons. It used to be more or less categorically stated that all amputations should be through the thigh because prospects for primary healing were better there than at lower levels. It was true that the increasing use of high amputations reduced the frequency of a number of amputations per person starting with the toe, the metatarsal joint, etc.; and primary wound healing became the rule rather than the exception. Of more importance, however, the degree of disability and invalidism among those who survived increased because of the loss of the knee joint. Elderly bilateral thigh amputees were rarely able to use prostheses, and only about half the elderly male, and very few of the elderly female, amputees were able to use an above-knee prosthesis effectively. Modern surgical and prosthetic techniques, coupled with adequate rehabilitation training programs, have definitely improved those statistics.

Although the objective of this chapter is to discuss the patient whose medical status is such that he already needs amputation, prevention of the problem before this stage should be considered. The physician should constantly promote health programs which include routine exercise and weight-control regimens as well as antiatherogenic diets when applicable, and cessation of cigarette smoking. Also, every effort should be made to avoid amputation if possible, and the use of sympathectomy, embolectomy, by-pass surgery, and/or arterial reconstruction should be investigated.

The basic indication for surgical amputation is either necrosis affecting the bone, tendon, joint, or joint capsule, as well as uncontrollable pain, or uncontrollable infection. One should be familiar with the fact that, at times, the process which is called *autoamputation* may take place.

In this situation, the affected part actually separates by itself. This is usually limited to the toe or the tip of a toe which is involved in dry gangrene.

If one evaluates the total picture, from need for amputation to final physical restoration and rehabilitation, there are five major areas which deserve discussion.

PREPARATION FOR AMPUTATION

Once the decision has been made to amputate a lower extremity, the physician must go through a careful evaluation of the patient's health status. It is necessary to make sure that there are no contradictory signs and symptoms of cerebral vascular disease, heart disease, or other things that may increase the risk for life during the surgery. Attention must also be paid to the extremity to be amputated. It is necessary to make sure that infection is controlled and that edema has decreased. This can be done by wet dressings and proper positioning of the extremity.

Of equal importance, however, is the preparation of the patient's psyche, because the loss of an extremity is usually a very traumatic experience. Most of these patients go into a fairly marked depression following surgery because they then view themselves as having a distorted body. Their apprehensions of losing physical ability, work ability, and personal esteem may become major problems in their rehabilitation process.

An example of this can be sited: A 64-year-old male worked in the accounting department of a rehabilitation hospital. Through his contacts with most of the hospital departments, he got to know, personally, most of the physical and occupational therapists and doctors. Many times he would sit down in the cafeteria and have lunch with the various ones, and he was always considered to be a very pleasant, personable individual.

One weekend, he was suddenly afflicted with pain and coldness of a lower extremity and was admitted to a general hospital. He was seen by a surgeon who appraised the situation and said, "Well, my friend, it looks like we'll have to cut this boy off, and I'll see you in the operating room tomorrow morning."

Surgery proceeded on schedule and following postoperative convalescence, the patient was admitted to the rehabilitation hospital where he had previously worked. He demonstrated, at this point, a total change in personality. He was very depressed, but more than that, he became rude and unmanageable. In therapy, he would yell at the therapist for immediate attention, and many times he would not follow through on treatment programs. He took the leadership of a group of amputee patients and attempted to instigate similar rebellion on their parts. Without anyone's knowledge, he arranged with a commercial prosthetic company to make him a prosthesis for which no prescription had been written. He finally signed out of the hospital, and while driving alone to the prosthetist to pick up this artificial limb, he was involved in an automobile accident and killed. This is obviously an extreme reaction to an amputation (but factual) and demonstrates to what length a patient may go if inadequately prepared and controlled emotionally.

When an amputation is to be done, this should be fully and frankly discussed with the patient so that he may have the opportunity to express his fears, his doubts, and to ask any questions which come to his mind. There should be a number of these sessions if possible before the actual surgery takes place. It is also wise to have another successful amputee patient, who is using his prosthesis well and who has finally adjusted to it and is happy about his result, come in and talk to the patient, so that the patient gets another viewpoint. He must be encouraged to realize that he will not lose the esteem of his friends, colleagues, and family, and that, with concentrated effort, he will be functionally mobile, and if not able to do all the things he has done before, certainly he will be able to do most of them. He must be made to feel that the efforts of all involved in his case are united to provide him with a pain-free, ambulatory, functional future.

SELECTION OF SITE OF AMPUTATION

It has become evident to the modern surgeon that the goal in any amputation is to operate at the lowest possible level, meaning in particular saving the knee joint whenever possible and at almost any cost. Whenever gangrene, edema, and infection are adequately controlled, the definitive amputation can be performed successfully at the next level proximal to demarcation, consistent with good function and provided that the skin at that level shows evidence of good nutrition and warmth.

There has been much discussion concerning the exact choice of the level at which to operate. Much must be based upon the surgeon's experience and knowledge. It has been demonstrated that the condition of the skin is the critical issue, and the presence or absence of bleeding from muscle is far less important in choosing the site. The better the peripheral circulation, the better the chance for primary healing. Existence of a palpable pulse at the next proximal level and the absence of ischemic pain are favorable assets; however, the absence of a popliteal pulse is not a contraindication to below-knee amputation.

Amputations may be done at the foot, the ankle joint, below the knee, and above the knee at about the mid-thigh level. It is possible to do supramalleolar guillotine amputations, but these are usually restricted to the patient who has an uncontrollable and extensive infection of the foot, and once the patient is out of his emergency situation, a formal below-knee amputation is then selectively performed.

Also, operations at the knee (knee disarticulation) are rarely indicated. It is important to consider, before making this type of decision, the technical problems the prosthetist might face in fabricating the best prosthesis possible for the individual. It is true that most prosthetists can make a prosthesis to fit almost every situation; the best results, however, are obtained with a good below-knee amputation or a good mid-thigh amputation.

Foot amputations are now indicated in a limited number of patients. They may be transphalangeal, transmetatarsal, or they may be done for transmetatarsal drainage. There is overwhelming evidence that the below-knee amputation is the most useful of all. Recent experience has shown that it can be performed successfully for most patients who have an ischemic occlusive disease. The main asset for performing at this level is that the knee joint is preserved, and this is of great importance for the geriatric amputee. It is suggested that the skin of the calf be spared, which will allow for a long posterior flap. An amputation level as high as the tibial tubercle is still preferred to an above-knee amputation; and if primary healing does not take place immediately, waiting for secondary healing may still be a better choice. However, a stump length of about 5 to 7 inches is preferable, because short stumps function poorly and very long stumps frequently break down in the available prostheses. Recent opinion also indicates that the desired stump shape is cylindrical rather than conical, hence a fibular length equal or almost equal to the tibia is recommended.

If it is impossible to provide a below-knee stump, an above-knee or mid-thigh amputation is indicated. Adequate length should be retained to provide efficient leverage for the prosthesis. Many patients requiring this procedure are so ill that the amputation must be as simple and as quick as possible.

POSTOPERATIVE MANAGEMENT

There has been a definite change in the routine to be used in the immediate postoperative period. In the past, the operative wound was closed and a simple application of soft dressing, or sometimes a compression dressing, was made. This made it easy to have access to the wound to inspect for infection. However, this procedure did not adequately contain the soft tissue of the stump and, at times, considerable swelling or discomfort occurred. Surgeons were also reluctant to allow too much handling of the stump so that traction or prone-lying to prevent flexion contractures of the hip or knee, and ace bandaging to provide shrinkage and shaping, were frequently not allowed for two to three weeks. In many instances, surgeons did not utilize this method of stump preparation at all.

The current procedure involves the utilization of a rigid plaster dressing at the time of surgery, followed either by an immediate preparatory prosthetic fitting, allowing immediate limited ambulation, or the application of a rigid plaster dressing, followed by an early temporary type of prosthesis after the sutures have been removed. Whichever method is used, the cardinal principle is to prevent swelling and discomfort of the stump, prevent flexion contractures of the hip and knee, and to start the shaping of the stump as soon as possible.

When the surgeon decides to do an immediate postoperative fit, the rigid dressing serves as a temporary socket to which a predesigned prosthetic unit with foot can be attached. See Figure 63. This does require a certain amount of training and experience on the part of the surgeon, because the technique of application must follow very closely known prosthetic principles. If this experience is not available, a qualified prosthetist probably should apply the original temporary prosthesis in the operating room. Again, the below-knee amputation lends itself most suitably to this type of procedure, but it can also be done utilizing a different prosthetic unit for the above-knee amputee.

When the prosthesis is not being worn, continuing shrinking and shaping of the stump or maintaining the stump may be done by the application of ace bandages. The procedures to be used in bandaging the above- and below-knee stumps adequately are as follows.

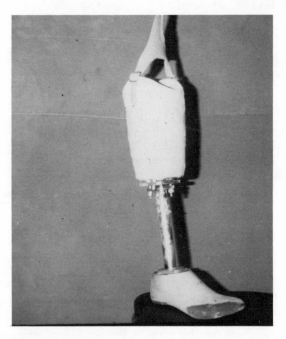

Fig. 63. Temporary prosthetic unit for immediate postoperative fitting of below-knee amputee.

Above-knee Stump Bandaging

One or two 6-inch bandages are used initially to contain the tissues of the stump, to provide a firm surface for the bandages to follow, and to anchor the bandages on the hip. They are not applied as tightly as usual, as the intention is not to shape or shrink. (The number used depends on the size and length of the stump.) The second bandage is a 4-inch, applied firmly in a figure-eight pattern; and the purpose is to shape and shrink the stump. Pressure is greater distally than proximally, and all wraps must be on the diagonal to prevent constriction of circulation.

BANDAGES

One or two (sewn end to end) 6-inch bandages and one or two separate 4-inch bandages. These may be of cotton elastic or spandex elastic.

POSITION

The patient may be positioned: (1) on his side with the stump on top. He must then abduct the good leg against the table to lift the pelvis off the supporting surface in order for the therapist to pass the bandages underneath. This position is necessary for bilateral above-knee (A/K) amputees and is preferable for bilateral AK/BK; (2) supine with nonaffected knee bent and foot on table. The patient then elevates the pelvis (bridging) while the bandage is passed around the hips; (3) standing on the remaining leg, near a support, e.g., bed or chair. This is a desirable position but cannot be easily maintained by elderly patients.

PROCEDURE

The 6-inch bandages are used first; the 4-inch bandage is always the last. The bandage is started in the groin and is brought diagonally over the lateral distal corner of the stump (Fig. 64A), then over the medial corner and brought back diagonally over the anterior stump to the iliac crest (Fig. 64B). It is then brought around the hips in a spica (Fig. 64C). It is important that the bandage be started from the medial portion of the stump so that the spica will pull the stump into extension. Care must be taken that the stump is not abducted at the same time.

As the bandage comes back around the hips to the stump, it is swung around the proximal portion of the stump high in the groin area from lateral to medial and around the hips once more (Fig. 64D). At this point, one 6-inch bandage will have been used and all the stump, except for a small part of the lateral distal corner, will be covered. If the stump is very flabby, the second 6-inch bandage is also started in the groin area but slightly more laterally so it can be brought around to cover the lateral distal corner in an oblique fashion. This second bandage is brought around in a hip spica, then around the proximal portion of the stump to another spica, in a similar manner as the first bandage. As the second bandage is brought around from its second turn around the hips, it should be brought across the stump as far laterally and distally as possible, to help keep the stump in adduction. In the average stump, both 6-inch bandages will

have been used at this point. If the stump cannot be adequately covered with two 6-inch bandages, a third one should be applied in a similar manner as the first two. While more of the first two bandages are used to cover the proximal aspect of the stump, care should be taken that the bandage does not cut off circulation. It has been found that bringing the bandage directly from the proximal medial area of the stump into the spica helps to keep the bandage over that area and prevents rolling to a reasonable degree.

The 4-inch bandage is used to exert the greatest amount of pressure at the distal end of the stump, to prevent "dog ears," and to achieve proper shaping for prosthetic fit. In all but very short stumps, it is not necessary to wrap this bandage in a spica. Thus, it is started at the lateral proximal portion of the stump, brought diagonally across the anterior stump, over the medial distal corner, and around the posterior stump to catch the lateral distal corner (Fig. 64E). Starting this bandage laterally brings the weave of the bandage across that of the previous bandage, thus exerting more even pressure on the stump. The bandage is continued in the usual figure-eight pattern, bringing most of the pressure to the distal end of the stump (Fig. 64F).

The finished bandage should provide for a well-shaped stump with the greatest amount of pressure at the distal end but with the proximal soft tissue well held within the bandage. The repeated hip spicas will assist in keeping the bandage in place for a longer period of time (Fig. 64G). Anchor the bandage with safety pins anteriorly to prevent pressure. Regardless of how well the bandage stays on, the stump must be rebandaged four times a day to maintain proper pressure and prevent skin problems from wrinkles.

BILATERAL ABOVE-KNEE STUMPS

The method of bandaging bilateral above-knee stumps is similar to that for all above-knee stumps, but to avoid undue bulk around the patient's waist, the following modification is made: two 6-inch bandages are sewn together.

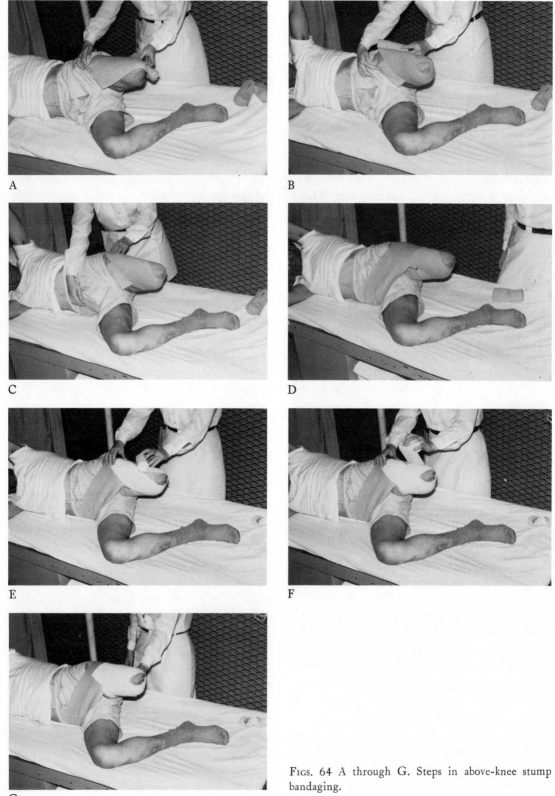

A

B

C

D

E

F

G

Figs. 64 A through G. Steps in above-knee stump bandaging.

With 6-inch bandage, start medially over groin area. Pass diagonally across over lateral distal corner, underneath, around in front, enclosing all tissue in adductor area (proximal medial). Pass laterally over anterior superior iliac spine (ASIS) and around pelvis (patient must roll to get bandage under him). Bring bandage around opposite hip, across body, across stump, and directly under (lateral and medial), keeping bandage high at this point (this will keep bandage on, particularly if patient is obese), and once again to enclose the adductor tissue. Be very careful to prevent any adductor roll. Take the bandage laterally and around pelvis once more. One bandage will usually end in groin area after second time around hips. Pin to secure. Continue with one 4-inch ace bandage on each stump as before.

BELOW-KNEE STUMPS

Care should be taken that there are no circular turns made in the bandage, which will choke the stump, cut off or slow the circulation, and lead to edema, sloughing, poor shrinkage, and bulbous stumps.

There is only one circular turn above the knee to anchor the bandage. All other turns are angular figure eights. In the average length stump, two 4-inch elastic bandages are necessary to shrink and shape the stump properly. Sometimes, in the early postoperative days, only one bandage is used if the stump can be adequately covered. In long or especially large stumps, three bandages are necessary for proper shrinkage.

FIRST BANDAGE

Start just above lateral tibial condyle; bring diagonally across anterior aspect of stump to medial distal corner (Fig. 65A). Then bring it back diagonally across stump posteriorly, across beginning of bandage, and anchor it with a circular turn above the patella (Fig. 65B). After a single anchoring turn above the knee, bandage is brought back down around medial tibial condyle and across posterior aspect of stump to lateral distal corner (Fig. 65C). Figure-eight

pattern is continued as shown, taking care to cross the crest of the tibia in an angular manner (Fig. 65D).

If semicircular turns are necessary to bring the bandage in proper position, they must always be on the posterior aspect of the stump in order to compress soft tissue without hampering circulation. Each figure eight should overlap the last so that the whole stump is covered with greatest amount of pressure on distal end. In a very short stump, it may be necessary to bring the bandage above the knee several times to avoid circular turns below the patella. The figure-eight pattern is proximal to distal to proximal, starting at the condyles and covering the stump to include both condyles and patella tendon. Only the patella is left free to allow free knee motion and free circulation in popliteal area. See Figure 65E.

SECOND BANDAGE

Wrapped like the first with following exceptions: it is started above the medial tibial condyle and brought across the anterior aspect of stump to lateral distal corner. See Figure 65F. With the first bandage, the line of stress is from proximal lateral to distal medial, pulling the medial distal tissue posteriorly and the lateral distal tissue anteriorly. In order to create uniform pressure for proper shaping, the second bandage is started medially, thus pulling the lateral distal tissue posteriorly and the medial distal tissue anteriorly. In a long stump, 6 inches or more, it is not necessary to anchor the second bandage above the knee; it can be anchored with a semicircular turn across the patella tendon.

With both bandages an effort is made to bring the angular turns across each other rather than in the same direction in order for the weave of the bandage itself to assist in exerting a uniform pressure on the stump (Fig. 65G and H).

BANDAGE PRESSURE

In the early postoperative days, the bandage is wrapped very loosely with minimal pressure distally and no pressure proximally. Gauze pads

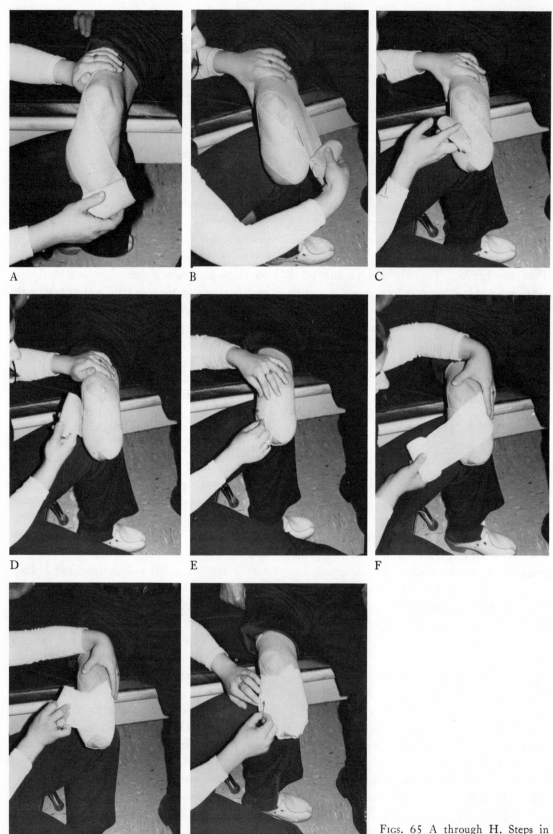

A B C

D E F

G H

FIGS. 65 A through H. Steps in below-knee stump bandaging.

are placed between the incision and bandage to absorb any drainage. After drainage has ceased, a single gauze pad is maintained between the sutures and the bandage so as to prevent pulling on the sutures. The pad is discontinued as soon as the sutures are removed, unless the stump has not yet healed primarily. Occasionally, primary healing is slowed by the vascular condition of the stump, and there may be an open area along the incision after the sutures are removed. In these cases, sterile, dry dressings are continued under the bandaging until the incision is completely healed. Bandaging and walking both aid healing, even with difficult cases, as they are deterrents to dependent edema and venous stasis.

As healing takes place and the sutures are removed, the pressure of the bandage is increased to the tolerance of the patient.

Because of individual differences, these procedures may have to be modified for some patients. The basic principles will *always* apply.

Patients who launder their own bandages should do the following:

1. Squeeze out bandages in warm, not hot, water using mild soap.
2. Rinse bandages well in more warm water.
3. Squeeze out excess moisture in towel. Do not wring or twist.
4. Lay flat—do not hang—to dry.
5. When dry, roll without stretching and smooth out wrinkles.

If the final prosthesis that the patient will receive is of a temporary type and does not require accurate total contact with the stump, one does not have to pursue the shrinking and shaping program to the ultimate degree.

REHABILITATION TRAINING FOR FUNCTIONAL GOALS

The actual measure of a successful amputee is as a functional prosthetic user. All the above steps can be successfully completed, but if in the end the patient remains in a wheelchair and leaves his prosthesis in a corner or closet, the final result is considered a failure.

For the elderly amputee, much more training is required to provide the security and the ease of management necessary to be a good prosthetic user. Their programs will vary considerably, depending upon the patient himself, other complicating illnesses, motivation, acceptance of the amputation, absence of stump complications, such as contractures, atrophy, or breakdowns, and the real, constant threat of possibly losing the remaining limb.

The type and number of amputations must also be taken into consideration. Generally speaking, the individual with the below-knee amputation on one side is the best candidate. If there are bilateral below-knee amputations, this is the next best situation. The above-knee amputation on one side has the third best potential; the below-knee on one side and an above-knee on the other side possess the fourth degree of potential, and the bilateral above-knee amputee, especially in the older population, in most instances, does not become a prosthetic user but can become quite independent with a suitable wheelchair.

Levels of achievement have been categorized into seven classes:

Class 1: Completely independent with cane or no assistive device.

Class 2: Independent in or out of home, including public transportation.

Class 3: Same as class 2, but not including public transportation.

Class 4: Independent in home with cane, crutches, or walker.

Class 5: Independent in home with wheelchair and independent in transfer activities.

Class 6: Same as class 5, but dependent in transfer activities.

Class 7: Totally dependent.

The program, as it is tailored for each patient, will depend upon the evaluation of all assets and liabilities. The strength of the upper extremities and the remaining limb, the strength of the stump, the patient's agility and sense of balance, and the patient's apprehension about falling, all must be taken into consideration. In most instances, progressive resistive exercises must be done with all extremities and stump to bring them up to a functional level to make it possible for the patient first to walk with crutches, or walker with the remaining limb, while the stump is being prepared, and finally, to take the first steps with assistive devices. With the below-knee (B/K) amputee, this process is helped by the immediate postoperative fit of a prosthetic unit, so that he can begin taking steps and bearing limited weight. See Figure 63.

For the above-knee amputee, a similar process may be undertaken, but there are commercially made *ambul-aiders* which come in three general sizes for left and right extremities with pelvic belts and hip joints which can be used for early weight-bearing and stump shaping. See Figure 66. One must be careful not to overdo training with this particular device, as it has no knee. This does not create a problem, however, if the elderly patient's final prosthesis is a laced thigh corset with a fixed knee; but if the person can progress to a mobile knee joint, he should not spend too much time developing what may be bad gait habits.

When the patient has achieved some mobility with crutches and assistive devices and has demonstrated his ability to use a prosthesis successfully, then a decision should be made as to the type of prosthesis to get. It is very important at this time to show the patient an example of the type of prosthesis which is being considered. No prosthesis looks exactly like a human limb, and there is a certain amount of rejection to all. However, there is much more rejection of the "temporary" types, and in many instances it requires a great deal of emotional support to get the patient finally to accept this prosthesis. This must be accomplished or else it is almost guaranteed that when the patient does go home, he will discard the prosthesis and remain in the wheelchair.

CHOICE OF PROSTHESIS

Modern prosthetists have developed a multiplicity of products. In choosing a prosthesis for the elderly, in particular, one must consider appear-ance, weight, ease of application, probable amount of usage, and cost. The type chosen will depend upon a number of factors, including the site of amputation, whether or not the person is a bilateral amputee, his overall medical and physical condition, his apparent powers and agility, and his motivation to become a functional user. The prostheses to be described are those most commonly used in the rehabilitation of the elderly, taking into consideration the above criteria.

For the unilateral below-knee amputation, there are two basic prostheses. The one which is now more popular and which seems to be more desirable for the majority of the patients is the patella tendon weight-bearing prosthesis (PTB), shown in Figure 67. This prosthesis is light-weight, easily applied, and has a simple knee suspension; and most patients, regardless of age, adapt to its use quite readily. Should there be additional problems of stability and support, then one might decide to use a temporary below-knee prosthesis, which has a laced thigh corset where most of the weight is borne, a leather insert for the below-knee stump, hinged knee, and sometimes even lacing of the lower segment. This is a much heavier prosthesis and much less cosmetically acceptable. See Figure 68.

For the above-knee, geriatric amputee, in many instances a temporary type above-knee prosthesis with laced thigh socket, drop-lock knee, hip joint, and pelvic belt may become the permanent prosthesis for that individual. Many elderly amputees find it much easier to utilize a prosthesis with a fixed knee so they have no fear of its bending and causing a fall. Also, the cost of this prosthesis is less. See Figure 69. For those amputees who demonstrate a much higher level of functional ability, one might prescribe a permanent type above-knee prosthesis which has a total contact quadrilateral socket (see Fig. 70), some type of friction knee, such as the Otto Bock (see Fig. 71) or Kolman, a silesian suspension (if the person has good pelvic stability) or, again, hip joints with pelvic belt may be employed. With this type of prosthesis, the patient actually

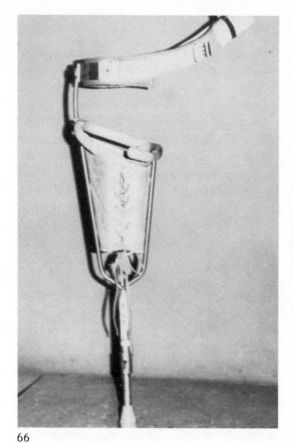

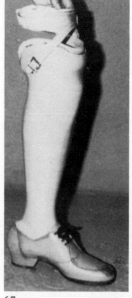
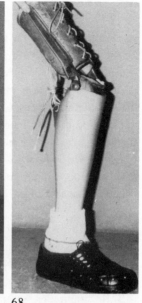

67   68

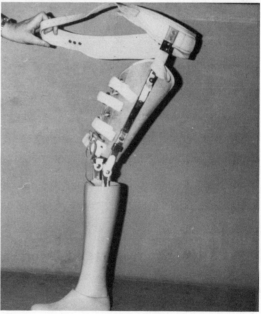

66

Fig. 66. Commercial Ambul-aider for early ambulation of above-knee amputee.

Fig. 67. Patella tendon (PTB) weight-bearing below-knee prosthesis.

Fig. 68. Temporary below-knee prosthesis with laced thigh corset and leather insert.

Fig. 69. Temporary above-knee prosthesis with laced thigh corset and fixed (locked) knee.

69

sits with his ischium on the posterior rim of the socket, and this is known as an *ischial weight-bearing socket*. See Figure 72.

A variety of ankle joints and feet are available. A common type of foot articulation for the elderly is the Sach foot, which is adequate in most instances and requires little maintenance or repair. See Figure 73. This prosthesis is more expensive but is much more cosmetically acceptable. It is possible to have a knee lock inserted if necessary.

Should the patient be a bilateral B/K amputee, it is possible, depending upon his agility, to make use of two PTB prostheses, as described, or two of the temporary type. If the patient has a B/K amputation on one side and an A/K amputation on the other, various combinations are possible; but in most instances, the person will function with a PTB on the B/K stump and a temporary type with fixed knee on the A/K stump. In extreme instances, the temporary type for the B/K may also be employed.

For bilateral above-knee amputees, in most instances, it is better to train them as wheelchair independent individuals. A special amputee wheelchair is available whose center of gravity is different, thus compensating for the absence of pedals. This allows the amputee to bring the chair directly up to the bed, toilet, etc., and to make his transfer back and forth quite easily. Training in this case is directed toward making the patient capable of making such transfers. Some chairs may be ordered with a zipper back to make it even easier for the person to transfer on and off a toilet. See Figure 74.

In a small percentage of cases, even an elderly amputee is able to handle what are called *stubbies*. These are short prostheses without knee joints but with some ankle action. They allow this type of patient to become ambulatory, usually with canes, and if he is a successful product, even to do stairs in each direction. See Figure 75.

A fair amount of space has been used to describe the pathways through which the elderly amputee proceeds. As noted, the final proof of the success of the program is whether the patient becomes a good functional user. The training program must be concentrated, comprehensive, and adequate.

In too many instances, the patient is fitted with a prosthesis, sometimes prematurely before the stump has been shaped, hardened, and strengthened; the patient has been given a few lessons, sometimes not even by a physical therapist; and he is expected to take it from there. In most of these cases, the prosthesis winds up in a closet or corner. It is necessary to provide exercises to strengthen all the extremities *and* the stump, because at first the patient may need to learn crutch walking or utilize a walker. None of this is easy and it requires expert supervision. The patient must then learn the proper gait with the prosthesis, and above all, security in its use. Patients are very apprehensive and require a great deal of practice in all phases —within the parallel bars, outside of the parallel bars with walking aids, up and down ramps, up and down curbs, up and down stairs—until they can do this as second nature. They must also be trained in car manipulation, if this is indicated, and in how to perform household chores standing with the new limb. This does not take place in a short period of time for many of these patients, but it is much better to invest the time in adequate training to ensure that they will become functional users.

A great deal can be learned about the problems of the elderly amputee by sitting down with groups of them and listening to them discuss how they see the whole situation. Such groups can be very effectively run and managed by trained social-service workers whose main purpose is to be supportive. This provides a medium through which a patient can discuss his fears, his anxieties, and his concerns regarding his future as an amputee. Frequently, the group members are seeking information on very practical matters which they do not wish to raise before professionals, because they think they will seem silly. They have many questions concerning phantom pain, why does it continue, will

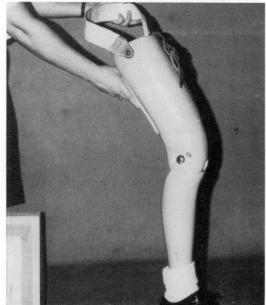

70

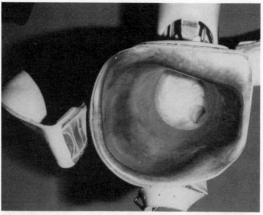

72

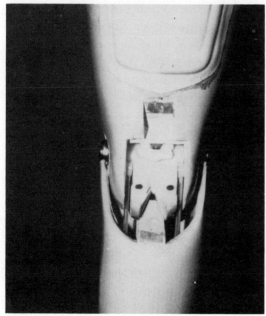

71

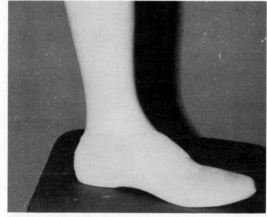

73

Fig. 70. Permanent conventional above-knee prosthesis with quadrilateral socket and friction knee.

Fig. 71. Bock friction knee mechanism.

Fig. 72. Quadrilateral ischial weight-bearing socket.

Fig. 73. Sach foot.

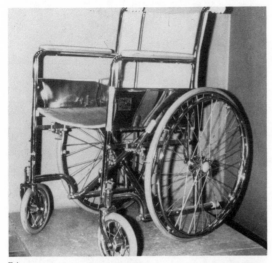

74

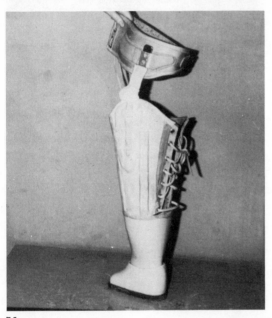

75

Fig. 74. Special wheelchair for bilateral above-knee amputee.

Fig. 75. Stubbies for very agile and strong bilateral above-knee amputee.

medication relieve it? In fact, many amputees wonder why the amputation was done in the first place, when actually the pain appears to them as severe afterwards as it was before. Many members of the group become mutually educated through these discussions, which lessen the feeling of isolation. It was found that group members often looked each other up between weekly sessions and continued the discussions of their problems privately.

Membership in the group seemed to facilitate socialization. Several patterns of discussion developed from these sessions. Initially, it was noted that all new amputees were extremely depressed, even to the point of being completely immobilized in certain instances. They often expressed feelings of wanting to die rather than continue to live without the severed limb. They reviewed events that led to the surgery and the mixed feelings that they experienced about agreeing to undergo this surgery. Group members of longer standing tended to be supporting of new amputees during this period. Another recurring pattern relates to the acceptance of the amputation by others. Amputees are concerned that other people, especially children, will be shocked and disgusted at the sight of the stump. The amputee frequently expresses fears that grandchildren, for example, will become terrified and reject them if they see them without a leg. This issue has been discussed at great length. Group members usually conclude that the way in which it is explained and presented to the child will greatly affect the child's acceptance of the situation. Also, attitudes of other family members will influence this acceptance.

Amputees also express the fact that in many instances the amputation was necessitated as a consequence of their own action. For example, if they had only followed their diabetic diet or stopped smoking they would still have the leg. They wonder if they can exercise enough self-control in these areas now so that they will not lose the remaining leg.

Once they become actively involved in group-therapy sessions, they often express the fear of not being able to "make it." They never expected therapy to be so difficult or take so long. Many surgeons tell their patients that rehabilitation therapy will take one or two weeks, and naturally the patients become upset when they see that this is far from the truth.

The greatest fear expressed by amputees is that, because phantom sensation persists, and because they have the feeling that the limb is still present, they will momentarily forget the amputation and attempt to walk without the prosthesis and injure themselves. Amputees often exchange ideas on how to train themselves not to act impulsively so that they can avoid this catastrophe.

It also develops that many times the surgeon, and even rehabilitation specialists, and family do not ask the amputee if he actually wants a prosthesis. It is assumed that he does and the amputee can become intimidated and made to feel guilty about refusing this "opportunity." Many, for instance, have stated that they would not mind spending the rest of their days in a wheelchair: at least, in this environment, the fear of falling is diminished. Falling is a fear that troubles all lower-extremity amputees. Several feel that bifocal or trifocal eyeglasses should not be worn while using the prosthesis. The different-strength lenses sometimes impair vision to the degree that safety is compromised. Also, many problems discussed are connected with the normal-life issues of people in their 60s and 70s. The issues of retirement, dependency, illness, death of friends and relatives, reduced income, and lack of meaningful activities are issues that confront people in this age group and have become even more meaningful since they are also now disabled.

Amputee groups can, therefore, be a medium through which information is exchanged, socialization encouraged, feelings and anxieties identified and discussed. It becomes one added reason why the amputee may have a successful final result.

Finally, the age of the patient should not be, in essence, used against the possibility of his becoming a functional prosthetic user. Each patient must be evaluated on his own merits by individuals who know their business and who have aggressive and optimistic philosophies. In the author's unit, a significant number of patients between the ages of 80 and 86 have been successfully fitted to prostheses; and, following adequate training programs, they have returned even to live alone in apartments and manage to shop and become functional members of their community.

REFERENCES

Committee on Prosthetic-Orthotic Education, National Academy of Sciences. *The Geriatric Amputee Principles of Management.* Washington, D.C.: National Academy of Sciences, 1971.

Procedure Manual. Cambridge, Mass.: Youville Hospital, 1972.

7

Spinal-Cord Injuries

Spinal-cord injuries (SCI) resulting in paralysis are of two basic types, those which affect the lower extremities (paraplegia) and those which affect all four extremities (quadriplegia). The former are commonly referred to as *paras* and the latter as *quads*. Both these conditions can be caused by such disorders as cerebral palsy, poliomyelitis, multiple sclerosis, spina bifida, basilar artery thrombosis, muscular dystrophy, syringomyelia, transverse myelitis, tumors, and even a ruptured intervertebral disc. This chapter, however, deals with those whose disability results from physical injury such as a fall, motorcycle, automobile, or diving accidents, and bullet wounds.

In paraplegia, the injury takes place in the thoracic or lumbar spine, whereas in the quadriplegic, the cord injury is in the cervical spine. The lesion can happen at various levels producing some variance in symptoms.

Since this is not a reportable condition, no one knows how many SCIs there are. The Department of Health, Education, and Welfare in Washington has announced that there are 200,000 Americans now disabled from SCIs, which have left them, to some degree, paralyzed. The increase of these individuals seems inevitable with highways becoming more densely crowded and accident-prone sports like hunting and skiing becoming more popular. Seventy-eight out of one hundred of these people are males, their more physically active lives making them more prone to accidents.

Today, paralyzed people make up a growing reservoir of manpower. One can imagine the waste if these 200,000 spinal-cord–injury victims today plus their future brethren remain helpless. Because of intensive efforts for their rehabilitation by the Armed Forces and Veterans Administration, paraplegic persons have become synonymous in the minds of many people with war casualties. There were, indeed, some 2500 cases of paraplegia in World War II. But the experience of the Veterans Administration hospitals shows that even though war casualties with paraplegia have been discharged, for every one of these there has been a nonservice-connected civilian paraplegic casualty admitted, and as a result the total case load has remained the same.

Paraplegia is thus distinctly a hazard of civilian life. It appears from comparisons of military and civilian series that the service group sustains about twice as many serious spinal-cord injuries, such as transection of the spinal cord and cauda equina, whereas paraplegia or paraparesis in civilians is more often caused by less serious spinal injuries. Therefore, on the whole, the final results of therapy should be even better in civilian patients than in veterans.

What is the outlook for the paraplegic patient of today? In World War I there were 400 traumatic paraplegic patients. The outlook for these patients was tragic because there were no adequate measures available to manage this serious disability, and there was a high mortality, especially from urinary infections and calculi. In World War II there were 2500 paraplegic patients. In these cases the outlook was entirely different, since much had been learned about the mechanism of paraplegia, the physiopathological changes it causes, and their management. Finally, it has been realized that the responsibility of the physician does not end with administration of the indicated surgical and medical measures but that it includes the responsibility for the patient's complete rehabilitation to ambulation, adequate bowel and bladder control, and the ability to compete in the economic struggle for survival. Since with the present improved methods for the control of urinary infections large numbers of paraplegic patients survive, a tremendous need for rehabilitation has been created.

Naturally, total rehabilitation does not mean in this case restoration of function of the paralyzed extremities. Here motion and control are lost forever. This necessitates the limitations imposed by the use of wheelchairs, braces, and crutches. With 24-hour control of bladder and bowels, however, the paraplegic person is able to lead a reasonably normal social life, live in a home that needs little special adaptation to his needs, and compete in the employment market with nonparalyzed workers. This is not ideal, but it is a good deal better than what the patient, his family, and friends (and often his physician) may expect when paraplegia first strikes. Since much too little is known about the true facts of paraplegia rehabilitation, the gloomy feeling usually pervades all concerned that the new paraplegic patient would be better off dead than alive.

It is hoped that the inclusion of this chapter on paraplegia may aid in filling the gap in general medical knowledge and may convince physicians that most of these patients have a right to demand that they be fully rehabilitated to the point where they are able to leave the hospital, without urinary or fecal incontinence or retention, and get about on crutches.

The paraplegic patient cannot be rehabilitated and cared for by any one man. No physician or surgeon, no matter how highly skilled, could be expected to handle alone the neurological, neurosurgical, urological, plastic surgical, orthopedic, physical, therapeutic, psychiatric, and social-service problems involved. A team approach is necessary, and it is usually best to obtain it in a center with considerable experience in this field. Even if such an institution is relatively far away from the patient's home, it will be more economical in the long run to arrange for his care at such a center than to take a chance of having the patient receive unskilled attention that results in only partial rehabilitation and possibly in serious complications.

The practitioner is of key importance in the team managing the paraplegic patient, since he is often the one who sees the patient first after the accident, and the one who has to obtain the patient's and the family's cooperation for the arduous task of rehabilitation. He often has to coordinate the work of the specialists and must interpret it to the patient. Finally, it is the practitioner who will periodically see the patient after he has been discharged to his home. He has to see to it that all goes well, and he has to anticipate or take competent care of complications.

FUNDAMENTALS OF MANAGEMENT OF PARAPLEGIA

THE ACCIDENT AND EARLY CARE

Overzealous first-aiders are often directly to be blamed for spinal or cauda equina transection rather than the accident itself, which may have caused only slight cord damage. There are cases in the literature where patients obviously did not have transected spinal cords until ambulance attendants placed them in a hyperextension position. One case has been described of a young flier injured in a crash landing. He had severe back pain but sensation and motion in both lower extremities until he was placed in overextension in the ambulance, where he lost motion and sensation in the extremities, obviously having had his cord severed during the trip.

Whenever a spinal-cord injury is suspected, as little motion as possible should be inflicted on the patient. All bouncing and jostling, as well as lifting, which inevitably causes spinal motion, should be avoided. Several men working together should roll the patient onto a stretcher, keeping back and extremities in the neutral anatomical position, and place him in a face-down position to minimize the danger of aspiration of vomitus.

The goal should be to get the patient to the qualified hospital or center for spinal-injury care within 2 hours. In some states, helicopters are used to accomplish this because the first hours are critical in the care of these patients. X-ray films should either be taken with the patient on the original stretcher or be deferred rather than risk further trauma. A firm, flat surface, such as a hair mattress with a foam-rubber mattress on top of it, should be used as a bed. A Stryker frame facilitates turning the patient frequently, which will be necessary to avoid bedsores.

Attendants must be carefully trained. A single, abrupt false motion may transform a reversible lesion into an irreparable spinal transection with permanent paralysis and anesthesia of the lower extremities.

It has been found by specialists in paraplegic rehabilitation centers that it often takes more time to overcome complications due to inadequate early management than to complete the total rehabilitation program. Damage can be done early within the first hours and days after the injury and while the patient is perhaps still in the care of the practitioner, who may have taken charge after the accident. The gravest consequences of early mismanagement are: accidental transection of the spinal cord, which was originally less severely damaged, urinary infection, retention, and calculus formation, malnutrition, development of pressures sores, contractions, and narcotic addiction.

Outside the United States, only 5 percent of these patients are treated surgically, whereas over 90 percent are operated on in this country. Since final results are comparable, it would appear that much unnecessary surgery is being performed. In the cervical region, the most effective approach is the reduction of the usually present dislocation and the application of traction.

The rehabilitation process should be directed by one physician who uses a team of consultants quite freely. He should not be a dictator but more like the conductor of an orchestra, demonstrating his knowledge of the complete score and his ability to bring in sections and instruments as needed. The patient must be an integral part of the ensemble.

Of paramount concern is the care of the urinary bladder. The paraplegic cannot normally feel a full bladder. When it becomes distended, the patient may perspire, get goose pimples, or a headache. This degree of filling should be prevented if possible.

There are three types of situations which can exist. The bladder may become automatic or reflex. In this case, the sphincter automatically relaxes when the bladder is full and the bladder empties itself. It is possible, in many instances, to train these bladders to empty at regular intervals on the toilet. Rubbing the abdomen, tapping over the bladder, or learning to credé may be helpful. Full cooperation from the patient is necessary.

The bladder may be spastic and respond to any mild stimuli, including leg spasms. This type of bladder is very unreliable and small amounts of urine will be voided at frequent intervals. It must be determined whether urine is being forced up into the ureters (reflux) because this must be prevented if at all possible. This is the start of a series of events leading to hydroureter and renal damage. If reflux is not present, an external drainage apparatus is indicated. In the female, catheterization becomes necessary, if absorbent pads and waterproofed pants are unsatisfactory.

The bladder may be flaccid with a relatively tight sphincter. In this situation, the bladder muscle cannot develop enough pressure to overcome the sphincter resistance, so it becomes stretched beyond its normal capacity and the urine backs up into the ureters and kidneys. A catheter is necessary to prevent this reflux.

When a catheter does not seem necessary, the residual urine must be checked periodically.

After the patient has voided, a straight catheter is inserted to see how much urine remains in the bladder. If the residual exceeds 3 or 4 ounces, the catheter may need to remain. A constantly high residual fosters infection and the formation of stones and may lead to reflux.

If catheterization becomes necessary, a Foley, no larger than size 16, with a 5 cc. bag should be used. These need to be changed every 1 to 2 weeks. Silastic catheters are now available which do not need changing for 4 to 6 weeks. The bladder should be irrigated three times per day. Several solutions may be utilized depending upon the purpose of the irrigation.

1. Normal saline in 100 cc. amounts.
2. Acetic acid 25 percent in 50 cc. amounts.
3. Neomycin in special situations 5 percent in 30 to 50 cc. amounts.
4. Renacidin 10 percent in 50 cc. amounts one to three times per day. This dissolves and prevents formation of sediment and calcium.

Numbers 2, 3, and 4 should be instilled, meaning that once the medication is in the bladder, the catheter should be clamped for 15 to 20 minutes, so that the medication can take effect. In contrast, the saline solution is allowed to run in and out freely. A spastic bladder should never be clamped.

A mild infection is always present when a catheter is in place. Suppression of high bacterial activity may often be accomplished using Mandelamine or Methianine. Both work better in an acid urine. Cranberry juice helps to provide this acidification. Banthene may be used for bladder spasms.

When out of bed, the patient should wear a leg bag. This should be alternated from leg to leg, to prevent pressure areas, and emptied every 4 hours. At night, the catheter should be re-attached to the constant drainage apparatus. It is most important for the operation of constant-drainage units to keep the entire system patent, closed to the air, and sterile. Most commercially available plastic setups work very well. A bottle

with the desired irrigation fluid can be incorporated by having the catheter attached to a Y tube. The irrigation bag is kept clamped off except when in use. The bladder drainage is constant, but some bladder tone is maintained by the placement of the Y tube at a level which requires the urine to travel upward before spilling over into the drainage bag. When irrigation is desired, the tubing to the bag is clamped off, and the irrigation fluid is permitted to flow into the bladder. This is then allowed to enter the drainage bag by releasing the lower clamp. This simple apparatus does away with the need for syringes, sterile trays, and frequent handling of the catheter. It therefore saves time for the person charged with the responsibility of the irrigations and decreases the probability of repeated infection by frequent handling of the catheter. The complete apparatus should be changed once a week.

These patients should be followed at intervals by urinalysis, urine cultures, intravenous pyelograms, and cystometragrams.

In certain centers, intermittent catheterization is preferred to constant drainage. This technique is responsible for a more sterile urine and fosters reflex voiding in 2 to 4 weeks. This is a more costly procedure, as it requires a skilled team who must preserve the asepsis of a surgical operating team.

There are other types of bladder management. At times, it may become necessary to do a suprapubic cystotomy when urethral catheterization becomes difficult. Recently, some urologists have favored a type of diversional conduit drainage called the *ileo-loop bladder*. In this process, a loop of ileum is isolated, preserving its blood supply, and severed in two places, making a separate loop. One end is sutured closed and the open end is brought through the skin to form an ostomy type of opening. The ureters are removed from the bladder and implanted into this loop. It serves as a reservoir and when full, spurts urine out into a bag which covers the opening. For some paras who have had to have a catheter and have had many problems with same, this becomes a much simpler way of management.

There are several ways to train a bladder when a catheter may be safely removed.

Method 1: Maintain fluid intake of 2400 to 4000 cc. the day preceding trial. Start trial early in morning so that it may be completed on the day shift. Take and record blood pressure. Inject Urecholine 7.5 mg. subcutaneously. Fill bladder by gravity flow with normal saline and remove the catheter. Encourage patient to void and stimulate voiding if necessary by tapping abdomen, stroking or brushing inner thighs, anal stimulation or by Credé's method. Encourage patient to drink 240 cc. of fluid every hour, and if he is still unable to void, repeat stimulatory techniques hourly for 2 hours. If not successful, a straight catheter should be inserted, the bladder drained, and the trial repeated. If voiding takes place, a catheterization for residual should be done, and if more than 100 cc., the catheter should be left in place.

Method 2: Intermittent clamping may be tried for nonspastic bladders. The schedule should be maintained throughout the 24 hours. Encourage patient to drink 240 cc. fluid every hour. Clamp catheter at 7:00 a.m. Instruct patient to notify nurse if cramps or discomfort develop. Release clamp at 9:00 a.m., allow to drain for 20 minutes, and reclamp. Gradually increase the clamping and releasing time, never exceeding 4 hours or an estimated capacity of 400 cc. When the patient reports the sensation of having to void, remove catheter and start a 2-hourly toileting schedule. Check for residual periodically.

Method 3: Tidal drainage accomplishes bladder rhythmic automaticity. It serves two purposes: it is an aid in the actual rehabilitation of the bladder itself, and it is a cleanser through the application of continuous irrigation. The underlying principle is siphonage.

A simple, inexpensive, effective tidal-drainage apparatus has been developed by the military. It consists of the following: two 50-cm. lengths of 6-mm. glass tubing (A) joined together by a

short length of rubber tubing and mounted beside a centimeter scale (B), which is marked off every 1.0 cm. on a cardboard strip. The zero level of the centimeter scale is set to correspond with the level of the patient's pubis, using an ordinary carpenter's level. See Figure 76.

At the top of the glass column there is placed a 23-gauge hypodermic needle (C) inserted into the rubber medicine-dropper cap (D). This enables the glass column to serve as an air vent, as well as part of both the irrigating system and the manometric arm of a cystometer.

An adjustable siphon loop (E) is suspended by a thumb tack at an appropriate level. Later, tubing 30 to 40 inches long with an internal diameter of 3/16 inch and a wall thickness of 3/32 inch is also needed.

The waste bottle (F) should have a two-hole stopper—one hole to receive the siphon tubing, the other to act as an air vent. A dispensing bottle (G), a screw clamp (H) to control the inflow at 60 to 90 drops per minute, and a

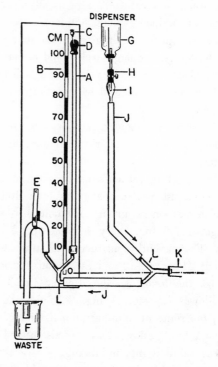

Fig. 76. A simple tidal-drainage apparatus (modified after Lyons).

Murphy drip of the sealed variety (*I*) are the necessary materials, along with latex tubing (*J*) 60 to 72 inches long with an internal diameter of ¼ inch and a wall thickness of 1/16 inch to complete the apparatus.

The catheter should be soft rubber and no greater in size than 16 gauge. Remaining connections are made with glass Y tubes (*L*). The entire apparatus can be conveniently mounted on a board fastened to a bedpost by clamps.

Attention to a few details will prevent failure of the apparatus. The usual cause of failure is a premature break in the siphon, resulting in either incomplete filling or incomplete emptying of the bladder. Air leaks cause this most frequently and may be due to the use of a Murphy drip of the unsealed variety, too great an internal diameter in the siphon loop, a hypodermic-needle air vent of too great or too small a caliber, kinks in connections, improperly placed clamps, occluded catheters, or formation of traps due to long catheter connections.

A common occurrence may be leakage of urine around the catheter. This usually develops because the position of the siphon loop is too high. In the early phases of drainage of an atonic urinary bladder, the siphon level should be set 2 to 5 cm. above the bladder level. Such leakage should never be remedied by inserting a larger catheter.

The stage of bladder recovery can be determined by the cystometric portion of the apparatus.

Method 4: In certain situations, a trial voiding period using Urecholine has been utilized. The medication is given subcutaneously at a dosage of 7.5 mg. every 4 hours for 2 to 3 days. The patient is instructed to strain while voiding. If successful, and the residual is below 100 cc., the dosage is reduced every 2 to 3 days as follows: 7.5 mg., 5 mg., 2.5 mg. At this time, the route of administration is changed to oral at a 75-mg. dose. This may also be reduced if successful to 50 mg. and 25 mg.

A successful bladder program provides definite benefits. It improves patient morale, lessens nurs-ing care, reduces linen laundry costs, and makes more possible discharge and acceptance at home.

PREVENTION OF PRESSURE SORES

It has been shown by metabolic studies that a great loss of body nitrogen (protein catabolism) occurs in the immediate posttraumatic phase and that this is one of the major contributing factors to the formation of bedsores (decubitus). It is therefore necessary to provide enough protein in the diet to compensate for these losses and also to provide enough energy by carbohydrates and fat so that maximal utilization of the proteins is possible. A 4000-calorie diet, containing 150 gm. of protein, should be provided. If this is impossible, protein hydrolysates and protein concentrates should be used as well as high-caloric fat emulsion, which may be given by mouth or intravenously. Severe hypoproteinemia may have to be corrected by plasma infusions. Protein anabolic agents have been of benefit in severe cases.

Good nursing is essential and should include moving the patient every 2 hours, light massage over pressure areas such as the sacrum, trochanters, and ischia, and the avoidance of such orthopedic devices as body casts and splints, which may cause long-continued pressure.

PREVENTION OF CONTRACTURES

Four to six times a day, all joints of the lower extremities should be moved passively through a complete range of motion. When it is not certain whether the cord has been severed, the hips should be moved as little as possible. Foot drop must be avoided at all cost. This can best be done by a footboard; a half-shell plaster cast or posterior splints are to be avoided. The feet should be kept at a 90° angle to the leg at all times. The sheets should be left loose over the foot of the bed or draped over frames* designed to hold up the bedclothes over the feet.

At the same time that the joints of the lower extremities are moved, active conditioning exer-

---

* Obtainable, for instance, at Lewis and Conger, Avenue of the Americas, New York, New York.

cises of the arms should be carried out, with special caution to prevent spinal motion. Triceps and finger flexors especially must be strengthened, since they are needed for crutch-walking. The customary trapeze or monkey bar facilitates movement but contributes nothing toward strengthening the triceps.

PREVENTION OF DRUG ADDICTION

The paraplegic patient who is addicted to narcotics is one of the most difficult medical problems. Every effort should therefore be made to combat pain without resorting to opiates or their derivatives. Pain is rarely an important problem in the paraplegic person, but if it exists and is severe enough to resist simple safe analgesics, it usually requires neurosurgical relief eventually. In most cases it is possible to control pain with salicylates, and this should always be tried intensively before resorting to agents that may cause addiction.

OTHER MEASURES IN THE EARLY PHASE

EARLY ESTABLISHMENT OF UPRIGHT POSTURE

Even before braces can be put on paraplegic patients, they (the patients) may be enabled to stand upright for considerable periods of time by the early use of a tilt table. Eight to 10 days after exploratory laminectomy, the patient may be fastened to such a table by means of straps around the chest, hips, and knees and can be tilted into the standing position for 1 or more hours every day.

This helps in preventing urinary infection and calculi, prevents later circulatory disturbances upon assuming upright posture, and improves the circulation in dependent parts of the body, thereby aiding in the prevention of pressure sores.

BOWEL CONTROL

Spinal shock may cause marked intestinal distention, sometimes marked enough to produce severe discomfort and to interfere with eating and breathing. Distention of this degree should never be allowed to develop. Prevention is often possible by omitting, at early signs of distention, all food and liquids by mouth and by inserting Levine and rectal tubes. Distention responds usually to administration of neostigmine (Prostigmin Methylsulfate) intramuscularly. However, some authorities (Munro) advise against it and suggest, instead, the use of rectal tubes and enemas. Sometimes Wangensteen suction must be instituted.

The ability to control one's bowel movements dependably is probably the single most important thing for most patients. Incontinency of defecation is a great source of embarrassment to the patient, and it also requires sterling fortitude on the part of all those who have to deal with it.

A successful bowel-care plan should:

1. Provide dependable bowel movement schedules.

2. Prevent constipation and frequent impactions. Fecal impactions occur easily and frequently in the geriatric population. They can present symptomatically, mimicking many situations, and can also actually be fatal.

3. Control incontinence.

4. Prevent decubitus ulcers and skin irritations.

5. Remove emotional stress.

6. Aid in the total rehabilitation process.

Procedure

1. A bowel-care plan should be worked out in cooperation with the physician and should be under his direction and orders.

2. Complete understanding of the nursing staff should be obtained and the full explanation of the entire goals of the program should be made. This should be done for all three shifts.

3. It is also necessary to obtain the patient's understanding and cooperation. Once the program has been adequately explained to the patient, he should be encouraged to cooperate and participate fully. One should assure him that bowel function can occur regularly, even without physical sensations.

Guidelines

1. A regular evacuation time should be established which, if at all possible, should correspond to the patient's pre-illness pattern. Some patients are used to daily bowel movements, others have them on alternate days. It should not be necessary for all patients to have a bowel movement each day.

2. Maximum mobility should be encouraged and exercises within the limits permitted by the physician and the capability of the patient should be routinely done.

3. Records are very important. All results should be recorded and observed on each shift.

4. It is necessary to assure an adequate fluid intake which helps to make a normally formed, easily evacuated stool. 2500 to 3000 cc. of fluid is recommended daily.

5. A well-balanced diet, served at regular times each day, should be provided. Roughage foods such as vegetables, fruit, and salads aid in preventing hard stools and help to stimulate peristalsis.

6. There should be adequate physical facilities for the patient to utilize, including toilets, adequate commodes, and above all, he should have privacy. The use of bedpans should be discouraged.

7. One must persevere in the program. One can anticipate that some relapses will occur during the first 7 to 10 days; one should not interrupt the program, however, for at least 4 to 6 weeks. Frequent changes only serve to make regulation more difficult.

8. There should be a continual review of progress or lack of progress with the physician, staff members on all three shifts, and the patient, as indicated.

Routine Techniques

1. At the time of admission, a complete history regarding past bowel habits should be undertaken with particular reference to food habits, fluid intake, use of laxatives, and regularity of movements. A digital examination should be performed and, if impaction is present, the physician should be consulted to determine whether manual removal or a soapsuds enema is indicated. It is necessary to start bowel training with a clean bowel.

2. Daily Program. Day one, insert suppository as far as finger will reach into the rectum past the internal sphincter and against the intestinal wall. Wait 45 minutes. Have patient massage his abdomen and attempt to defecate while sitting in privacy in as normal a situation as possible. If no results, disimpact. Day two, same as day one. Day three, if still there is no voluntary bowel movement, give a tap-water enema. Day four, start procedure over again. If bowel movement on second day, then on the third day, consider it the first day in the procedure and start over again.

3. Close observation and good recording must be undertaken. Note time lapse until the patient has the desire to evacuate after insertion of the suppository; note the place of evacuation—whether commode, toilet, or bedpan. Also note consistency of the stool—whether it is normal, hard, soft, or watery.

4. Medications. There are a number of approaches that one can make to this problem through medication.

a) Suppository: As a general rule, suppositories should not be refrigerated, because refrigeration makes it take longer for them to act. They should be kept at room temperature unless they show a tendency to melt. Dulcolax suppositories are being used more and more frequently. They provide good results; however, they are expensive, they overstimulate the bowel, and sometimes, the patient may tend to leak the melted suppository, which has the appearance of mucus. Dulcolax suppositories may also tend to make the stool very loose; therefore, their usage must be closely supervised. They should not be lubricated before insertion. Glycerine suppositories do need lubrication; they do not dissolve, and they have the advantage of being cheap. It will take the patient a little longer to establish his program, in some instances; therefore, it is desirable to start with the Dulcolax regime and then switch to the glycerine.

b) Colace, 100 mg. bid or tid and in some instances qid may be used as a stool softener. One should not keep the stool too soft, however, because it is difficult for a bowel with decreased tone to expel stool which is very soft.

c) Milk of magnesia, 30 cc. HS is also a common mild laxative. It should be remembered that patients cannot always control a laxative and laxatives are often unpredictable.

d) Should the stool become too soft, then Metamucil 15 cc. bid may be given to provide bulk to the stool and absorb excess water.

Things to Remember

1. If the patient starts training while he is a bed patient with little activity, one should expect, when he starts getting out of bed, that he will be using more abdominal muscles and may have more bowel accidents. If this happens, the bowel program should be changed on an individual basis. It may require decreased bowel medication, either stool softener or laxative, or it may be necessary to change the suppository to every other day.

2. A patient does not need to have a daily bowel movement but should not go more than three days without one.

3. The constant use of enemas or harsh laxatives should be discouraged. They tend to cause loss of bowel tone which will eventually lead to consistent distention. Selectively, however, at times, especially in individuals who are impacted with stool high up in the colon, a high-colonic or high-irrigation enema may be indicated. This may be accomplished by inserting a lubricated rectal tube slowly into the rectum; hold enema can level with the buttock, let the solution run into the colon *slowly*. If the patient complains of being uncomfortable, or if water starts to leak around the tube, the can should be lowered below bed level, thus letting the solution run back into the enema can. One should not force the solution into the colon. This will only cause the bowel to spasm and force the water out. Rectal tube should be inserted about 4 to 6 inches. This procedure takes about 45 minutes to an hour.

4. Digital stimulation of the anal sphincter may also be utilized when necessary to get the evacuation mechanism started.

Termination of Program

The program should be continued daily for 6 to 7 weeks. If unsuccessful, report to physician for possible readjustment of routine and medication. If successful, one can try gradual withdrawal of the suppository as time goes on.

The benefits of a successful program are:
1. Improvement in patient's morale.
2. Restoration of patient's dignity and self-respect.
3. Reduction in nursing care.
4. Reduction in linen and laundry costs.
5. Most important, a guarantee that the patient will probably be able to return home to family and community.

FUNDAMENTALS OF LONG-TERM MANAGEMENT AND REHABILITATION

The eventual aim of treatment is total rehabilitation, which has been described by Munro as being predicated "by full ambulation within the limits imposed by the use of braces and crutches, twenty-four hour control of the bladder without the need of a urinal, twenty-four hour control of the bowel, and no significant pain or spasm." These achievements enable the paraplegic person to live a reasonably normal life and to compete successfully for jobs with nonparalyzed workers. Rusk has formulated this somewhat more succinctly as rehabilitation aimed at "training the patient to live and work within the limits of his disability but to the hilt of his capability." He also observes that "most of these paraplegic patients face life with a strong desire to live it as fully as possible" and that "they logically turn to the medical profession, which has saved their lives, for help in living their lives."

Two considerations must be paramount in the philosophy of retraining: (1) that "the doctor's responsibility does not end when the acute illness is ended; it ends only when the patient is retrained to live and work with what he has left," and (2) that "the patient must be forced to make himself a maximum effort to take an active part in the group that he lives and works with, and his initiative must not be continually sapped by the understandable desire of the community and his family to relieve him of the burdens that would otherwise annoy him."

To achieve the aims set by this philosophy the patient is made a most active member of a rehabilitation team that works with him rather than for him. A 5-hour working day is mapped for each patient, including exercises and occupational therapy, preparing the patient directly for the needs of his daily life. The individual program is largely determined by a thorough initial inventory of the activities of daily living still possible for the patient before rehabilitation, and by a muscle test. The program for rehabilitation varies considerably from patient to patient, but, for example, it may include general conditioning exercises, which are best done on a mat on the floor with a group of other paraplegia patients. The various muscle groups of the upper extremities are strengthened by specific exercises designed for each muscle group. Balance while sitting is learned on the mat. Sawed-off crutches are used for push-ups from the sitting position. Ambulation is taught when braces have been fitted, beginning with standing between parallel bars, followed by instruction in a swing-to gait, and then a swing-through gait while still between the bars.

The use of crutches follows, first in the bars, then with the help of an attendant, and finally unaided. Two hours daily may be spent in learning the activities necessary for daily living, one of the hardest of which for the paraplegic person is, for instance, getting in and out of a bus. An hour may be spent on vocational counseling, and in the evaluation and assistance in problems of emotions, social relations, and vocation.

Such a program is best carried out in groups

by specialists, but obviously some of it may still have to be continued after the patient returns home, and its coordination may well become the responsibility of the practitioner.

MANAGEMENT OF BEDSORES

The nutritional and general nursing measures outlined in the sections on the early phases of treatment will eliminate the causes of most bedsores. These must be considered a preventable, and therefore unnecessary, complication. However, particularly in military series, there is still a high incidence of bedsores in paraplegic patients.

If bedsores have developed in the paraplegic patient, they may represent an extremely difficult and stubborn problem. Various hospitals have a variety of techniques which have been tried. As in most things, the marked diversity of some of the treatments, from sugar instillation to electrical stimulation, lets one know that there is no one good treatment. There are some cardinal principles to follow:

1. Pressure should be removed and shearing forces avoided. The patient should be taught to change his position at regular intervals, whether in bed or wheelchair. If this is not possible (i.e., a quad), staff or attendants should be charged with this duty.

2. Localized infection should be cleared. Frequently, halogen type compounds, such as Iodiform gauze or Dakins-solution irrigations, do better than specific antibiotics.

3. Debridement of dead tissue should be carried out as frequently as needed.

4. Ultraviolet treatments may stimulate granulation.

5. Necessary regulation of abnormal medical situations, such as anemia, malnutrition, and hypoproteinemia should be accomplished.

6. When indicated, surgery should be considered. Some feel that bedsores are primarily a plastic-surgical problem and that all major bed-

sores in paraplegic patients should be treated by wide excision of the ulcer and regional scar tissue, excision of regional new-bone formation, together with the underlying bony prominence, rotation of a flap of muscle over the exposed bone, and closure of the wound by the use of a flap of skin and fat rotated to the area of the decubitus, placed so that suture lines and resultant scars are not over the site of the previous decubitus. A free graft of skin is then used at the point from which the flap was elevated. The resection of underlying bony prominences has increased the percentage of success in the operative closure of decubiti. Full success can now be obtained in more than 80 percent of the cases. Surgery of this nature, of course, will interfere with the rehabilitation program; and more conservative and yet effective methods for the treatment of decubitus ulcers must be sought.

MANAGEMENT OF SPASMS

Spasms and mass reflexes occur once the period of spinal shock has passed. They are a common accompaniment of transection of the spinal cord at any level, except in a pure cauda equina injury. According to the most recent investigations, the presence of these mass reflexes or spasms in quadriplegic, quadriparetic, paraplegic, and paraparetic patients has no prognostic significance whatsoever. About one-third of the patients with proved transections of the cord never have mass reflexes or spasms; on the other hand, such spasms can occur in patients with only partial cord injury.

Spasms, if bearable, can be a help as well as a hindrance. Often they keep tone in muscles which would otherwise waste away. Some patients learn to use these spasms to help them in such functions as turning in bed and transferring from wheelchair to car and back. They may be a blessing in disguise. It is Munro's belief that a large majority of patients with spasms will need rhizotomy before they can be rehabilitated. Only about 12 percent of patients with spasm had

spontaneous regression or relief from spasm without surgery. This was only partial, and complete recovery from spasm without active therapy occurred in only 2 percent. Surgical relief of severe spasm is best accomplished by the transection of the anterior dorsal and lumbar roots, from the eleventh dorsal through the first sacral segment on both sides.

AUTONOMIC CRISES

These rarely happen if the injury is below T5. Those with injuries above that level are apt to get them. They are due to malfunctioning of the autonomic nervous system, which is involved in blood-pressure regulation. In a crisis, the blood pressure rises suddenly, causing a blinding headache, sweating, and excitement. Things such as severe constipation, catheter changes and blockage, and enemas are the most frequent precipitating causes. A physician should be called at once.

MENTAL AND EMOTIONAL ADJUSTMENT

As may be expected, depression is a realistic component of spinal-cord injury. The emotional shock of sudden or prolonged helplessness is unimaginable. Howard Rusk said it all when he wrote, "Physical disability constitutes a threat to a way of life. It may cause intense anxiety, depression, and rage. It may be interpreted as punishment for sins, real or imagined. It may represent a threat to omnipotent strivings or a normal mastery and may produce feelings of helplessness and panic. It may unloose previously controlled psychopathology, such as paranoid ideas, and create intolerable interpersonal relationships. On the other hand, the disability may be organized into neurotic strivings, such as dependency and fear of competition, and be unconsciously welcome as a way out of a conflictive struggle.

"Finally, the disability removes the individual from normal social experiences and from work situations—the two major sources of satisfaction and self-esteem. Disruption in family life and friendships, separation from loved ones, economic problems, shattered ambitions and dreams —all of these lead to serious threat and damage to the socially functioning human being."

Paralysis that destroys bladder and bowel control may affect the ability to have sexual relations. However, spinal-cord injury does not guarantee sexual incapacity. The vast majority of disabled men can have erections, up to 70 percent of those with incomplete cord damage can ejaculate, and most of them, given a patient and knowledgeable partner, can have coitus. Females have become pregnant and delivered normally, or more often, by Caesarean section.

Many physicians are not equipped to deal with the sexual problems of the physically handicapped. Frequently, the disabled person is handicapped by his own taboos and fears. Where there is a will, however, there is a way, and males who have no sexual feeling to instigate an erection can still accomplish this reflexly in a number of ways which provide friction. Seventy-five to ninety-five percent can thus achieve erection.

More emphasis needs to be placed upon this problem. The National Sex and Drug Forum has tackled this head on with an explicit film concerning the sex life of the paraplegic, entitled, "Touching." This is a good resource for the education of physicians, allied health personnel, and patients themselves.

RECREATION AND SPORTS

Many paras and quads are young. Sports such as bowling, wheelchair basketball, wheelchair archery, and wheelchair square dancing are done with enthusiasm. There are many excellent basketball teams who participate in vigorous league competition throughout the country. It is an invaluable experience to have such teams play for the new and uninitiated para or quad, as it points out the skills of wheelchair maneuverability which may be attained by many. There are also worldwide wheelchair Olympics which take place periodically!

REFERENCES

EDWARD, W. H., SCHWEIKERT, H. A. *An Introduction to Paraplegia*. Washington, D.C.: Paralyzed Veterans of America, 1966.

FROST, A. *Handbook for Paraplegics and Quadriplegics*. Chicago: National Paraplegic Foundation, 1964.

KRENZEL, J. and ROHRER, L. M. *Paraplegic and Quadriplegic Individuals—A Handbook of Care for Nurses*. (3rd ed.) Chicago: Paraplegic Foundation, 1969.

LITTLE, J. *How to Get Help If You Are Paralyzed*. Chicago: National Paraplegia Foundation.

Management of Spinal Cord Injuries. Durham, N.H.: New England Center for Continuing Education, Conference Transcript, 1971.

MUNRO, D. The rehabilitation of patients totally paralyzed below the waist, with special reference to making them ambulatory and capable of earning their own living. I. Anterior rhizotomy for spastic paraplegia. *New Engl. J. Med.* 233:453, 1945.

Policy and Procedure Manual. Cambridge, Mass.: Youville Hospital, 1972.

RUSK, H. *Patient Publication #1. Primer for Paraplegics and Quadriplegics*. New York: New York University Medical Center, Institute of Physical Medicine and Rehabilitation, 1960.

SALTMAN, J. *Paraplegia: A Head, A Heart and Two Big Wheels*. Public Affairs Pamphlet #300. New York: Public Affairs Committee, 1965.

Sex and the Paraplegic. *Medical World News*, Jan. 14, 1972.

SILLER, J. Psychological situation of the disabled with spinal cord injuries. *Rehabilitation Literature* 30:290, 1969.

Spinal Cord Injury, Hope Through Research. Information Office, National Institute of Neurological Diseases and Blindness.

8

Complications of Chronic Illness

Many of the complications of chronic illness are not simply the consequence of a progressive malady but also result from a combination of adverse circumstances which, often triggered by an accident and ensuing trauma or by an acute illness, lead to vicious circles that are difficult to break.

Thus, the aged person in apparently perfectly good health may fall, fracture a leg, and, a few days after having become bedridden, develop respiratory complications. This in turn may lead to a prolonged stay in bed which will cause osteoporosis from disuse and delayed healing. During the enforced rest, appetite is lost, and malnutrition results; the resistance to infection is consequently lowered, and urinary-tract infection becomes bothersome; this leads to incontinence and wetting of the bed, and soon decubital ulcers develop. Thus, without any new major illnesses, a patient with just one difficulty at the start may become a chronic invalid or a terminal case.

For each of the most frequent complications of chronic illness, there are methods of prevention and treatment, and when these are properly used much distress can be prevented. The cardinal rule to remember is to keep the chronically ill, and especially the elderly, out of bed, active, and self-reliant as long as possible. If complications prevent their walking, let them lead an active wheelchair existence; if this is impossible, they should spend most of their time in a comfortable chair and only some time in bed. If complete bed rest is required, they must be taught to exercise in bed and to move about and change position as often as possible. In this chapter, some of the most common complications of chronic illness are discussed.

URINARY COMPLICATIONS

CHRONIC URINARY INFECTION

A survey of urinary sediments and cultures taken in any chronic-disease hospital reveals signs of urinary infections in a large percentage of the patients. These vary all the way from bacteriuria with occasional white cells to frank pus in the urine. Most of these infections are asymptomatic. They are especially prevalent in women, but men are by no means free from them, and, indeed, if prostatic smears were taken, a large number of asymptomatic chronic prostatic infections would also be discovered.

It is not clear what causes this situation in bedridden and debilitated patients. Many of them may have been infected at one time or another by catheterization, and perhaps the presence of cystoceles, prostatic hypertrophy, and atonicity of the bladder favor stagnation of urine and bacterial growth. Many of these patients have irregular bowel function, varying from constipation to diarrhea, and it is entirely possible that bacteria travel from the intestinal into the perivesicular lymphatics, and so into the blood stream, and thence into the urine. By similar mechanisms, chronic cervicitis may be a causative factor for urinary infection in women. These foci of infection are an ever-present threat to the chronically ill patient. Any episode of malnutrition or generally impaired resistance may call forth bouts of cystitis, pyelitis, prostatitis, or pyelone-phritis.

The urine of patients who are bedridden for extended periods of time should be watched carefully. Cleanly voided specimens should be examined weekly if possible, and when suspicious sediments are found in women, catheterized specimens should be obtained for sediment and culture. In men, catheterization is not necessary for this purely diagnostic purpose. The Gram stain* of sediment smears is of key importance in the diagnosis of urinary-tract infections. Since at least 100,000 organisms per milliliter of urine must be present for them to be visible on a Gram stain, their presence in such preparations confirms the existence of urinary-tract infection even when symptoms are absent.

A negative Gram smear, on the other hand, even in the presence of a positive culture, may indicate one of three things: (1) there may be no urinary infection, and the organisms grown in the culture may be contaminants; (2) there may be a ureteral block with pyoureter or renal lesions causing the typical symptoms but no organisms in the urine; or (3) there may be a urinary infection caused by cocci, which grow less abundantly in the urine and therefore may not be detectable on Gram preparations.

This *preventive* system of urine examinations should be carried out in all chronically ill patients, even if they have no symptoms referable to the urinary tract. When the possibility of urinary infection is kept in mind in the case of any patient confined to bed for long periods of time, urinary infections may be prevented with considerable success by the adoption of some quite simple measures.

* *The Gram stain.* The urine is spun down, the supernatant portion discarded and the sediment smeared out on a slide. This is dried in the air and fixed in the flame of a Bunsen burner. Gentian violet is applied for ½ to 1 minute (5 gm. gentian violet in 10 ml. of 95 percent alcohol, 2 ml. aniline oil, 88 ml. distilled water) or until preparation is black. Wash and allow to dry. Decolorize with 95 percent alcohol or acetone until no more violet washes off. Counterstain with dilute carbolfuchsin (1 part in 10 parts of water) for 1 minute or until the smear has the color of the counterstain.

First of all, a reasonably large fluid intake—about 2 liters of fluid per day, or enough to result in at least 1000 ml. or more of urine in each 24-hour period, depending on the specific gravity of the urine—should be maintained. It is desirable to keep the specific gravity between 1.005 and 1.008, since at this high dilution urine becomes an unsuitable medium for growth of some bacteria. The pH of the urine should be checked when the weekly sediments are studied and should be kept close to neutral. If it is alkaline or acid, a regimen should be instituted using either ammonium chloride (to lower the pH) or sodium bicarbonate (to raise it). This can also be accomplished by suitable dietary measures, employing a ketogenic diet to obtain a more acid, or a vegetable-fruit diet to obtain a more alkaline urine. *Pyocyaneus* is very sensitive to low pH, while *Escherichia coli* grows well even at pH 4.5. At the slightest sign of urinary difficulties, mild urinary disinfectants, such as Pyridium (phenazopyridine) or Mandelamine (methenamine mandelate), should be given. In the average case this will clear up the disturbance.

Mandelamine is given in daily doses of 3 to 9 gm. Higher doses may sometimes cause nausea and bladder irritation. During Mandelamine treatment the urine pH, as measured by Nitrazine paper, must be kept at pH 5.5 or below. Mandelamine may be given intermittently in courses of 1 week with a 1-week interval, or continuously as long as necessary.

If signs of infection persist, whether in the form of clinical (frequency, dysuria, fever) or laboratory evidence (such as pus or positive smears and cultures), definitive treatment becomes necessary. This treatment will be of one of two possible types, depending upon whether facilities for urine cultures and bacterial sensitivity studies are available (the scientific method), or not available (the empirical method). The empirical method is often quite sufficient, because sulfonamides and Mandelamine, the old standbys, are quite effective against a broad range of organisms usually present in urinary infections.

Gantrisin (sulfisoxazole) or preparations of

triple sulfonamides, especially those containing the pyrimidine type of sulfonamide, such as sulfadiazine, sulfamerazine, or sulfamethazine, are the sulfonamides of choice, because of their high solubility and the resulting unlikelihood of their causing renal complications. These are given daily in divided doses. If there are accompanying signs of colitis, due in all likelihood to *E. coli*, this should be treated simultaneously by Sulfasuxidine, 12 gm. daily in divided doses, or Sulfathalidine, 4 gm. daily in 4 divided doses. Because of their poor absorption, Sulfathalidine (phthalylsulfathiazole) and Sulfasuxidine (succinylsulfathiazole) cannot be expected to act directly upon the urinary infection although they will lessen the colitis. In women, concurrent trichomonas, vaginitis, and chronic cervicitis should be treated effectively to avoid prompt recurrence of urinary infection.

In the empirical method of treatment, antibiotics should not be used lightly but only if the therapy previously described has failed. When the offending organism is unknown, the choice of the appropriate antibiotic is difficult, and blind antibiotic therapy is to be condemned, since it may produce resistant strains of bacteria in the host so treated. Chloromycetin in particular should not be used without compelling indication, since serious side effects have been reported.

The scientific method identifies the causative organism by stain and culture and determines the choice of the best antibiotic by sensitivity studies. Today such studies are carried out quite simply by the use of commercially available disks impregnated with antibiotics which, if effective against the organisms studied, will clear the agar plate around them of culture growth.*

The antibiotic that has proved to be most powerful in vitro is then used in the patient. The correlation between sensitivity determinations and clinical effectiveness is not always perfect, but in nearly all instances this laboratory procedure is a good guide for chemotherapy.

* Widely used, for instance, are Bacto Sensitivity Disks, produced by Difco Laboratories, Detroit, Michigan.

Urine Retention

In chronically ill patients, particularly the elderly and senile, disoriented subjects, urine retention with distention of the urinary bladder may occur and go unnoticed unless thought is given to this possibility. It is advisable to have nursing personnel keep close supervision of excretory activity in these patients and to report immediately to the physician any unusually low output of urine or failure to void.

In warm climates and during summer heat the sweating of bedridden patients may cause considerable dehydration, with small urine volumes. This must be corrected by increasing fluid intake during such periods. Electrolyte balance should be maintained by giving salt tablets.

When failure to void is noted, the bladder should be percussed, and if distended, the patient should first be encouraged to void. Men should do so in the standing position and in privacy where possible. If this fails, catheterization should be performed, emptying the bladder slowly but completely. The cause of the retention must be found and corrected. This should be done as soon as possible. If no anatomical cause for the retention is found, the patient must be catheterized every 6 to 8 hours, fluid intake being restricted, and normal urination may then resume its course. It may sometimes be necessary to place such patients for a temporary period of time on constant drainage.

Every patient who has to undergo repeated catheterization is likely to become infected, and the preventive and curative measures for urinary infections described above take on added significance in these patients.

Incontinence

Dribbling incontinence in men may actually be overflow through the sphincters from a distended bladder, usually due to prostatic hypertrophy. This calls for diagnosis and treatment of the underlying condition. In any case of incontinence one should, of course, first ascertain whether there is an overflow seepage or true incontinence.

It is, therefore, good policy to catheterize incontinent patients to determine the volume of residual urine.

It has been suggested that some forms of urinary and fecal incontinence in debilitated men might be due to atrophy of the levator ani muscle.

Urinary incontinence occurs in paraplegic patients, whose problem has been discussed, and in other neurological conditions accompanied by atonic bladders. It is also found in men and women in senility with personality deterioration and may present a serious complication of debilitating disease. Wetting by urine constitutes a serious hazard to the skin and favors the development of bed and pressure sores.

If long survival is anticipated, some of these bladders can be retrained by tidal drainage and bladder training, depending on the degree of cooperation that may be obtained and on the devotion of the nurses. When this is impossible or incontinence is a terminal phenomenon, constant drainage may be instituted in order to keep the patient dry. A closed system is best and less likely to lead to infection.

Irrational patients must be restrained from removing the catheter. Indwelling catheters of the Foley type may be used, but they are not indispensable. Urine sediments must be examined frequently and infections treated. Small catheters, no larger than 14 French, should be used in men, to avoid necrosis of the urethral mucosa, prostatitis, and other complications. Catheterization should always be performed gently and in the same manner which the operator would like to have used upon himself if he were in the patient's place. Stylets, urethral sounds, and such surgical instruments should be used only by the experienced urologist. It is important to check periodically to see that catheter and connecting tubing are in place and that urine flows freely. Bladder irrigations should be carried out three to four times a day if it is anticipated that constant drainage will last more than 1 week. The urine should be kept at a neutral pH and the flow at least 1 liter per 24 hours.

STRESS INCONTINENCE

One special form of incontinence in women that is amenable to surgical therapy is stress incontinence. This occurs relatively frequently in women approaching or past the menopause, and consists in loss of sphincter control at the slightest stress, such as laughing, coughing, or sometimes merely talking. This condition is due to a relaxation of the perineal musculature and to ptosis of the bladder neck. Stress incontinence may, of course, occur in bedridden patients as well as in ambulatory ones, and may be a serious problem in chronically ill women because of the complications that go with the urinary wetting of the skin in such patients. At best it is an annoying nursing problem, and at its worst it may endanger the health of the bedridden patient. One must carefully weigh the problems of the necessary plastic surgery against the nearly certain benefits and come to a decision in the light of the anticipated length of invalidism necessitating bed rest, the gravity of the primary disease, and the outlook for the patient's life expectancy. Occasionally this form of incontinence may be relieved by relaxing the detrusor muscle with atropine, 0.6 mg. three times a day, and by retraining the pelvic musculature by systematic exercise.

If it is decided to perform surgical repair for the correction of stress incontinence, the physician must make certain that this will be done by an experienced specialist able to select and perform whatever type of operation may be best suited for a given case.

Sometimes vaginal plastic correction alone is not sufficient, and care must be taken to resuspend the bladder neck in its physiological position by any one of a number of possible techniques. Unless this is done the failure rate may be around 20 percent.

The chronically ill woman should not be deprived of the benefits of effective therapy for stress incontinence merely because she is suffering from a primary chronic disease, since the correction of the incontinence may be an even more important procedure for her than it is for the otherwise healthy woman.

NOCTURIA

Nocturia—another special type of incontinence —should not be misinterpreted as simple incontinence, since it may often be due to quite specific causes. It may represent, for example, the first sign of otherwise asymptomatic cardiac decompensation. Cardiac nocturia is produced by a number of factors, such as the influence of the recumbent position, which favors reabsorption of edema fluid, even though edema may not be clinically apparent. There are many other causes for nocturia, which occurs fairly frequently in older patients, especially in men. It may be physiological, due to an excessive fluid intake late in the evening or during the night; psychological, conditioned, for example, by a pattern of frequency which may have been caused by prostatism and which may persist and become apparent during the night long after the original cause for it has been removed. It may be renal, in cases of real insufficiency in which the ability of the kidney to concentrate is reduced and the volume of urine is enlarged, and it may be urological, caused by any obstructing lesion of the bladder, or by diseases which reduce the bladder volume.

The management of nocturia in chronic patients is, of course, urological when the cause is urological; otherwise it calls for the remedy for various underlying causes. In the case of psychological nocturia, however, retraining may be possible if the patient is sufficiently intelligent to cooperate, and if the physician and nurses are persistent enough to undertake this arduous but important task.

GASTROINTESTINAL COMPLICATIONS

NAUSEA AND VOMITING

Nausea is a frequent complication of a variety of chronic diseases. It is defined by Webster as "any sickness of the stomach, like seasickness, with a desire to vomit; qualm, a feeling of distress associated with loathing of food." This broad definition indicates the multiple causes and mechanisms that may be involved in the sensation of nausea. It is not always easy to distinguish between dizziness—a sensation of whirling— and nausea, since the two terms may be confused in many patients' minds and since the two difficulties are often experienced simultaneously.

True nausea may be produced by numerous causes. It may originate in the central nervous system, as in the case of motion sickness, and the nausea accompanying brain lesions, or it may be caused by metabolic disturbances such as uremia, diabetic coma, insulin shock, and the aftermath of certain types of anesthesia. There are reflex causes for nausea, such as intense pain from coronary attacks, gallbladder attacks, renal colic, "acute abdomens," gastric distention, or intestinal occlusions. The last of these is sometimes caused by simple fecal impaction, especially in the aged. Complex mechanisms also enter into play in the case of nausea of radiation sickness, pregnancy, and some rarer forms of nausea, which are poorly understood.

Whenever the cause or the mechanism is known, elimination of the cause will rapidly relieve the distress of nausea. Cranial decompression for inoperable brain lesions, short-circuiting operations for palliation of intestinal occlusion, gastric or intestinal suction, analgesic therapy of pain in colic or angina attacks, all may cause cessation of nausea occurring in these situations. When removal of the precipitating factor is not possible, the necessity for symptomatic treatment arises, which presents a difficult problem.

A host of therapeutic agents have been proposed for the palliation of nausea. These include the antispasmodics, on the theory that the vicious circle of nausea may be interrupted by checking the antiperistaltic waves of the stomach, and by drying up salivary and gastric secretions.

Many antihistamine drugs such as Dramamine (dimenhydrinate, U.S.P.) have been proposed for the purpose of suppressing nausea. Unfortunately, all these drugs are not generally effective in many types of nausea. Since some of them may be useful in perhaps half the cases, they may be tried, but not too much should be expected. Thorazine, Compazine, and Sparine are quite effective.

When nausea is accompanied by vomiting, these agents should be given subcutaneously, since oral medication is often vomited before it can be absorbed.

In nausea of reflex or central-nervous-system origin, simple sedation is often most effective. This can be accomplished by giving barbiturates, such as Sodium Amytal (amobarbital) or Nembutal (pentobarbital), subcutaneously. When there is adequate nursing and medical coverage, this can be combined with scopolamine or Pantopon (soluble hydrochlorides of the total alkaloids of opium). Care must be taken that sedation is not so deep as to interfere with the deglutition reflexes, since this presents the danger of aspiration of vomitus should vomiting occur in spite of these measures. When there is intracranial hypertension, opiates and their derivatives are, of course, contraindicated.

The phenothiazines and related compounds (tranquilizers) are general nervous depressants with less effect on the sleeping centers than that of the barbiturates. In our hands, they have been remarkably effective in controlling nausea and vomiting in patients with advanced cancer and have shown few side effects. Somnolence, however, does occur with materials of this structure.

When vomiting cannot be controlled and occurs with great frequency from any cause, attention must be paid to the patient's electrolyte balance. In this situation the amounts of chloride and water lost may be considerable and must be replaced by intravenous fluids or hypodermoclysis.

CONSTIPATION

Sluggishness of the bowels is one complication of any period of immobilization, which cannot be avoided without proper management, and may lead to serious and distressing complications

if allowed to continue for any length of time. These complications include fecal impaction, ulcers in the rectum, and extreme discomfort upon the expulsion of dry fecal masses. All this may be prevented by common sense, before true constipation is allowed to become established. In patients with cerebral vascular accidents, hypertension, or aneurysms, where straining at stool must be avoided, mineral oil is indicated. In all patients who must face extended partial or complete immobilization, the dietary management *must* include provisions for sufficient bulk, and occasionally bulk laxatives may have to be used.

In the chronically ill patient as well as in the sedentary elderly subject, constipation is frequently caused by immobilization combined with soft diets of small bulk. While it may not be possible to avoid the lack of exercise, the deficient bulk of the diet can be provided by suitable selection of foods such as cereals (bran), fruit (prunes, etc.) muffins and cookies containing bran, and by a sufficient fluid intake.

A regular habit pattern of bowel evacuation should be formed and adhered to. In such patients it may not be necessary to have a bowel movement every day. If a well-formed, reasonably large stool is passed twice a week, this may be perfectly sufficient.

Aged and debilitated subjects, who quite often show signs of impaired thyroid function, may greatly benefit, so far as their constipation is concerned, from small doses of thyroid, since this improves the tonus of intestinal musculature. In nervous patients with evidence of colonic spasticity, atropine sulfate in small doses or tincture of belladonna may have beneficial effects.

When facing the problem of constipation in the aged or the chronically ill, one must first of all decide whether or not there are organic causes. In elderly people constipation should never be treated on the assumption that it is functional. Instead, organic causes must first be sought and ruled out. It is most discouraging (and it happens all too often) to discover eventually an incurable carcinoma of the sigmoid in a patient who has been treated during previous months for constipation. No older patient should be treated for persistent constipation before a complete study of the gastrointestinal tract has been made and a thorough search for organic causes has been carried out.

When the diagnosis of functional constipation has been made on a sound basis, then it is well to attempt bowel training first, before using the cathartics. The stools should be made soft and bulky by dietary adjustments, as outlined above, and glycerin suppositories or small mild soapsud enemas should be used at those times when evacuation is desired. Gradually a spontaneous pattern of bowel function may develop.

In general, the cathartics should and can be avoided, or should be reserved for those cases where they may be indicated temporarily, such as in the postoperative period, during pregnancy, or following cerebral vascular accidents. When it is necessary to use the irritants to break a vicious circle of established constipation, these should be used only to reactivate bowel movements and should then be followed by the milder dietary management.

It must be remembered that once the patient has been purged it may take some days before another bowel movement can be expected, and that it may take weeks of bowel training to establish sound and regular habits in a person changing from an active to a sedentary or immobile way of life.

Diarrhea

Diarrhea can be an irritating complication of chronic illness. In the aged and debilitated subject diarrhea may be a consequence of a faulty diet, deficiencies of gastrointestinal enzymes or other secretions, or difficulties in mastication. Two types of modern drugs are causing diarrhea in some cases and apparently more frequently in elderly patients than in younger subjects. These are some antibiotics and the metabolic antagonists, such as the antifolic agents used in cancer chemotherapy. In these situations the antibiotics must be changed, and the chemotherapeutic agents should be discontinued if diarrhea occurs.

Diarrhea in the older age group, particularly when alternating with constipation, is sometimes a sign of lower-intestinal cancer and should *always* arouse the physician's suspicion of the presence of this disease. Also in the aged a frequent cause of diarrhea is loose feces bypassing fecal impaction. In institutions, diarrhea epidemics may occur and are either of bacterial or amebic origin, or may precede epidemics of infectious hepatitis.

It is thus quite clear that not all patients with diarrhea should be treated symptomatically, but a search for the cause should be made. However, even while the cause is being investigated, the intestinal loss of electrolytes and the discomfort of diarrhea must be stopped whenever possible. Food by mouth should be omitted for 24 hours and nourishment and fluid provided intravenously or by clysis, if necessary. This should be combined with a variety of symptomatic measures.

Among the simplest and most innocuous of these are the adsorbents, which act by providing an inert substance to adsorb bacterial agents, gases, and toxins. Such substances are activated charcoal (U.S.P.), kaolin, bismuth subnitrate, bismuth subcarbonate, and bismuth subgallate. Of course, such adsorbents also adsorb nutrients, enzymes, and vitamins, but the temporary and partial loss of these is a minor consideration if the diarrhea can be stopped. Kaolin is used in doses of 10 to 100 gm. after each liquid bowel movement. The bismuth salts are used in hourly doses to 0.65 to 1.5 gm. until diarrhea ceases. The adsorbents should be continued for some time after diarrhea has ceased.

When there is severe pain, opiates or morphine (0.015 gm.) may be used. Such drugs should, however, be withheld in the early stages until the bowels have been well emptied. Following this, 1 teaspoonful of paregoric (camphorated tincture of opium, U.S.P.) may be given in water after every bowel movement until diarrhea ceases. Paregoric can also be combined with the adsorbents. In most cases, however, paregoric will be effective after a few doses.

For the bedridden patient with a chronic illness, diarrhea can be a most distressing complication and should be treated vigorously. From the very beginning of diarrhea, increased attention must be given to cleanliness. After each bowel movement the perineal region should be carefully washed with cold water, and it may be necessary to apply some anesthetic ointment or bland petroleum jelly (Vaseline) to prevent anal discomfort. The skin over the buttocks and the sacrum must be kept even more scrupulously clean than usual, and soiled bedclothes must be changed immediately. In the colostomy patient diarrhea can be a serious complication, upsetting irrigation routines and calling for prompt treatment by adsorbents and opiates, prompt definition of the cause, and effective causal therapy (such as sulfa drugs or antibiotics) if necessary.

BED AND PRESSURE SORES

In the not too distant past bed and pressure sores were the dreaded and practically unavoidable accompaniment of all chronic illness, occurring in the majority of patients who had been confined to bed for any length of time exceeding a few weeks. It has always been realized that good nursing care can contribute much to prevent or at least delay the appearance of decubital ulcers. However, only since the importance of good nutrition and the maintenance of adequate plasma protein levels has been realized has the prevention of most pressure sores been possible.

Today, in well-organized hospitals for chronic disease, the development of decubitus ulcers is the exception rather than the rule. They still occur, but usually only in the late and terminal phases of prolonged illness. In that stage ulceration of the skin at pressure points is an expression of a general breakdown of tissue, failing circulation, and deficient nutrition.

The prevention of pressure sores involves the following measures, which must be adopted as a routine in the management of all patients who are bedridden or immobilized in wheelchairs for any length of time:

The skin must be maintained clean to decrease the dangers of infection. The patient must be bathed daily with soap and water or with a mild detergent and water. The skin should be rubbed mildly with rubbing alcohol after the bath and then greased with a lanolin cream. Talcum powder should be applied to the back, the buttocks, and the skin folds of the genital areas, to the armpits, and to creases about the breasts and, in the obese, about the abdomen. Daily or more frequent changes of bed sheets are a necessary part of cleanliness. Sheets must be replaced whenever they have been wet by urine or soiled by feces.

Throughout the day the position of the patient should be changed frequently—not less than once every hour—so that no single area keeps bearing weight for any extended period. This does not involve turning the patient entirely from side to side. Minor changes of position are sufficient to accomplish the desired alternation of pressure areas. The wheelchair patient, for instance, may be trained systematically to acquire the habit of shifting his weight in the chair from one buttock to the other at regular intervals without much moving about. In bed foam-rubber pillows, which can be placed under the side of a patient in the manner of wedges, are helpful in positioning patients in such a way that a slight displacement of the pillow will shift pressure to other portions of the body.

Most commonly, decubitus ulcers develop over the sacrum, the buttocks, and the back of the heels, all areas that are under constant pressure if patients are allowed to rest on their backs. These are the areas to be watched most carefully and upon which as little continuous pressure as possible must be permitted. However, in emaciated patients pressure sores sometimes develop even over the iliac crests and the knee-caps from pressure of clothing and bedclothes.

In severely emaciated persons it is therefore wise to construct light frames of wire mesh or wood to keep the weight of bedclothes away from the protruding areas of the body.

Any superficial skin infection must be treated as soon as it appears. Vioform cream (iodochlor-hydroxyquin, U.S.P.) and permanganate soaks are useful for this purpose, as are Mercuro-chrome (merbromin) or a number of newer and widely used surface disinfectants. Care must be taken to use such agents in weak solutions in order to avoid skin burns. Dusting with sulfa-drug powders or antibiotics must be done with discrimination. Some of these powders are rather gritty and may be irritating, especially in skin folds or where there is unavoidable rubbing contact of clothing.

Dressings, especially those applied with adhesive tape, should be avoided as long as possible. The bulk of gauze, cotton, or any dressing material causes additional friction on the surrounding skin. A plastic liquid dressing containing 10 percent vinylite in alcohol, which may be sprayed on the skin, provides the best covering for minor skin lesions. The plastic film, which must be applied to the cleansed and dry skin, remains in place for 12 to 24 hours. Thereafter it peels readily and may be replaced by new spraying.

Nutrition is most important in preventing decubitus ulcers, and, depending on the state of nutritional debilitation of the patient, protein requirements may be quite high. The adequate feeding of such patients may present a difficult problem. This is discussed in the last section of this chapter.

If decubitus ulcers develop in spite of cleanliness, the prevention of undue pressure and skin infection, and with adequate nutrition, they are usually a terminal phenomenon and will progress in spite of all therapy unless the patient's general condition improves. On the other hand if decubitus ulcers have arisen from neglect of any of the measures designed for their prevention, then they may respond well to conservative therapy consisting of intensive application of the same means as those outlined for the prevention of ulcers.

Before this regimen is begun, the ulcer must be cleaned surgically or by the use of protcolytic enzyme preparations (streptodornase or streptokinase). At the time the ulcer is debrided and cleaned, a decision must be made whether conservative measures or the surgical method should be used. This depends on a great many factors. In paraplegic patients experience has shown that surgical excision of the ulcer with removal of underlying bone prominences may be the treatment of choice. This may also be the case for decubitus ulcers in debilitated bedridden patients, and perhaps the conservative attitude toward bedsores should be changed. A great deal of pain could be spared these patients by operative treatment of decubiti, and the nursing problem could be simplified. On the other hand, there are situations in which one has to treat a decubitus ulcer by the conservative method, and often healing can be obtained by debridement, relieving pressure on the area, and proper nutritional management.

After the ulcer has been cleaned as described above, all dead tissue should be removed, great care being taken to reach the point where profuse bleeding of viable tissue starts. Bacterial cultures of the lesion should then be taken. If the cultures reveal the presence of organisms, or if obvious acute infection has set in, the ulcer site should be treated with warm, wet saline dressings followed by the application of a specific antibiotic ointment, in order to sterilize the field. Once the ulcer has become sterile, it should receive daily exposure to ultraviolet radiation, and the lesion should remain exposed to the air during certain periods of the day. This procedure will generally promote gradual healing of the ulcer. In some cases, when the defect does not heal completely, skin grafting may be indicated, in which event it is important to make sure that scar tissue, or granulations which might put inner pressure on the grafted skin, have surely been excised.

Regardless of what may be done to the ulcer locally, it must be remembered that decubitus is not merely a local disease, but an expression of a state of debilitation that must be corrected if healing is to take place and recurrence of decubitus is to be prevented.

CONTRACTURES

True contractures, which may follow in the wake of paralysis, immobilization, or amputation, comprise one of the most difficult problems seen in the care of the chronically ill. Perhaps it may be well first to define what is meant by a *true contracture*, since there are many contradictory opinions. The joint, the tendon, and the muscle are basically involved. When a joint is immobilized because of pain, paralysis, or prolonged immobilization, or when there is an imbalance of muscles and tendons around the joint, the fibers of the involved muscles and the tendons shorten and atrophy, causing a limitation of the range of motion of the joint. The true contracture cannot be stretched by manual manipulation, even under anesthesia, without the help of surgical intervention, prolonged persistent mechanical stretching, or softening by injection of corticosteroids. Contractures involving the shoulders are most common, especially in patients with paralysis due to a stroke, or in persons who immobilize the shoulder themselves because of pain, as in bursitis.

Flexion contractions of the hip are seen frequently in patients who have above-knee amputations, and in patients with arthritis who keep their legs in certain set positions because these are more comfortable. Flexion contractions of the knee are common in arthritis and stroke patients, especially when a well-meaning but uninformed person puts a pillow under the knee and keeps it in a bent position. Contractures of the ankle in plantar flexion (foot drops) are also seen in stroke patients.

It is most important to realize that all these contractures are actually preventable and that, with modern methods of active nursing care, they should not occur. The time required for a true contracture to develop depends on many known and unknown variables. In the shoulder joint, for instance, a contracture will develop in a very short period of time. Contractures develop most rapidly in joints that are paralyzed, as in the case of hemiplegia, paraplegia, or quadriplegia. Contractures rarely develop in healthy joints or muscles immobilized by plaster casts, and if they occur, this requires a long period of time. In a study of ten rabbits whose hind legs were immobilized by splints, it was found that fairly solid contractures developed within 2 weeks. However, in a series of twenty dogs, the time required for contracture was at least 4 months in about a third of them, 6 months for another third, and the final third never developed clearly irreversible contractures. This study further demonstrated that, if for any reason the cast was removed, allowing the leg to move or bend, even only temporarily, formation of contractures was prevented. This is one of the two cardinal principles that should be utilized to prevent contractures. When a person is paralyzed or immobilized for any reason, all joints that are not in casts should be put through their complete range of motion four or six times a day. This can be done by the patient himself, by a nurse, by a member of the family or, indeed, by anyone who has received simple instructions on how to bend and stretch all joints to their full capacity to keep them supple.

The second important principle to be remembered is that inactive joints should be properly positioned and splinted. This means for the patient who has suffered a stroke, for instance, proper positioning of the shoulder with a pillow placed under the affected axilla and the arm in abduction and external rotation, the use of footboards to maintain the ankle at a right angle, sandbags to prevent external rotation of the hip, and night splints as necessary for the hands and fingers to prevent flexion contracture deformities.

By using frequent, periodic mobilization of the involved joints and proper positioning and splinting when at rest, contractions can be prevented. Once they have been allowed to occur, it requires a very strenuous, prolonged, and usually painful course of physical therapy to restretch these limited joints, and frequently it is necessary to employ surgery or steroid injections, or both, to break or soften the tendons, in order to improve function.

COMPLICATIONS ORIGINATING IN THE CENTRAL NERVOUS SYSTEM

RESTLESSNESS AND INSOMNIA

The patient who is condemned to a bedridden existence or a sedentary, confining life has every reason to experience restlessness and to find it difficult to fall asleep at night. To go to sleep may be particularly difficult for those who are institutionalized, since the noises of the night in most hospitals and nursing homes are many and disturbing. The temptation is great for the physician to write an order for phenobarbital *pro re nata,* and to let it go at that. This, of course, is not the proper way to cope with these problems.

Many aged people, particularly those who have retired from or are physically incapable of their accustomed daily activities, find it difficult or impossible to settle down for a good night's rest, or if they can find sleep at reasonable hours, they may awaken unduly early in the morning.

The total care of the chronically ill patient as well as the aged in fairly good health must include a thorough consideration of the patient's needs for a regular waking-sleeping cycle. The physician must consider several phases in a program aimed at assuring sound sleep for the patient:

1. Alleviation of daily worry, anxiety, and pressure.
2. Maintenance of some measure of diurnal activity.
3. Assurance of restful and comfortable surroundings for the evening and night.
4. Prescription of suitable drugs when needed.

ALLEVIATION OF DAILY WORRY, ANXIETY, AND PRESSURE

To some extent any aged person, and to a greater extent every bedridden or invalid person, has worries and tensions that are justified and often inevitable. It requires skill, intelligence, and maturity for the physician to alleviate these concerns as much as possible and to help the patients to adjust to the situations that worry them. The aged and chronically ill rarely have anyone to whom they can turn with full confidence that that person is doing all that is humanly possible to alleviate their plight. They are all too often left to themselves, except when some disaster, such as an acute infection, a vascular accident, or a trauma which they have sustained falling out of bed, or some other such accident, renders them an acute medical problem.

Many a chronic patient who does not require much professional attention, since his or her status is stabilized, has nevertheless grave concerns about the problems of every day. If given an opportunity to discuss these matters from time to time with a competent and sympathetic medical man, these patients will do so and will greatly benefit, if not physically, at least in their minds. The physician who accepts responsibilities for chronically ill patients must realize that although this simple psychotherapy is often all he can offer, it may mean much to the patient, and it may be more powerful than the most potent drug.

The guiding principle for such discussions must be to listen, rather than to talk, but to guide the conversation so that important points can be made. These points of emphasis must take into account the patients' intelligence and must be so phrased as to be understandable to them. It is important to be honest. No patient who is ill for extended periods of time can be deceived for long. No man or woman of 75 can be led to believe that he or she is 40 years of age. Unjustifiable hope should never be held out. There is nothing worse than to insist upon how much better a patient is, when in effect his state is becoming worse.

What has to be expected in the light of the physician's experience should be stated in terms to which the patient can adjust. The challenge of long-term rehabilitation work, for instance, may spur patients on rather than depress them, if it is explained to them what they may hope to achieve. Like any drug or surgery, however, such talks are dangerous weapons and must be handled skillfully and wisely, lest they do more harm than good. Nothing can be worse and cause more apprehension, however, than to be the patient by whose bed pass the best physicians— without stopping—as happens day after day to so many patients in chronic-disease hospitals.

Alleviation of pressures of daily living includes trying to maintain harmonious relations between patients and persons with whom they have daily contacts. This is particularly important in those cases in which patients live within their family groups. The care of an aged or semi-invalid person is a burden for any family and always creates serious problems for all concerned. This situation may cause in the patient a feeling of being resented and of being a nuisance to everyone around him. If such an atmosphere prevails, it is sometimes better for all concerned, including the patient, to arrange for institutional care rather than to have him remain in the home. On the other hand, where a harmonious relationship can be brought about between patient and family, home care is infinitely preferable and far more economical.

The physician can be of very great help in guiding the families of patients in the solution of their home-care problems. He should be able to define the amount of attention that is actually needed from the family and to outline to a patient to what degree he may be able to be active and helpful even though confined to the house. The doctor should know about home-care programs in the community, if such exist, and be familiar with the home services which visiting-nurse associations and district nurses may be able to render.

The family physician must assume the functions of the social worker where there is none available to help, or he must secure the aid of social service if this is indicated and available.

In institutions for the chronically ill it is important that attention be paid to the way in which patients get along with their fellow patients. Concern with these social problems is often amply recompensed by the resulting elimination of unnecessary pressures and the correction of much nervousness and sleeplessness.

MAINTENANCE OF SOME MEASURE OF DIURNAL ACTIVITY

Two important considerations weigh in favor of the maintenance of some sort of activity during the day, even for chronically immobilized patients, who should be few in number if rehabilitation techniques have been fully used. First, physical fatigue following a day's work or routine walk is the best inducement for sleep during the night, and second, the feeling of usefulness which goes with the performance of a set daily task contributes to the peace of mind necessary for sound sleep.

It is, therefore, important to attempt to develop programs of some useful activity for even the most handicapped and bedridden patients, whenever possible. In an institution this is the task of the occupational therapy department. At home the devising of such plans may tax the imagination of the family and the physician, but some solution can usually be found if the problem is adequately considered.

In principle it is important that the tasks devised for the chronically ill person give the impression to those who perform them that they are not mere motions to be gone through to pass the time of day, but that they serve a useful purpose. Hospitals have succeeded in putting some patients to work in clerical capacities; inventions have been devised and developed by bedridden patients; useful objects are being produced and sold by some departments of occupational therapy; switchboards for message services are being operated by incapacitated bedridden patients; and businesses are being run from the homes of paraplegic or otherwise confined patients. Obviously it may be easier for the previously skilled person to devise tasks to keep busy while incapacitated. However, there are a great many manual skills that can be acquired by the unskilled, making use of their time during enforced immobilization. The important thing for the physician is to convince his patients that there may be serviceable ways of filling their time, rather than to avoid the subject. Surprisingly useful developments may then take place. At the same time the patient will probably become better adjusted and more confident of the future if kept busy during the day.

ASSURANCE OF RESTFUL AND COMFORTABLE SURROUNDINGS FOR THE EVENING AND NIGHT

This prerequisite for sleep may be easier to fulfill at home than in the hospital. The nightly hospital routine and the unavoidable activities in the halls and on the wards render sleeping difficult in most institutions. Also, the hospital bed is not always as comfortable as it should be, and other patients may be restless and make it hard for fellow patients to fall asleep.

Quiet, darkness, fresh air, and a sense of being protected are conducive to sleep, and every effort should be made to provide these conditions. In the home, patients should have their own rooms if possible, especially if they have previously been accustomed to this. While there, they should be left quiet and in the dark, but it must be made clear to them that someone is always within calling distance. If such patients can help themselves enough to get up if necessary during the night unaided, low-intensity night lights should be left on to keep the path from bed to bathroom well lit at all times. Cheap, reliable plug-in fixtures of low wattage and with shields which direct the beam in the desired direction are readily available.

PRESCRIPTION OF SUITABLE DRUGS WHEN NEEDED

A little alcohol before retiring may go a long way toward preparing the patient for a good night's sleep. Brandy is said to be a good vasodilator for the coronaries, in addition to its central-nervous-system effects, and whiskey has long been used for this purpose and is also the cheapest and safest peripheral vasodilator. These beverages are thus indicated in moderation for older people. In addition, they have rightly been dubbed "night caps."*

HYPNOTICS

The oldest hypnotic and perhaps still the cheapest and the best, particularly in geriatrics and in the management of chronic disease, is chloral hydrate. This can be used in doses of 1 to 2 gm. as a hypnotic, except in patients with liver or kidney disease, in severe cardiac cases, and in the presence of gastritis, where it may be given in enteric-coated capsules or in oil-retention enemas. Chloral hydrate should not be given in solution with alcohol, since in that combination it acts as knock-out drops.

A false-positive reaction for sugar may be found in the urine of patients receiving chloral hydrate. Habituation to the drug develops rarely. Chloral hydrate, though much neglected today, has such good therapeutic properties that it should always be tried first when sleeping difficulties of the elderly or chronically ill require drug therapy.

Perhaps the most widely employed hypnotic drugs are the barbiturates. Tolerance to barbiturates develops and these drugs are habit-forming. The danger of developing dependency on barbiturates, however, is relatively negligible in aged and chronically ill persons, compared with the alternative of innumerable sleepless

* We are aware of the fact that the therapeutic use of alcohol is a controversial subject. However, in the aged or chronically ill, its psychological and pharmacological advantages outweigh the danger of alcoholism which precludes its medicinal use in people with longer life expectancy.

nights. This danger may be further minimized by alternating barbiturates with chloral hydrate. As has been mentioned above, chloral hydrate should always be tried first. A more serious danger with barbiturates, as with any hypnotic, is that of accidental death by overdosage, which may happen when a patient under the influence of barbiturates forgets that he has already had his dose and sleepily grabs his barbiturate bottle and swallows a fatal overdose. It is a wise precaution to instruct the patient to leave each night only that dose of barbiturate within reach which is intended for that night and to place the remainder in a less accessible place.

The choice of the barbiturate depends on the type of sleeping difficulty. If it is a case of extreme difficulty in dropping off to sleep, a short-acting barbiturate will suffice; if the patient has the habit of awakening during the night, even though medication may not be needed to induce sleep, a long-acting preparation may have to be employed.

When the difficulty of falling asleep is due entirely or in part to pain, barbiturates alone will not suffice, and analgesics must be used. The analgesic action of salicylates, pyrazolone, and paraminophenol is potentiated by barbiturates. Some caution is indicated when barbiturates must be combined with opiates, particularly for elderly patients.

There are few contraindications to barbiturates except renal or hepatic failure and Parkinsonism, where muscular rigidity may be aggravated by barbiturates.

Another useful hypnotic is paraldehyde, which can be given in doses of 15 to 30 ml. or more by mouth, or mixed with oil as a retention enema. It is nontoxic and most effective, and is contraindicated only in pulmonary disease, because much of it is excreted through the lungs. This last factor also renders its use inconvenient in ambulatory patients, because of the characteristic odor of their breath, which lingers long after a dose of paraldehyde.

The establishment of a total plan of combined measures which ensures a patient a good night's sleep may take some time and considerable thought. A great deal of individual variability exists in terms of sensitivity to the action of hypnotics. Every physician gradually evolves from personal experience his own scheme of management for the problem of insomnia, which will undergo modifications according to the patient's reactivity to these drugs. It will usually be found that with the use of one or another of the drugs mentioned, combined with common-sense measures discussed earlier, and with analgesics when needed, the problem of insomnia of most older people and chronically ill patients may be overcome. It should be remembered, however, that the hypnotics are not cure-alls for insomnia and must be combined with intelligent psychotherapy and provisions for the necessary sleeping comfort.

SEDATION

In the elderly person and in many patients who are confined for long periods, insomnia may not be the only problem; they may also suffer from a continuous tension, fretfulness, and varying degrees of agitation. Here, again, the total care includes sympathetic psychotherapy that goes beyond the niceties of bedside manners. The use of sedative drugs is often indicated and may supplement the psychotherapeutic efforts directed toward helping the patients to adjust themselves to their plight. The sedative dose of the barbiturate is about one-third of the hypnotic dose. Such sedative doses may be repeated during the day as necessary in each individual case. Unless hypersensitivity is encountered sedation with barbiturates is simple, safe, and effective. The tranquilizers (of the phenothiazine type) are of use in the sedation of agitated senile patients with various degrees of anxiety, sleeplessness, and so forth. In doses varying from 30 to 150 mg. per day, in divided doses taken by mouth or given by intramuscular injection, these drugs are useful in the less manageable patients. During the first few days of therapy, agitation in these patients may become aggravated, but their mental state improves dramatically in most cases after a few days of this therapy, and they continue to feel better and to behave more normally on maintenance therapy.

A wide list of tranquilizers is now available and many of them may be useful in the care of aged or chronically ill patients. However, it must be remembered that, especially when used for long periods of time, there are side effects such as drowsiness and dryness of the mouth that may be merely disagreeable, and other manifestations of toxicity, such as Parkinsonlike syndromes, that may even be severe. Tranquilizers, therefore, are not a panacea but must be used with due care, sparingly, and only when specifically indicated.

DEPRESSION

The first reaction of any sensitive person to the depression so often encountered in the chronically ill is to consider this as perhaps the only possible attitude; and what hope, indeed, is there in many of these situations? However, since the main function of medicine is to alleviate suffering, be it physical or mental, by maintaining and restoring health, an effort must be made to remedy this trying symptom. It cannot be expected that one will be able to transform a depressed and despondent patient into a happy, well-adjusted person overnight, but much can be done to improve the situation. First of all, the availability of a physician who is willing to sit down and listen is most helpful to some of these patients, and the same principles should guide these discussions as were outlined in the preceding section. Second, drugs helpful in brightening a patient's outlook are available.

REFERENCES

URINARY COMPLICATIONS

CONN, H. F. (ed.). *Current Therapy.* Philadelphia: Saunders, 1953.

COUNCIL ON PHARMACY AND CHEMISTRY, *American Medical Association.* Chloramphenicol. *JAMA* 154:144, 1954.

KINCAID-SMITH, P., BULLEN, M., FUSSEL, U., MILLS, J., HUSTON, N., and GOON, F. The reliability of screening tests for bacteriuria in pregnancy. *Lancet:* II(7350):61–62, 1964.

LICH, R., JR. Urinary stress incontinence in the female. *J. Geront.* 7:555–558, 1952.

MIKUTA, J. J., and PAYNE, F. L. Stress urinary incontinence in the female: a review of the modern approach to this problem. *Amer. J. Med. Sci.* 226:674–687, 1953.

ROSE, D. K. Geriatric management of prostatism. *J. Geront.* 7:71–76, 1952.

RUBIN, S. W., and NAGEL, H. Nocturia in the aged. *JAMA* 147:840–841, 1951.

VLAVIANOS, G., SEAMAN, G., and VLAVIANOS, M. A further clinical study of anabolic steroids in incontinence. *Amer. J. Psychiatr.* 118:539–542, 1961.

OTHER COMPLICATIONS

CLARK, A. B., and RUSK, H. A. Decubitus ulcers treated with dried blood plasma: preliminary report. *JAMA* 153:787–788, 1953.

FOX, H. M., and GIFFORD, S. Psychological responses to ACTH and cortisone: a preliminary theoretical formulation. *Psychosom. Med.* 15:614–631, 1953.

FRIEND, D. G., and CUMMINS, J. F. New antiemetic drug: preliminary report. *JAMA* 153:480, 1953.

GOODMAN, L., and GILMAN, A. *The Pharmacological Basis of Therapeutics* (2nd ed.). New York: Macmillan, 1955.

HOMBURGER, F. An accurate method for the quantitative study of surface wounds. *Science* 118:272, 1953.

HOMBURGER, F., and SMITHY, G. The use of chlorpromazine (Thorazine) in the management of patients with advanced cancer. *New Eng. J. Med.* 251:820–822, 1954.

MACK, M. Y. Personal adjustment of chronically-ill old people under home care. *Geriatrics* 8:407–416, 1953.

MILLER, J. M., GINSBERG, M., LIPIN, R. J., and
  LONG, P. H. Clinical experience with Streptokinase and Streptodornase. *JAMA* 145:620–624,
  1951.
ROSENFELD, E. D., EGER, S., AXELROD, J., and
  MARGOLIN, E. Hospital care goes home. *Geriatrics* 6:112–116, 1951.

VARTIAINEN, O., VENHO, E. V., and VAPAVUORI, M.
  Influence of various alcoholic beverages on coronary flow. *Ann. Med. Intern. Fenn.* 42:162, 1953.
WINKLEMAN, N. W., JR. Chlorpromazine in the
  treatment of neuropsychiatric disorders. *JAMA*
  155:18–21, 1954.

II
General Principles

9

The Modern Physician: A Dynamic Approach to Total Care

PREVENTIVE MEDICINE

Some of the chronic diseases and more of the complications of aging can be warded off by intelligent preventive medicine employing all the knowledge available today. This is a point of view that, although realistic, is often still ignored. The attitude of many physicians, when faced with an aging person, is often one of resignation and lack of interest. Yet these patients present some of the most rewarding opportunities for preventive as well as curative medicine.

It had been hoped that with the youth rebellion of the 1960s, attitudes perhaps might change. Along with the advent of long hair, beards, cries for peace, and changing styles of living patterns came the cries for equality, the right to medical care for all, and improvement in minority status. When the chips are down, however, the poor—the ghetto minorities and the aged—fare little better in their medical care than before. The vocal, liberal, new-image, medical student still usually seeks his internship, residency, and, finally, his fortune in urban America, and the words formerly espoused become empty as the time for action arrives.

The life expectancy of a person turned 80 is more than 5 years. Does this not present a challenge for medicine to render these years as agreeable as possible? The patient over 50 who presents aches and pains, and who may have senile osteoporosis, will be either a shriveled, weak, unhappy person or a well-preserved, active one a few years later, depending entirely upon whether or not the physician knows how to handle his problem and does so aggressively and effectively, or whether he dismisses the situation as just another price to be paid by the patient for growing old.

The dyspeptic elderly person who is depressed and loses weight, and whose uneven temper is hard for those around him to bear, may benefit a great deal from a searching study into the problem, from a dietary readjustment, and from thorough evaluation of life situations and some intelligent psychotherapy. It is, of course, bad medicine to give pills for dysfunctions that arise in older people just because they feel lost, useless, and lonely; but it is equally poor medical judgment, simply because a person is old, not to try to seek and find those difficulties that may respond to therapy.

Many difficulties can be observed and treated relatively early in life, which otherwise will present later disaster and chronic disability. Hypertension is a good example of this. Contrary to many lay people's belief, early hypertension is usually asymptomatic. Yet most individuals who, in later life, develop coronary artery disease or stroke give a past history of high blood pressure. In view of the fact that cardiac disease is the nation's number one killer and stroke is the nation's number one crippler, adequate control of hypertension is most important. Unfortunately, many cases discovered and initially treated again become active because the patient stops his medication and salt restriction under the false premise that he cannot feel his blood pressure elevated at that time. Diabetes, too, should be detected and controlled early, rather than allowed to go unheeded for a long period. Many patients with stroke and coronary disease will also have a history of diabetes, and it is frequently found in the background of those who require lower-extremity amputations. Urinary infections can be eradicated and mechanical difficulties in the urinary tract can be corrected so that later renal damage and some types of hypertension will be forestalled.

Nutritional fads that, if uncorrected, may lead to dietary deficiencies, gastrointestinal difficulties that may interfere with the proper maintenance of the nutritional state through denture troubles, achlorhydria, deficiencies of pancreatic enzymes, biliary-tract dysfunction, and chronic constipation may all be correctable; and their treatment may contribute to the improved well-being of the patient. Great emphasis has been placed for years upon the possibility of the early diagnosis of cancer, and certainly much misery and economic loss can be prevented if neoplasms are found early and treated adequately. Surely, however, it does not require the dramatic impact of cancer upon a person's life to impress upon people how important it is to search for diseases in early stages and to prevent them. Other and considerably more frequent and tractable diseases require early treatment or prevention before they become apparent, if the patient is to remain well.

Preventive geriatrics requires a broad approach to people as persons with potentials for degeneration and dysfunctions existing all along the line of medical possibilities, including the infectious, neoplastic, cardiovascular, metabolic, degenerative, and geriatric diseases.

Periodic examinations of their motor cars, teeth, and eyes have become accepted procedures and integrated acts of the daily lives of most people. Broad preventive health examinations, however, are the exception rather than the rule. This may be so because up to very recent times, the discovery of most diseases and dysfunctions meant only trouble, and little could be offered for their correction. Today, many diseases can be controlled and are more readily manageable when discovered early. This concept of periodic

medical examination is not universally accepted, however. The federal government, through the vehicle of Medicare and private insurance companies, as exemplified by Blue Cross/Blue Shield, will not pay for routine, periodic physical examinations. There are also those physicians who feel that there are not enough members of the profession available to treat all the sick, therefore, that check-ups of the well should be given low priority. Attempts to combat this deficiency have begun on different fronts. The computer is being used and electronic analysis of data is taking place in certain areas. The new role of the physician's assistant is emerging. These individuals are often former military corpsmen who receive 3 to 12 months' training in subjects related to medicine. They are used to take histories, do physical examinations, perform specific procedures, and even to establish certain diagnoses.

The family doctor is, of course, the one who should be most competent and alert in these matters. Fortunately, there has been a swing in medicine back toward the generalist. The age of specific specialization seems to be waning. The establishment of the Academy of Family Practice has given stature and impetus to this, and the elderly can only benefit by this trend. It is still difficult, in many areas, for the aged to be serviced by house or, in particular, night calls.

Prenatal visits to the obstetrician are an accepted procedure, and so are regular pediatric follow-up examinations. During adolescence and mid-life, regular health examinations become less fruitful because the incidence of unsuspected diseases is low during that period of life. After 40, however, insidious dysfunctions that may become serious in old age begin to appear, and to give them attention will pay immense dividends in terms of good health, longer and better years of life, and peace of mind.

This seems a simple, reasonable point of view, but in effect, it requires a new state of mind which has to be developed in the present generation of medical students, who still are inclined to consider a patient over 50 years old, with only minor complaints, an "old crock," and a patient of 70 as someone for whom "nothing can be done anyway."

Statistics indicate that as life expectancy increases, due to better control of infectious disease and advances in medicine, the problem of chronic disorders in the aging population also increases and thus constitutes a continuing challenge to the medical profession.

While approximately 38 percent of our population under age 65 suffered from some form of chronic ailment, in the group which included persons aged 65 and older, 83 percent (more than twice the number of the younger group) reported at least some chronic condition. To add to the seriousness of the problem of chronic illness in our aged population, the number of chronic conditions per aged patient is also more than double that of the younger patient. Of those who have chronic conditions that *substantially* limit their activities, 40 percent are 65 and older, and 34 percent are between 45 and 64 years of age.

Effective prevention of many of these disabilities is possible with present-day knowledge. There are, however, important areas where adequate knowledge is not yet available and which represent challenges for research. Such is the case for arteriosclerosis and for the problems of regressive aging changes in tissues. It is conceivable that new knowledge developed through research will make available preventive measures, nutritional or pharmaceutical in nature, which will allow us to slow down or to eliminate so-called degenerative processes that today are accepted as inevitable.

CARE: KNOWLEDGE OF MODERN METHODS

The same antiquated medical attitude that holds society back from reaping the potential fruits of good preventive geriatrics also renders it difficult for many aging people and patients with chronic diseases to find sympathetic medical understanding and competent care. Few physicians like to deal with patients who have vague complaints and are "simply getting old," and for whom they feel they can do little or nothing. It is extremely wearing, time-consuming, and unglamorous to care for chronically bedridden patients, and it is often economically unrewarding. As a result, there are innumerable elderly "nuisance patients" who go from doctor to doctor and receive little more than some polite conversation and largely ineffective medication, if any.

This lack of American medical supervision is glaringly critical in long-term care facilities, such as chronic-disease and mental hospitals and nursing homes. It has been almost impossible to find physicians so enlightened that they would dedicate themselves to the care of the institutionalized aged and chronically ill. Because of this default on the part of the American physician, the medical coverage in many of these facilities has been left to the foreign medical-school graduate. Herein lies another paradox. There are hundreds of thousands of chronic, disabled, institutionalized patients; there are few American physicians available and fewer interested; many foreign medical-school graduates are available; many have adequate training and have been taught in the English language; yet, required qualifying examinations to enter even into formal training programs in this country effectively keep many of them from passing. Even worse, once the foreign graduate has successfully passed his examination, he mimics his American counterpart and proceeds to enter the specialties of general medicine and surgery, as he departs from chronic care—usually for good.

Medicine has often been guilty of procrastination in bringing to the patient the fruits of new knowledge, and it continues to procrastinate once more in the management of the ills of old age and long-term chronic illness. A physician who did not learn in medical school how to manage effectively the problems of a paraplegic patient, for example, should not pass up the opportunity that now exists to gain this knowledge. He owes it to his patients at least to know the possibilities and to find the specialists who are interested in the modern management of the difficulty, rather than to dispense pessimism. He should know that a colostomy is no calamity but can enable the patient to function so that a normal life is possible. He should know that the stroke that fells a patient may not mean the end of active life. He should know how to select those patients who can be rehabilitated, and he should either rehabilitate them or refer them to someone who will do so.

He should know that the aches and pains of old ladies must no longer simply be taken as inevitable but that they may be osteoporotic in nature and can often be cured. He should know that his gouty patients' attacks may be prevented and their metabolism kept fairly normal by modern management. He should know that the arthritic patient must no longer be allowed to become a helpless prisoner of his joints without a heroic medical struggle employing all the weapons in the present-day therapeutic armamentarium. Even degenerative bone and joint disease may benefit in varying degrees from modern management and, failing this, may often be correctable by surgery. He should know this and much more, lest he be like a man trying to manage diabetes without insulin or pernicious anemia without liver extract or vitamin B_{12}.

In addition to knowledge of the possibilities of preventive and curative geriatrics, the planning and carrying out of medical and nursing care of aged and chronically ill persons requires consideration of the following cardinal points:

1. A thorough knowledge of the patient, including his hidden, latent problems.
2. Cooperation between physician, social agency, and patient's family.
3. The patient's physical and mental capabilities must be determined.
4. A bit of daring must be included in the shaping of any program of active care and rehabilitation, and this calls for faith in the physician's own abilities and in the patient's motivations and potentials.
5. The patient must be made to feel wanted and loved.

The importance of these considerations cannot be overemphasized.

THOROUGH KNOWLEDGE OF THE PATIENT

The physician should also do more than give passing interest to the elderly "nuisance patient." He can evaluate from all possible angles the nature of the many complaints and outline a program of total care, rather than get rid of such patients only to leave them unhappy and ready to move on to the next practitioner.

The investigation of such aged or chronically ill patients includes a thorough evaluation of life histories. What changes has aging brought into the lives of the patients? What are their interests, their social contacts? Just what is the routine of their daily lives? What are their family problems, their business or working difficulties? How well are they oriented in time and space? What do their family and their friends think of them? What do they eat? Why do they fail to maintain reasonable feeding and living habits?

The examination must be as thorough as in the most interesting case of acute disease. What is the nutritional status? Are there signs of early deficiencies? What is the cardiovascular status? What is the metabolic and endocrine situation, especially with respect to diabetes, renal function, thyroid function, sexual function?

The laboratory studies must be thorough and include, as a minimum, blood studies (complete red-cell and white-cell counts, stained smears, hematocrit, sedimentation rate), thorough urine studies including sediment, and, at the slightest suspicion of chronic urinary infection, Gram stains and cultures on cleanly voided specimens. The stools should be examined not only for occult blood but also for undigested fat and meat fibers.

Blood chemistries should include fasting blood sugar, urea nitrogen, calcium, and phosphatase (also, acid phosphatase in men). A glucose tolerance test should be carried out, and T3, T4, and radioactive iodine uptake should be studied when necessary.

The cardiac status should be checked by electrocardiography and exercise tests, and the status of the blood vessels should be evaluated by eyeground examination and by visualizing the aorta and heart by roentgenography or fluoroscopy. Particular attention must be given the vascular status of the extremities.

Only after such a minimal check can a physician sit down and decide on a program for the patient. Such a program should include a survey with the patient of all phases of his life, medical history and findings, and clear prescriptions for useful changes of and additions to his established habits. Far from rendering them hypochondriacs, such a plan of total care will give patients a challenge, something to live up to, and it will show them clearly that for once someone, their doctor, is really interested in them.

This does not end the physician's function. It merely starts a program of continued supervision and patient participation, which should continue, ideally, until either the patient or the physician dies. This plan represents the ideal patient-doctor relationship, which is so much talked about but so rarely found in practice. The family practitioner is not the only one who can, if he makes the effort, offer his patients this type of total care. It can be organized in clinics, provided that the same patients are seen always by the same doctors, and that a thorough report is passed on from one doctor to another whenever medical personnel changes.

Simple and reasonable as this sounds, it is rarely today a part of outpatient clinic organization, and patients soon become disgusted with changing from one doctor to another until they know nearly all the professional personnel of an outpatient department and can practically predict which doctor will prescribe what medicine, the choice usually being between phenobarbital, belladonna, and aspirin.

The medical profession is not alone to be blamed for sketchiness and superficiality. In clinics as well as in private practice the patients tend to seek out the specialist: for a headache, the neurologist; for gastric upsets, the gastro-enterologist; for urinary difficulty, the urologist; for palpitations, the cardiologist.

The splitting of the medical profession into the atoms of specialties has brought great progress and developed supreme skills, but it is time to put the puzzle together once more, for the emergence of the supraspecialist—the competent practitioner who can treat and likes to treat the patient as a whole, and not merely so many cases of this or that.

The medical profession has learned more and more about less and less, and it must attempt to provide medical men and women who know a lot about everything if the fruit of specialization is to be reaped and its benefits brought to all patients. This is particularly urgent in geriatrics, and in treating chronically ill patients, where many things can go wrong all at one time and all the time.

The pathologists are well aware of the fact that the bodies of old patients are often truly pathological museums, exhibiting many diseases. The pathological diagnoses on such patients often read like the table of contents of a treatise of medicine and surgery. The good practitioner in geriatrics and chronic disease must be able to foresee, forestall, discover, and treat all these difficulties, or at least know where he can get them treated. This is what the aging patient population has a right to expect of its doctors.

COOPERATION BETWEEN PHYSICIAN, SOCIAL AGENCIES, AND PATIENT'S FAMILY

The families of these patients expect even more. Not only do they look to medicine to prevent and cure the ills of their loved ones, but they also expect help and advice in coping with the practical problems that arise. When must a patient be placed in an institution for the care of long-term sickness rather than being left as a charge to his family? Just exactly what are the chances that he will be able to take care of himself by himself, and how long will his rehabilitation take? Where can it best be accomplished?

There is no set method of handling these

problems. Here is a tremendously urgent and fruitful field for social, psychological, and psychiatric research. For the present, the physician must rely on his judgment, his philosophy, and his heart.

From a practical point of view, he should know the social agencies in his community and their officers, so that he may guide the patient's family to those places where they will find the aid they need. However, the families of these patients have a right to expect physicians to be willing to discuss these problems with them and to give them whatever help they can in making the necessary adjustments and in taking practical measures where needed. Cooperation between physician, social agencies, and family of the chronically ill or aged patient will lead, in many instances, to the effective use of facilities and services that are today available in many communities for the dynamic and successful care of these patients.

PHYSICAL AND MENTAL ABILITIES

The best nursing care in the world, the application of the most modern rehabilitation techniques, and the strictest attention to the clinical aspects of a case go a long way toward speeding the patient back to recovery; but the ultimate success of a case may hinge on whether or not due consideration has been given to a less apparent, but equally important, phase of nursing care— the patient's need for physical or mental activity, or both. Thus in undertaking the care of an invalid, one should first determine what his specific needs are in this area. The patient with a hip fracture, for instance, may become permanently immobilized if suitable exercises are not prescribed for his uninjured leg, as well as for his arms. Similarly, unrelieved bed rest and inactivity can be devastatingly detrimental to stroke victims, or to patients with paraplegia or arthritis, all of whom may be mentally alert. These patients must be encouraged and taught to use first a wheelchair and then other aids to mobility, as rapidly as possible and to the greatest extent of

their capabilities. If this concept impresses the reader as being somewhat drastic, he should bear in mind that it is no kindness to make the invalid so comfortable, so completely dependent, that he loses all initiative and the desire to do for himself. Physical activity, then, is one of the keys which opens the door to maximal independence and a speedy return to as nearly normal a routine as is possible.

Physical activity is a means of retaining independence in the aging individual who enjoys good health but who, when left to his own devices, neglects this important phase of his daily regimen. Thus, a well-balanced geriatrics program, whether formally administered in the hospital or rehabilitation center, or worked out informally at home, should include a judicious amount of exercise tailored to the specific needs of the individual.

By the same token, mental stimulation is a must for both the incapacitated and the healthy oldster, and every effort must be made to provide material suited to his temperament and inclinations. Aside from the cost of materials, this type of therapy is the most inexpensive and, at the same time, the most effective means of promoting the patient's sense of well-being.

A DARING THERAPEUTIC PROGRAM

A bit of daring may (and often should) be injected into a proposed therapeutic program, since generally accepted, conservative methods of management often fail to provide the patient with enough motivation, activity, defect repair, and security. In this case, there should be no hesitation in trying new approaches, new mechanisms of action, the most modern of equipment, and improved therapies. If this sometimes requires daring, let it be remembered that failure to make a bold approach may spell the difference between the patient's recovery and his shattered hopes.

Faith, which sometimes accomplishes the seemingly impossible, is another essential factor in successfully caring for the invalid. Persons directing this type of care must have faith in themselves and in their patients. Such confidence in one's knowledge and skill—one's ability to deviate from accepted methods intelligently and at the right time—will be communicated to the patient, who in turn will develop motivation, put forth the effort to achieve his goal, and eventually, in many cases, achieve the seemingly impossible.

THE NEED TO FEEL WANTED AND LOVED

Besides this self-confidence, persons caring for chronic invalids need the capacity to love and the ability to project this love. The patient who suddenly finds himself in the new role of a helpless invalid is suffering severe emotional shock. Weak, seemingly alone and frightened, he must reconstruct his relationship to family, friends, and society; he is at the lowest ebb in his life and his behavioral pattern may be at its worst. He needs love and understanding desperately, and those striving to work successfully with him must not only offer all the ingenuity at their command but also cultivate tolerance; they must set forth for him a shining goal, never accepting defeat in the pursuit of that goal—and in so doing, they will offer both love and charity which these patients need.

RESEARCH ON CHRONIC DISEASE AND AGING

In the management of aging and chronically ill patients, everyday problems often occur for which there is no adequate solution. This indicates the need for intensive and carefully planned research.

There are, of course, those who still take the point of view that some problems will just never be solved, and who frown on research efforts in areas that are uncharted and difficult. Explorers have always been few, and the complacent and unenthusiastic too many. Progress is due always to the pioneer, never to the doubtful. There will always be curious and enthusiastic research men who will explore the various facets of aging and chronic disease and gradually assemble new knowledge, but they need broad support. Research, particularly that dealing with patients' problems, is expensive and time consuming.

Enlightened self-interest of the people demands ever increasing financial support for research on chronic disease and old age. No matter how good the medical care may be, no matter how many hospitals are built for the chronically ill, no matter how much money is appropriated for the care of the aged, the problem cannot be solved without research! This must provide the methods and means to keep aging people healthy and out of the hospital, self-supporting and productive much longer than is now possible. It must produce solutions for the more effective management of chronic disease, so that those patients who are now hospitalized for long periods may be rehabilitated and brought out of the hospital and back into society.

If the interest of the young generation of medical students in problems of aging and chronic disease could be aroused, if enlightened laymen and politicians (in the best sense of the word) would realize the need, it could be done. Otherwise, without intensified research, this country may well become a giant nursing home, and the aged a financial burden on the shoulders of their offspring.

The directions for such research are many. Much more must be learned, at the basic science level, about the processes of degeneration than we know at present. Such fundamental physical-chemical problems as the behavior of mucopolysaccharides, proteins, and lipids, and other constituents of the supporting interstitial tissues of the body, require study in the test tube and under the electron microscope. Aging must be studied in simple, primitive organisms to learn about the basic aging changes of cells.

The effects of heredity, nutrition, and other factors such as environmental conditions on the longevity and aging changes of various animals used in laboratory work require study. Surprisingly enough, little is known, for example, of the aging process in mice, rats, and hamsters because it requires much time, money, and laboratory space to study aging in these animals, even though their life-span is relatively short. Slowly, but progressively, we acquire some knowledge on the causes and mechanisms of arteriosclerosis. Nutrition and hormones emerge as important factors besides heredity and may eventually offer means not only for the understanding of this major aging change but for its prevention and control.

A dismal lack of knowledge still exists on the integration of the aging or ill persons into their surroundings. In therapeutics much is as yet empirical, and little is known about the mechanisms of action of some of the important therapeutic agents. There is practically no end to the possibilities for the intelligent probing of an abundance of problems, and there is a great dearth of interested and qualified men and women.

The system as labeled by the modern generation is also making the attainment of these goals, at times, most frustrating. During the last half a decade, the physician has found himself to be more and more a pawn in a federal chess game. Although many of the new programs initiated were done in good faith and aimed for less expensive, more inclusive, and better total medical care, their planning and establishment left much to be desired. Medicare, which was to provide for all persons over age 65, has continuously cut back on its services because of the cost. Medicaid did not learn from Medicare's problems and created another program of runaway costs for those states which took on all or most options. The poor in other less dedicated states received far fewer benefits. Both required more and more paperwork, thus allowing the physician to spend less time with his patient. The process of requiring each physician periodically to recertify that his patient required hospital care was established and created the need for extensive utilization-review committees, record-review panels of fiscal intermediaries, and retroactive denials of bills. These procedures have markedly impaired the efficiency of long-term fa-

cilities which care for most elderly and disabled people, and by requiring more clerical help, physician coverage, and overhead expenses for watchdog review panels and appeal boards, they have paradoxically increased the cost of medical care and certainly have not improved upon it.

The physician faces more challenges to come. The Nixon administration is pushing the establishment of Health Maintenance Organizations (health-care units) to provide for the patients' total needs. Already many hospitals, stung by decreased bed utilization, retroactive denials, delayed payments from Medicaid, and overcompetition are joining this bandwagon in spite of the fact that it is also a program which has not been well planned, organized, or studied and which some observers claim will be even more costly to the American public.

Other physicians, in an effort to stave off federalization, are creating medical foundations which will attempt to provide the required services on a private basis. There are others who are promoting the use of a problem-oriented record, which aims to ensure that attention be given to all the patient's health problems and that each be studied and followed until controlled or cured. This requires a massive reeducational process for all physicians, record librarians, and hospitals.

Where will it all end? Because the modern physician has received criticism from his public, his government, and even his colleagues, peer review is being strongly pushed by medical organizations. Private records, treatment documentations, and ongoing educational experience must be bared to the scrutiny of others. Yet, who is to set the standards? Again, no agreement, because most groups propose systems to their own liking. Some favor periodic recertification examinations, others feel mandatory attendance at educational courses each year is indicated; neither can actually guarantee that better care will be provided to the patient at the grass roots. The American Medical Association, although castigated by most lay people and physicians alike, has a sensible solution in its Physicians' Meritorious Service Award. For this, a physician may accumulate points toward a required total from all areas of experience which encompass his educational life. These include formal courses, teaching of medical students, presentation of oral scientific papers, written publications, exhibits presented, meetings attended, etc.

The vast majority of physicians are dedicated people. They certainly want to see and participate in providing all the superlatives of medical care at a reasonable cost. The challenge for the immediate future and next half a decade becomes clear. The principles and attributes of honesty, sensitivity, concern, dedication, courage, creativity, and independence must never be compromised. The physician of today must provide some exciting and adequate answers to these problems or someone else will do it for him. He must be involved in the creation, planning, organization, study, and implementation of a reasonable, effective, adequate, acceptable, total medical-care program for all people. The support for such a program must come from many resources—government, private, and voluntary. Then, and only then, will medical care for the people attain the projected heights envisioned and perhaps as a corollary, prestige, respect, admiration, and love may return for the physician and the profession for which he stands.

REFERENCES

U.S. National Health Survey *Limitation of Activity and Mobility due to Chronic Conditions, United States, July 1957–June 1958*. U.S. Public Health Service: Washington, D.C., 1958 and 1959.

Facts on Major Killing and Crippling Diseases in the United States Today. National Health Education Committee, New York, 1961.

10
The Nurse

Nursing is a profession which concerns itself with helping individuals who have health problems. The aim of nursing is to enable people to maintain their health or to attain a level of health whereby they can function at their best potential. When the health status of an individual has deteriorated to the point where life is no longer possible, the nursing practitioner is interested in providing all the measures which are necessary to guarantee a peaceful death. Therefore, nursing has two components: (1) maintaining or improving the health of individuals, and (2) assisting people to die with ease. Nursing practitioners must recognize their responsibility in both these components of care and must realize that each requires the utmost knowledge, skill, and compassion.

Nurses are educated and prepared to identify the needs of individuals at moments of crisis or difficulty. Individuals with health problems vary in the way they react. Some need much assistance from others when the initial impact of the illness is too overwhelming. Many ill people are distressed by the health problem, for it usually means a modification of their life style, and they need time to talk and to plan their activities. A few accept disability with unusual resignation and are eager to continue functioning at any level possible. Occasionally, an individual cannot accept the severity of his health status, particularly if it means many restrictions, and he either lives life fully as best he can—hastening his death —or he does not wait for death to come and takes his own life.

These various reactions to health problems present challenges to nursing practitioners, for they must come to know the individual and the reasons for his behavior. The nurse often sees the individual at times of great conflict, stress, and pain, when symptoms of the disease interfere with his usual functioning and with his ability to be himself. Gradually, as the acute episode of the illness diminishes, the individual becomes more himself and demonstrates his capabilities. Most people want others to understand when they cannot be themselves, and they ask for patience, support, encouragement, and, most importantly, acceptance. The nurse should attempt to display all these responses. It is imperative for her to realize that the illness is disturbing and that it provides anxiety which leaves many individuals feeling threatened. She tries to help them feel more comfortable by rendering services which give some relief to the physical distress, while at the same time her pleasant manner helps to reduce the fears so that relaxation finally comes.

Acceptance by the nurse of the person and his health problem is crucial. Physical, emotional, social, and spiritual needs must be met to a minimal degree for comfort and security. Also, the nurse must realize that she cannot be all things to all patients, and it is well to seek the expertise and assistance of other health-team members whenever necessary. The individual must be encouraged to do for himself whenever possible and must be taught that activity is helpful rather than harmful. Being able to do some activities helps the person to feel: *independent* (all of us like to retain our independence), and *capable* (for he can perform some activities without difficulty or distress and he enjoys doing them even if they take a long time). The nurse is cognizant that an individual is happy and content when he is doing, when he is involved, when he senses that he belongs, and when he feels someone cares about his existence.

The nurse is a valuable member of the health team that cares for the aged and the chronically ill. The physician directs the medical plan of care, and the nurse provides much of the care and services that the patient receives. Her presence is viewed favorably by the patient, for she is always available to meet his needs at all stages of the illness. She is regarded as a source of security and warmth, and while she knows illness can make a person dependent, she does not encourage this. Excessive dependence is not an uplifting process. It causes many problems for the patient and does not enhance his self-image. The nursing practitioner is aware that the aged and the chronically ill need a number of rehabilitative measures to keep them functioning at their optimum level. They will be encouraged and supported by the whole health team, but the motivation to accept and to perform the activities which will enhance their health must come from themselves. The patient may need assistance in reaching his goals, but the greatest contributor is the patient himself. The physician, nurse, chaplain, and therapists intervene to relieve his discomfort, but the acceptance of the condition and the necessary treatments come from the patient. The nurse must help him to work toward these goals for health.

Nursing the aged and the chronically ill requires many qualities, because the learning process can be long and tedious, depending on the patient and his handicap. The nurse therefore must possess not only patience, but also tolerance, understanding, ingenuity, and humor. She must be able to direct, encourage, or cajole the patient into efforts that ultimately grow into achievements measured by independent daily activities. To accomplish these ends, she must be able to demonstrate her belief in the patient as a person; she must have knowledge concerning the principles of learning; she must have an understanding of human behavior and its relationship to the physiological changes taking place in the patient; and finally, she must have mastered the necessary technical aspects of the rehabilitation procedures to be used.

PATTERNS IN NURSING EDUCATION

Nursing is an applied science, for it draws on the basic biological, physical, social, and philosophical sciences to help an individual attain or maintain his health. A variety of nursing programs have been developed and each educates and prepares men and women to practice nursing. The nursing programs meet the educational requirements set by the states where they are located. The complex professional, technical, and psychological task of nursing practitioners today requires that their nursing education have a liberal arts and a professional component. "There are 1,355 state approved programs for professional nurses, which graduate some 43,639 students each year." A breakdown of the various education programs that prepare professional and practical nurses follows:

THE ASSOCIATE DEGREE PROGRAM

This program may be completed in two academic years or in two academic years with a summer session. These nursing programs are offered in junior or community colleges and grant an Associate Degree (A.S.C.N.). The graduate takes the state-board examinations upon completing the program to obtain her registration to practice professional nursing. Graduates of the programs are prepared to assume beginning positions in nursing and function under the direction of an experienced professional nurse or physician.

THE DIPLOMA PROGRAM

The diploma program is conducted under the control of a hospital, and the student earns a diploma in nursing upon graduation. The length of the program varies from twenty-eight to thirty-six months. When the student graduates, she takes the state board examinations to obtain her registration to practice professional nursing. The number of diploma nursing programs in the United States has decreased in recent years because of the trend to prepare nurses in educational settings, i.e., in junior colleges and universities. Today the hospital programs continue to prepare the majority of professional nursing practitioners to assist with the administration of health care.

THE BACCALAUREATE PROGRAM

The basic baccalaureate program is usually completed in four academic years. A few schools offer five-year programs. These programs are found in universities or colleges and may be administered by a separate school or by a Department of Nursing within the university. Graduates earn a baccalaureate degree in nursing and are eligible to take the state-board examinations to obtain their registration to practice professional nursing. It is expected that the graduates of this program can function in any area of nursing concerned with direct patient care and that they can advance to positions of greater responsibility without much difficulty.

PRACTICAL NURSING OR VOCATIONAL NURSING PROGRAMS

"There are 1,134 state-approved programs for practical nurses which graduate some 37,128 students each year." The programs in practical (vocational) nursing prepare men and women to practice the basic skills of patient care, and these graduates function under the direction of a registered nurse and/or physician. The length of the program varies from 12 to 18 months. The graduates take the state-board examinations upon graduation to receive their license to practice practical (vocational) nursing. The licensed practical nurse is an accepted and valuable member of the health team in our hospitals, clinics, extended-care facilities, and other institutions.

The American Nurses' Association is the largest professional association for registered nurses in the United States, with a membership of 204,704. The National League for Nursing is an organization whose membership is composed of individuals (professional nurses, licensed practical nurses, physicians, educators, businessmen, etc.) and agencies interested in nursing, with a membership of 21,157.

Practical and registered nurses may carry out their work as private practitioners and make themselves available, through registries of nurses, for home care and work with private patients in institutions. In addition, nurses may be employed by hospitals, physicians, nursing schools, visiting-nurse associations, state or federal public-health services, or the armed services.

COLLABORATION WITH HEALTH TEAM

A rehabilitation program becomes truly meaningful and effective when each member of the team not only understands and utilizes his own contribution to the effort but also understands the interrelationships of the other team disciplines, which together meet the ever-changing needs of the patient. The nurse must acquire the concept of the team approach to total patient care, and she must comprehend her role on the team. She should not be the weak link on the program because much depends upon her strength and ability. The nurse must be perceptive and able to discover the needs of the patient and refer them to the team member best able to meet them. In her role, she is in a good position to interpret the functions of the other team members to the patient and the family, as well as the patient's problems to the team. The more the patient is involved as an active participant on the team, and the more he understands the program and goals, the greater will be his satisfaction and the harder he will work toward recovery.

The nursing practitioner is able to collaborate with others when she is skillful in her nursing practice and sensitive to the needs of the patient. She is observant of the patient as she renders care or unusual responses to the illness; administration of drugs and treatments are also reported and recorded. She is willing to admit to a difficult problem, which requires a team approach for a resolution, rather than pretend that all is well. The nurse understands the objectives of the plan of care and she incorporates the patient's preferences whenever possible.

The contribution of the nurse as a member of the team is great. She is with the patient for longer periods of time than any other team member and as a result sees the patient during various daily activities and time cycles. She is aware of his total response to the illness—during the day, evening, and night and can discuss his care without difficulty. Other team members expect her to inform them of new problems as they develop or they want her to report a chronic problem that also needs their consideration.

NURSING CARE

The actual nursing care of the chronically ill patient and/or the aged can be complex, challenging, and at times, difficult. The patient may have lived with his disability or disease for a period of time and often needs support, assistance, and encouragement to continue with the medical regime. He becomes upset as the symptoms or disability increase and realizes he will need help from others to maintain his equilibrium. He is dependent and he wants to be independent, yet his illness is too incapacitating, and he cannot manage alone. It is extremely hard for a patient to accept help from others, and this situation is aggravated when there is no family or no one else who cares. The patient feels rejected and it is up to the health team to win the trust of the individual so he will accept their help.

One needs to reflect on the impact of chronic illness and aging on an individual. The person is not able to be himself, he fatigues early, he cannot respond quickly, he often experiences pain or discomfort, and he requires assistance to

perform some routine activities of daily living. He is concerned with his self-image and strives to keep the effect of his illness or aging from others; he is unwilling to be a bother to them. The chronically ill and the aged need time, interest, and nursing care, so that they will feel wanted and comfortable as they continue living and functioning, using their best potential.

LEVELS OF CARE

The following categories of patient care are given as guides for nursing practitioners involved in caring for the chronically ill and the aged. Each level of care will be discussed in detail so that the nursing responsibilities will be highlighted. Patients will, at various times in their illness, be at one level of care. Nursing practitioners must recognize the needs of the patient at a particular level of illness and attempt to meet those needs as completely as possible. The nurse must accept the individuality of patients, respect their dignity, and provide nursing care which reflects the best knowledge, skill, and utmost compassion.

The classification of patients that follows is an attempt to define the different levels of care patients require in daily practice. Very often, nursing care is considered to be the same for all people. It is indeed different and unique for each individual. On any clinical unit, in any health-care agency, one will find people in various stages of health and illness. The classification should make the management of patient care easier.

THE COMATOSE PATIENT

The comatose patient is totally dependent upon the medical and nursing staff for his existence. He cannot survive without their care and intervention. His basic needs are managed so that he will not develop unnecessary complications. His condition is constantly being evaluated so that he will have every chance for survival. When coma continues and deepens, so that his response to stimuli is minimal, the plan of care must reflect a respect for the dignity of the person. Too often, the patient in this condition is referred to as "a vegetable" and this label connotes no worth. It is true that because of a physical or emotional problem, the patient's condition has deteriorated, yet he is a human being who requires care until he recovers or until death occurs.

The patient is unresponsive to the care given and he cannot interact with the environment, so the responsibility to be thorough in nursing care is paramount. One cannot afford to allow the care of the patient to become routine. As the nursing tasks are performed, the nurse should observe the patient, talk to him in a gentle voice, and be concerned with providing him privacy. Conversation while in his presence should consist of dialogue which one would not mind being repeated. It is a known fact that comatose patients can hear, therefore, give them stimuli that is worth hearing. The same interest, attention, and effort that are given to other patients are also needed by the comatose patient. His response to good care may be living another day. This level of living requires the type of care which will prevent numerous complications such as contracture, bedsores, dehydration, etc.

Nursing practitioners need to accept the comatose patient and his needs. They must practice as well as help others to demonstrate care, concern, and respect for him. Contact should be meaningful. When the patient is thirsty, it is necessary to give him something to drink, or mouth care so that his lips and tongue will not be coated. When he is uncomfortable, his position should be changed, his skin rubbed to give him some relief, and when he needs treatments, one should be gentle and careful in approach.

In addition to accepting the responsibility of patient care, the nurse is concerned with assisting the family members to cope with him. It is difficult for the family to visit, attempt to communicate and not be able to share themselves with the patient. The visits are made easier when a member of the nursing staff stops by to be with the family member for a while, or when they can share a cup of coffee together in the visiting room or solarium. The family requires assistance to accept the comatose state of the patient and to prepare themselves for the death when it comes, particularly when the patient's condition continues to deteriorate. Members of the family have questions and will welcome a gesture on the part of the nurse which allows them to raise questions or sometimes just to talk. The nursing practitioners can help them to prepare for the death of the patient and to accept it as the final process of life. Time should be allowed for them to be with the person, to assist in some nursing measures if possible, to talk, to be quiet, to visit with a member of the clergy, and to know that the medical staff is observant and aware of the patient's condition at all times. The nurse must be supportive, patient, gentle, willing to listen, and finally, communicate to others how the family member accepts the status of the patient.

The nursing literature has not paid much attention to the reactions of family members to patients who are comatose. They should be included in the plan of care for the patient.

THE CUSTODIAL PATIENT

This patient may be described as one who has a physical or emotional problem which prohibits him from fully participating in his own care. He may be able to do some activities for himself, i.e., some bathing, eating with supervision, dressing with assistance, and ambulating with direction or guidance. He cannot be left alone for long periods of time, and measures to ensure his safety are necessary. He may or may not be mentally competent; he may or may not be able to communicate; he may be incontinent; he may be an observer of activities rather than a true participant. Yet he is alert, has awareness, and can receive some sensory input. He tries to respond to the stimulation of others, i.e., a greeting, an attractive photo, a special food, music, or visits from those he knows well.

Life is difficult for this patient, for in a sense he is a captive. He is not able, because of pathophysiological conditions, to be himself and demonstrate his potentials. He can only show his capabilities in some areas and he needs assistance in others. He usually cannot be as expressive as he would like. He knows he has limitations and tries to adjust to them. He realizes he has to be dependent upon others for some, or much, of his care. He has tried to maintain his independence as long as possible and now accepts the results of the disease process. The frustrations he feels are difficult to comprehend. One can only be sensitive to his needs, allowing him to be himself whenever possible, and provide the measures which ensure his comfort and well-being.

This patient has need of warmth, affection, and concern. He does not want to be passed by without an acknowledgment. One should make a comment about him, his dress, his room, or his activity. Take time to let him respond to a question, or spend time with him if others have company. Be courteous—permit him to make as many decisions as he can. Continue to involve him to whatever degree it is possible. Be supportive to the family and help them to participate in his care. Be willing to try to stimulate him, to offer diversion, rather than accepting the status quo. Realize that he will lose whatever capacity he has unless he is provided with opportunities to use it. Accept his ability to observe activities rather than enforcing his participation. He can enjoy pleasures without having to participate. Grant him an occasional day of not cooperating, of wanting to retreat, of not caring, for he must have great difficulty in accepting his current status, and discouragement comes easily. Be willing to extend oneself to help him regain his composure so that he might confront his existence. Attempt to know the person he *was* and incorporate *his* likes into the plan of care. Help him to maintain his dignity; give him the assistance he needs whenever necessary. Never make him plead or wait to have a nursing measure provided that would ease his discomfort. Take care to learn about him, his needs, and his pleasures. Learn to accept his health status. Wishing it to be different does not help the patient. If one has a trying day with the patient on

one occasion or even several occasions, remember that he lives with the disability daily and needs support not rejection.

THE REHABILITATIVE PATIENT

The patient with a chronic illness or one who is aging can often be helped to live up to his optimum potential by an adequate and effective rehabilitation program. The rehabilitative patient is one with a disabling health problem who needs the services and skill of a team of experts to help him reach a maximal functioning potential. They may also help him to adjust and live with his illness. He needs assistance and guidance to regain his functions and ability. His confidence and self-esteem may be damaged, therefore the health team needs patience and understanding as he attempts the rehabilitative process. His progress should be noted and encouragement given as he achieves independence in any particular area of daily living.

The aim of any rehabilitation program is to help the person attain his maximum level of health and independence. The patient is encouraged to do the activities of daily living (i.e., bathing, dressing, eating, ambulation, social and work activities) for himself. He is helped gradually to assume responsibility for his own care and to exercise his body so that he can manage these activities without difficulty. The process can be slow and drawn out and is often impeded by complications. However, the team keeps their objectives for the patient uppermost in their minds so that when complications arise they can be managed easily. The patient must accept the goals that the team has established, for without the patient's consent and effort, the best plans will fail.

It takes the patient some time to adjust to the severity of his illness or the aging process and to accept the limitations that are imposed. The nurse must continually encourage him to do his exercises, to walk the corridor, to dress himself, to maneuver his wheelchair, to care for his prosthesis, to take his medication, and gradually to leave the dependent state; and the patient must detect a desire on the part of the nurse for him to be himself to the best of his ability.

The entire nursing staff must be informed of the goals for the patient so that they can contribute to his progress. The channels of communication between all shifts (tours of duty) must be open so that the needs of the patient are met. If the patient has difficulty doing his exercises in the evening because of fatigue, this fact needs to be reported, so that his plan of care can be modified. If the patient has anorexia, it should be reported, so that proper nutrition can be ensured. If the patient has been unable to communicate with the staff, one person (if this is possible) should be assigned to him to gain his trust and help him to begin to relate to others.

The patient with rehabilitative potential grieves for a while because illness or aging has caused a modification of his life style. He needs empathy and support, but most importantly he needs direction so that he may see a way out of the darkness that has engulfed him. Often, he needs strength because his is waning. The nurse has seen and cared for many patients with major health problems. This serious illness may be the patient's first encounter with disability, and he cannot be objective. He is overcome by the enormity of the medical, surgical, and emotional problems, and so, needs the assistance of others at this moment of stress. The nurse may have to be direct, firm, insistent, and organized, so that the patient will perform all his activities and become involved in his plan of care. These actions are necessary for his well-being. He does not need someone to pamper him, for he is pampering himself.

CONTINUITY OF CARE

In the nursing care of the chronically ill and the aged, one of the prime responsibilities of the nurse is to be concerned with coordinating the activities of the patient. Very often, the medical plan of care includes a variety of services or treatments designed to help the patient, but the nurse can ensure that the treatments are provided. She realizes the objectives or goals of the health team and knows that if the patient is to attain his maximum level of health, he requires assistance from the nursing staff. Nursing personnel see the patient daily for longer periods of time than any other members of the health team. They reinforce the teaching, the goals, and philosophy of the team members. It is important for all the nursing practitioners to be informed of the plan of care for the patient, so that they can implement the care without difficulty. The patient is less anxious and cooperates more fully with the staff when he senses that the nurse is confident and knowledgeable about his care. When he can detect a similarity in the way all members of the nursing staff communicate with him, care for him, and encourage him, then relaxation and acceptance come.

The patient who is striving to achieve his maximum level of health requires the services of others on a continuing basis. It is important that his care not be fragmented or sporadic. Usually, the patient receives particular treatments, medications, and exercises on a regular schedule, i.e., daily or several times a week. In order for him to maintain his health status or to progress to another level of health, it is essential that he have his care planned so that he will be on time for appointments with the various therapists, diversional activities, and any other services which contribute to his well-being. The nurse is often the person who helps him to accept the daily schedule of activities which are necessary for rehabilitation to occur. She observes him, cares for him, listens to him, encourages him when he experiences fatigue, and communicates to the other team members his progress or problems.

Continuity of care means that all the services required by the patient will be provided over a period of time without interruption. This concept may have to be interpreted to the patient and his family members. An initial explanation should be given to them and it should be reinforced whenever the need arises. Usually, as the patient responds to the therapy and becomes more independent in his daily activities, he is eager to participate and follows the daily schedule without difficulty. Gradually, the patient and family, or the patient with the health team, begin to discuss plans for discharge.

Usually the patient has had at least a day or weekend away from a long-term health-care facility before such plans are activated. Since the time of admission, the patient, health team, and family have planned their activities so that discharge could be possible. Discharge could be to the home, a small apartment, a boardinghouse, or a facility for the aged. The essential factor is that the patient has received quality care and achieved his best level of health, so that discharge from the acute or chronic hospital has become a reality. The nurse and the social worker work closely together to provide the continuity of care necessary to meet all of the patient's needs.

EVALUATION OF NURSING CARE

Nursing practitioners must be concerned with the quality of their nursing practice. In order to determine the effectiveness of their care, evaluation is necessary. The evaluation process relates to the nursing goals established for the patient and final analysis to determine if the objectives have been met. Nursing practitioners need to ask themselves:

How effective was their management of the patient?

Are his problems less troublesome?

Is his health status unchanged?

Did he develop unnecessary complications?

Could his recovery have been achieved without nursing interventions?

Was the physical status of the patient considered primarily and other needs ignored?

Did the patient have an active role in the rehabilitation process?

Was the family included in the plan of care, and were they informed of the need to allow the patient to do activities for himself?

The process of evaluation helps identify the measures which are helpful to the patient as well as those which are not effective. One can learn from both results. Too often, however, failures are ignored and only successes discussed. The examination of failure can help to identify a better way to plan the care of the patient, a new approach to a treatment, or a different manner of relating and communicating. It fosters thoughtfulness, knowledge, purposefulness, and skill.

The patient, the team, the other nursing personnel all benefit by this process.

REFERENCES

BIER, KATHRYN S. Guthrie-Smith Apparatus: Its construction and use in rehabilitation. *Phys. Ther.*, 28:227, 1948.

BLUMBERG, JEAN, and DRUMMOND, ELEANOR E. *Nursing Care of the Long-Term Patient.* New York: Springer, 1963.

BONNER, C. D., JOHNSON, M., LYFORD, B. E. A portable sling suspension apparatus. *Phys. Ther.* 49:47, 1969.

CALNAN, MARY, and HANRON, JANE. Young nurse —elderly patient. *Nurs. Outlook* 18:44, December, 1970.

CUMMING, ELAINE, and HENRY, WILLIAM E. *Growing Old—The Process of Disengagement.* New York: Basic Books, 1961.

DRUMMOND, ELEANOR E. Communication and comfort for the dying patient. *Nurs. Clin. North Am.* 5:55, March, 1970.

ELWOOD, EVELYN. Nursing the patient with cerebrovascular accident. *Nurs. Clin. North Am.* 5:47, March, 1970.

FIELD, MINNA. *Aging with Honor and Dignity.* Springfield, Ill.: Thomas, 1968.

GASPARD, NANCY J. The family of the patient with a long-term illness. *Nurs. Clin. North Am.* 5:77, March, 1970.

GUTHRIE-SMITH, OLIVE F. *Rehabilitation, Re-education and Remedial Exercises.* Baltimore: Williams & Wilkins Co., 1943.

JOHNSON, M. M., BONNER, C. D. Sling suspension

techniques, demonstrating the use of a new portable frame. Part I. Introduction, definitions, equipment and advantages. *Phys. Ther.* 51:524, 1971.

Johnson, M. M., Bonner, C. D. Sling suspension techniques, demonstrating the use of a new portable frame. Part II. Methods of progression in an exercise program: The upper extremity. *Phys. Ther.* 51: 1092, 1971.

Johnson, M. M., Bonner, C. D. Sling suspension techniques, demonstrating the use of a new portable frame. Part III. Treatment of motor disabilities: The lower extremity. *Phys. Ther.* 51:1288, 1971.

Johnson, M. M., Ehrenkranz, C., Bonner, C. D. Sling suspension techniques, demonstrating the use of a new portable frame. Part IV. Treatment of motor disabilities, neck and trunk. *Phys. Ther.* 53: 856, 1973.

Kintzel, Kay C. (Ed.). *Advanced Concepts in Clinical Nursing*. Philadelphia: Lippincott, 1971.

Lyford, Bernice E., Bonner, Charles D. An improvised method for sling suspension exercise. *Phys. Ther.*, 39:530, 1959.

National League for Nursing. *State-Approved Schools of Nursing—L. P. N.—L. V. N.* New York: National League for Nursing, 1971.

National League for Nursing. *State-Approved Schools of Nursing—R. N.* New York: National League for Nursing, 1971.

O'Brien, Maureen J. *The Care of the Aged: A Guide for the Licensed Practical Nurse*. St. Louis: Mosby, 1971.

Porath, Thomas. A caring philosophy of the aging. *Hosp. Progr.* 52:53, June, 1971.

Schmieding, Norma Jean. Relationship of nursing and the process of chronicity. *Nurs. Outlook* 18:58, February, 1970.

Sorensen, Karen, and Amis, Dorothy B. Understanding the world of the chronically ill. *Am. J. Nurs.* 67:811, April, 1967.

11

The Physical Therapist

Physical therapy is a dynamic, growing profession which offers much to aged or chronically ill patients. A therapist, acting upon the referral of a physician, has many tools and skills at hand to evaluate and treat a variety of medical problems. Early descriptions of this profession, which included the therapeutic use of heat, light, water, and electricity, no longer provide a truly accurate picture of the skills a physical therapist can offer today.

The physical therapist:

1. Evaluates the patient by performing specific tests which help determine neurological, musculoskeletal, respiratory, and cardiovascular status.

2. Plans a treatment program based upon the results of the evaluation.

3. Utilizes physical measures and instructs the patient as part of the overall treatment program.

4. Instructs nonprofessional workers, members of the patient's family, or family substitutes in carrying out specific procedures and also supervises their activity.

5. Communicates and cooperates effectively with other health workers in the total rehabilitation effort.

6. Functions in the prevention of disabilities, particularly of the musculoskeletal system.

Education and practice prepare the therapist to assume these responsibilities. This involves a 4-year baccalaureate or 2-year postgraduate program with extensive training in the basic sciences, in the normal and abnormal functioning of the human body, and in supervisory human-relations skills. Graduate education is also available for the physical therapist who wishes to specialize in administration, education, or research. In addition to this university-based education, a therapist receives a vast amount of clinical training in a hospital setting.

EVALUATION

Evaluation begins at the time of the physician's written referral, which should include the patient's diagnosis and emphasize any precautions to be taken. Usually, more than one system is assessed, for the geriatric or chronically ill patient frequently demonstrates concurrent neuromuscular, musculoskeletal, circulatory, or respiratory symptoms. Motivational and emotional states are also important to assess, for a successful treatment program is often dependent upon the cooperation and motivation of the patient. Evaluations are done upon admission, at specified time intervals throughout treatment, and at the time of discharge. Follow-up evaluation after the patient is at home is also important in order to determine whether or not his level of functioning has been maintained since discharge. A physical therapist routinely uses a number of specific procedures and standardized tests to evaluate the patient. These can best be understood if considered in relation to the presenting symptoms.

Pain

Pain is a frequent complaint in the type of patient population discussed in this book. Inflammation, muscle spasm, and protective muscular splinting are all assessed as possible contributing factors. Visual inspection, palpation, and active and passive movement generally reveal a great deal about the pain status of the patient.

Edema

The degree of edema present is determined by visual inspection, palpation, and girth measurements. The swelling is noted at different times during the day and after certain activities to determine the effect of varied positions upon it. Elevation of the part and massage can reduce the edema which is caused by the effects of gravity.

Restriction of Range

Restricted range in any motion is often caused by bony blocks, soft-tissue changes, or by excessive muscular holding. Palpation of the area surrounding the joint can usually reveal whether adaptive shortening of the muscles and ligaments has occurred. Protective muscular splinting as a limiting factor must also be considered. An improvement in range can generally be noted after using relaxation techniques. These techniques can also be used to obtain temporary relief in spasticity.

The most frequently used instrument to measure joint range of motion is a goniometer which consists of a protractor with extended, movable arms. The center of the protractor is aligned over the anatomical center of the joint while the movable arms are aligned over the lever arms of the joint. Measurement begins with the anatomical position as the starting point and continues throughout the range to the point of restriction. Active and passive ranges are taken as needed. Reliability is higher if the measurements are repeated by the same examiner. Often, subtle differences in placement from one therapist to the next can cause measurements to differ as much as 5 to 10 degrees.

Other forms of measurement are used in the assessment of specific joints. For the hand, therapists have recently been using office copying equipment to determine joint range and de-

formity. These photocopy records have proved to be simple, accurate, and economical.

Muscle Weakness

The primary causes of muscle weakness are disuse and peripheral nerve disruption caused by injury or disease. Central nervous system insults can also produce secondary weakness which can be accompanied by changes in muscle tone. Instability resulting from an imbalance of muscle power can also create significant weakness. It is important for the therapist to pinpoint the precise cause of weakness in order to plan an appropriate treatment program.

Most muscle tests utilize the Lovett method, which includes the use of gravity and resistance as its basis for grading. The patient is asked to perform various motions which are believed to test the function of specific muscles or muscle groups. Standardized positions are used to minimize differences in kinesiological conditions from one testing situation to the next. A typical manual muscle-test form is given on pages 161–163.

A muscle receiving a grade of zero exhibits no evidence of contractility and is unable to move the body part. A *trace muscle* responds with a slight evidence of contractility but is still unable to move the body part. A *poor muscle* is capable of completing the range of motion with the effects of gravity eliminated. A *fair muscle* moves the body part through full range against gravity and represents a definite functional threshold. Muscles receiving a good grade can complete the range against gravity while taking some resistance against the motion. Finally, a *normal muscle* is able to tolerate a normal amount of resistance throughout the range.

Reliability of the muscle examination is also higher if the same therapist repeats it. Because subjectivity enters into the grading, especially with the good and normal grades, two therapists may record different grades or degrees of the same grade as indicated by a plus or minus. The resistance given must also reflect the norms for the patient's size, sex, age, and occupation.

Numerous other, less standardized measures

MANUAL MUSCLE TEST

Name: _____   Birthday: _____

Diagnosis: _____   Onset: _____

LEFT				Examiner's Initials:			RIGHT		
				Date:					
				NECK:					
				Sternocleidomastoid Accessory	C2-3				
				Ant.Vertebral flexors	C1-2				
				Extensor Group	C1-6				
				TRUNK:					
				Rectus Abdominus	T5-T12				
				Rt.Ext.Obl. ⎰ Rota- ⎰ Lt.Ext.Obl. / Lt.Int.Obl. ⎱ tors ⎱ Rt.Int.Obl.	T7-L1				
				Extensors Thoracic	T1-T9				
				Extensors Lumborum	T10-L5				
				Quadratus	T12-L3				
				HIP:					
				Iliopsoas	L2-3				
				Gluteus Maximus-Inf.Gluteal	L5-S2				
				Gluteus Medius-Sup.Gluteal	L4-S1				
				Adductors-Obturator	L2-4				
				Internal Rotators	L4-S1				
				External Rotators	L3-S3				
				Sartorius-Femoral	L2-4				
				Tensor Fasciae Lata-Sup.Gluteal	L4-S1				
				KNEE:					
				Quadriceps-Femoral	L2-4				
				Biceps Femoris-Sciatic	L4-S2				
				Semitendinous/Membranous-Sciatic	L4-S2				
				ANKLE:					
				Gastrocnemius Tibial	S1-2				
				Soleus Tibial	L5-S2				
				FOOT:					
				Peroneals S.Peroneal	L4-S1				
				Tibialis Ant. D.Peroneal	L5-S1				
				Tibialis Post. Tibial	L5-S1				
				TOES:					
				Ext.Dig.Longus Peroneal	L4-S1				
				Ext.Dig.Brevis Peroneal	L4-S1				
				Flex.Dig.Longus Tibial	L5-S2				
				Flex.Dig.Brevis Plantar	L5-S1				
				Intrinsics-Lumbricales	L5-S1				
				Interossei-Plantar	S1-S2				
				Interossei-Dorsal	S1-S2				
				HALLUX:					
				Ext.Hall.Longus Peroneal	L4-S1				
				Abd.Hall. Plantar	L5-S1				
				Add.Hall. Plantar	S1-S2				
				Flex.Hall.Longus Tibial	L5-S2				
				Flex.Hall.Brevis Plantar	L5-S1				

LEFT				Examiner's Initials:		RIGHT		
				Date:				
				SCAPULA:				
				Serratus Ant.　　　　L.Thoracic　　C5-8				
				Middle Trapezius　　Access.　　C2-4				
				Upper Trapezius　　Access.　　C2-4				
				Levator Scapulae　　　　C3-5				
				Lower Trapezius　　Access.　　C2-4				
				Rhomboids　　D.Scap.　　C5				
				SHOULDER:				
				Ant. Deltoid　　Axillary　　C5-6				
				Coracobrachialis　　Musculo.　　C5-6				
				Middle Deltoid　　Axillary　　C5-6				
				Posterior Deltoid　　Axillary　　C5-6				
				CL.Pectoralis Maj.-Ant.Thor.　　C5-C7CL.				
				St.Pectoralis Maj.-Ant.Thor.　　C5-C7St.				
				Int. Rotators　　C4-T1　　C5-8				
				Ext. Rotators　　C4-C6				
				Latissimus Dorsi-Thoracodorsal　　C6-8				
				Teres Major　　C5-7				
				ELBOW:				
				Triceps　　Radial　　C6-T1				
				Biceps Musculocutaneous Brachials　　C5-6				
				FOREARM:				
				Supinators Radial/Musculocut.　　C5-6				
				Pronators　　Median　　C6-T1				
				WRIST:				
				(Ext. Carpi Rad. Brevis-Radial)　　C5-8				
				(Ext. Carpi Rad. Longus　　）				
				Ext. Carpi Ulnaris-Radial　　C7-8				
				Flexor Carpi Radialis-Median　　C6-C7				
				Flexor Carpi Ulnaris-Ulnar　　C7-T1				
				FINGERS:				
				Flexor Sublimis 1st Median　　C7-T1				
				"　　"　　2nd　"　　C7-T1				
				"　　"　　3rd Ulna				
				"　　"　　4th　"				
				Flexor Profundus 1st Median　　C7-T1				
				"　　"　　2nd　"				
				"　　"　　3rd Ulna				
				"　　"　　4th　"				
				Ext.Digitorum Communis 1st Rad.　　C5-7				
				"　　"　　"　　2nd　"				
				"　　"　　"　　3rd　"				
				"　　"　　"　　4th　"				
				Lumbricales 1st Median　　C7-T1				
				"　　2nd　"				
				"　　3rd Ulna　　C8-T1				
				"　　4th　"				
				Dorsal Interossei 1st Ulna　　C8-T1				
				"　　"　　2nd　"				
				"　　"　　3rd　"				
				"　　"　　4th　"				
				Abductordigiti Quinti Ulnar　　C8-T1				

	LEFT			Examiner's Initials:		RIGHT			
				Date:					
				Palmar Interossei 1st Ulna	C8-T1				
				2nd ''					
				3rd ''					
				Flexor Pollicis Longus Median	C7-T1				
				Abd.Pollicis Longus Radial	C7-C8				
				Abd.Pollicis Brevis-Median	C6-7				
				Opponens Pollicis-Median	C6-T1				
				Flexor Pollicis Brevis Median & Ulnar	C6-8				
				Adductor Pollicis-Ulnar	C8-T1				
				Extensor Poll.Brev.-Radial	C7-8				
				Extensor Poll.Longus-Radial	C7-8				
				Facial					

KEY:
N — Normal — Complete range of motion against gravity with full resistance.
G — Good   — Complete range of motion against gravity with moderate resistance.
F — Fair   — Complete range of motion against gravity.
P — Poor   — Complete range of motion with gravity eliminated.
TR — Trace — Evidence of slight contractility, no joint motion.
O — Zero   — No evidence of contractility
S —   Spasticity
C —   Contracture

Double Grades: Range/Strength — to use when lack of ROM or spasticity limit full range, but PT is able to take resistance, e.g., F−/G+

Facilitation Grade — to use when patient has zero grade but when facilitation technique is used, PT is able to move part, e.g., O//F−

COMMENTS:

are also employed in the evaluation of muscle weakness. A functional examination reveals weakness as it interferes with the activities of daily life. This evaluation is especially important for adequate treatment planning. Lacking specific measures to cure many of the chronic diseases, a therapist must assist the disabled to live and to work as effectively as their remaining physical abilities allow. A functional evaluation is the basis of this training.

This most often includes an analysis of activities in three main groups: self-care activities, ambulation activities, and hand activities. Self-care activities of eating, dressing, and toileting are commonly evaluated by the occupational therapist and the rehabilitation nurse in greater detail. Gait analysis entails close investigation of muscle function at each joint during both swing and stance phases. The patient is also observed during stair climbing, outdoor walking, and other traveling activities. Evaluation of hand activities includes the management of wheelchair pedals and brakes, braces, clothing, and other appliances the patient may be using.

Muscle function in patterns of movement is another important way in which to assess weakness. Since the brain essentially controls groups of muscles acting in patterns to produce coordinated movement rather than isolated motions, an inability to function in these patterns may be more indicative of dysfunction with a central-nervous-system lesion than the standardized muscle test. In addition, many therapeutic exercises used today are based upon these basic patterns of movement.

ABNORMAL MUSCLE TONE

The evaluation of abnormal muscle tone presents the physical therapist with one of the most difficult symptoms to assess objectively. Spasticity, or hypertonicity is graded as slight, moderate, or severe, depending upon the amount of resistance to movement which is felt by the therapist. Spastic patterns of movement, presenting with certain postures or changes of position, are

also important to note. Since abnormal tone is in a state of constant flux, the patient may demonstrate different gradations of spasticity and posturing within the same day. For this reason the manual muscle test is not appropriate for use with the spastic patient suffering from an upper motor neuron lesion. Upon examination, the spastic muscle demonstrates an initial resistance to movement which is then followed by muscle relaxation. This is known as the *clasp-knife phenomenon.*

Rigidity is another form of hypertonicity and is characterized by excessive holding by antagonistic groups of muscles. Thus, there is resistance to movement in any direction. Cogwheel rigidity offers a release in tension at various points throughout the range whereas lead-pipe rigidity is felt as constant tension throughout the motion.

Hypotonic muscles feel soft and flabby and offer less than the normal resistance to movement. In patients with marked hypotonia, the joints are often hyperextended.

SENSORY DISTURBANCES

Sensory input plays a key role in the initiation and control of movement and therefore must receive close attention in the physical-therapy evaluation. This includes testing proprioception from the muscle spindles and joint receptors and exteroception from the skin and subcutaneous receptors. Visual and auditory influences upon movement are also considered. An inability to perform various gross motor activities may be indicative of impaired function. Proprioception has been found to be particularly important in sustained, postural activities whereas exteroception appears to be more related to complex or rapid movements of the limb.

Specific tests to assess receptor integrity are also performed. Kinesthesia, or awareness of body part and position, is used to assess the integrity of the joint receptors. Vibratory sense, reflex response to stretch, and coordinated activities of an unconscious nature are used to determine the effectiveness of the muscle receptors.

Touch, pressure, pain, and temperature are usually evaluated on the basis of the patient's ability to perceive stimulation applied to the local receptors. This examination usually reveals specific areas of hypersensitivity and hyposensitivity or analgesia, according to nerve distributions or dermatomes. Stereognosis, or the ability to judge consistency and shape, is tested by having the patient distinguish different objects without the assistance of vision.

Although an accurate sensory evaluation is time-consuming and often difficult to obtain, it is, nevertheless, essential to a therapist's understanding of the patient's motor difficulties. It is also vital for effective treatment planning, because the use of sensory stimulation to facilitate movement seems to be a central tenet of therapeutic thought today. Without an accurate evaluation, many of these measures may become ineffective or even harmful.

TREATMENT

On the basis of the evaluation, the therapist plans an appropriate treatment program designed to relieve the presenting symptoms and to increase the patient's functional capacities. A typical program might include the use of modalities and electrotherapeutic measures in addition to therapeutic exercises. The therapist can choose from a number of traditional exercise regimes, or she may employ some of the many sensorimotor stimulation techniques found in the newer approaches to exercise. Whatever the program, it must be individually structured to meet the patient's specific needs.

Reduction of Pain and Edema

The most frequently used modalities in the treatment of the aged or chronically ill are hot packs, whirlpool baths, paraffin, and ice packs. They act to relieve pain and muscle spasm by increasing circulation to the affected area. Moist hot packs provide a convenient and effective method of local application which can be applied to most areas of the body. Paraffin dips are used to cover the more irregular body surfaces, such as the hands and the feet. Although initially more unpleasant, ice packs provide a similar relief of pain through their reflex vasodilation action. They have also been used to obtain temporary relief in spasticity through their inhibiting effect on the muscle spindle. Whirlpool baths are most often used to treat body segments. In systemic body conditions, such as rheumatoid arthritis, the patient is immersed totally in a hubbard tub. Exercises can then be performed while the patient is still in the water, because the buoyancy force creates an effective exercise medium. Measures to reduce edema consist of manual massage, bandaging, or the application of intermittent compressive devices, such as the Jobst unit.

The most frequently used electrotherapeutic measures are ultrasound and diathermy, depending upon one's orientation. Ultrasonic machines pass sound waves through the superficial tissues, producing heat, increased absorption of fluids, relief of pain, and stretching of scar tissue. This has been found particularly useful in traumatic and inflammatory conditions. Diathermy consists of the use of a high-frequency, alternating current which passes through the tissues without stimulating motor or sensory nerves. It has seen less usage since the advent of more modern techniques. Both shortwave and microwave diathermy machines are now available, although the latter provides the more effective, deeper heat.

Decubitus Ulcers

The use of ultraviolet rays is an effective treatment procedure for the alleviation of decubitus ulcers, commonly found in the bedridden or wheelchair patient. Prolonged healing time can often be greatly reduced with effective application and dosages. Ultraviolet acts specifically to increase blood supply, destroy bacteria and in-

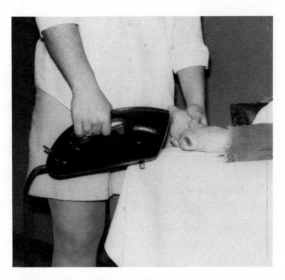

FIG. 77. Aero-Kromeyer ultraviolet gun used in treatment of decubiti.

dolent tissue, and stimulate growth of new tissue. It has also proved useful in the treatment of other types of indolent skin conditions or infected wounds. See Figure 77.

RANGE OF MOTION

The physical therapist acts to maintain the patient's normal range of motion and to restore it when limited. Often, this entails instructing the patient and other health workers in range-of-motion techniques. Unless these techniques are performed regularly throughout the day, the efforts directed toward maintaining range may prove useless, especially if the patient has marked spasticity. Passive range-of-motion exercise is performed to prevent contractures in the patient with partial or complete paralysis. Selective stretching is done in patients who might benefit from some residual tightness. In the quadriplegic, for example, the function of the hand may be dependent upon the tenodesis effect. If the hand is completely stretched out, this effect is lost.

Other types of stretching exercises include active and active-assistive exercises. For these, voluntary activity and cooperation of the patient are required. The therapist may choose to use mechanical aids which assist in independent exercise or to employ inhibition techniques which assist the patient in gaining increased range. Pulleys, slings, and sling suspension setups provide effective mechanical assists. The newer approaches to therapeutic exercise offer a number of different procedures aimed at increasing range.

MUSCLE REEDUCATION

A therapist can choose from a number of different traditional exercise programs designed to improve strength, range, and coordination. Muscle reeducation usually begins with active assisted movements. The therapist supports the body part while the patient responds with an active contraction. Once the patient is able to accomplish this task, the therapist then removes her support. The patient must now overcome the resistance of gravity while performing the desired motion. After proficiency is obtained in this task, resistance is added against the motion. As the muscle's strength and endurance increase, the resistance also increases. The improvement noted following this type of exercise program results from specific gains made in mobility, strength, control, and endurance. Throughout this progression of exercises, the therapist encourages the patient's responses through the use of manual contacts, verbal instructions, and repetition.

Progressive resistive exercises, PRE, are designed to obtain increases in muscle strength, bulk, and endurance through the use of weights, either as assistive or resistive forces. Various piece of equipment provides accommodating revide this type of resistance. These include the Delormé table (see Fig. 78), ankle exerciser, shoulder wheels, barbells, sling-suspension setups, and recently, the isokinetic exerciser. This last piece of equipment provides accommodating resistance to the patient's maximum abilities throughout the range, at controlled speeds. This principle of varying the resistance throughout the range enables the muscle to be loaded to its maximum throughout the exercise.

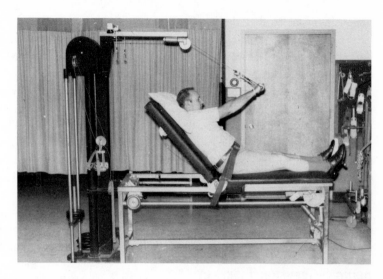

FIG. 78. Patient performing load-resisted shoulder extension on De-lormé table.

Faradic or modified direct currents can also be used in a program of muscle reeducation. These electrical currents facilitate contractions in specific muscles or groups of muscles. Thus, they are used with partially denervated or weakened muscles. In cases of temporary paralysis, such as Bell's palsy, they can be used to maintain muscle bulk and strength while the patient is recovering. Electrical stimulation can also be used to alleviate spasticity in certain cases. The stimulation is given to the antagonistic muscle, and through the effects of reciprocal innervation, the spastic muscle is inhibited. With the advent of the sensory-stimulation techniques, found in the newer approaches to exercise, the above procedures have become less widely used in physical therapy today.

TRADITIONAL EXERCISE REGIMES

Specific exercise regimes have been developed over the years to achieve a variety of goals. Pendulum exercises of Codman or Chandler were developed to improve the range and strength of the shoulder-girdle musculature. Buerger-Allen exercises were developed to improve the peripheral circulation of the legs. H. S. Frenkel developed his program of exercises to improve problems of incoordination and ataxia. Patients with low back problems were usually given a

program of Williams flexion exercises. Relaxation exercises were designed to promote relaxation and release of residual muscle tension.

Most of these exercise programs were originally proposed as specific routines which were not to be altered greatly from patient to patient. This approach is not widely held in therapeutic thought today, however, because exercises should be devised on the basis of an evaluation which is designed to meet each patient's individual needs rather than trying to fit any patient into a specific exercise program.

PHYSICAL THERAPY FOR PULMONARY CONDITIONS

Physical therapists act to improve breathing patterns and alleviate respiratory distress in patients with various pulmonary conditions. Deep and relaxed breathing with a rhythmical cycle is often a primary goal of treatment. In certain patients, segmental or unilateral breathing patterns are sought. Progressive endurance activities are given if the patient experiences shortness of breath following only slight activity. This is often seen in the patient with chronic obstructive lung disease whose breathing capacity has become markedly decreased. Postural drainage is given to assist the patient in clearing his lungs of excessive secretions. The patient is placed in various positions so that the involved segment is in the up position, enabling the mucus to drain into a larger trunk, eventually reaching the trachea. Postural drainage is always done in conjunction with deep breathing and coughing. Various techniques are available to assist the therapist in promoting adequate drainage. These include percussion or clapping over the involved area and vibration or shaking during exhalation. Mechanical percussors can also be used. These breathing exercises and drainage procedures are carefully selected by the therapist to meet the specific needs and diagnosis of the patient.

SLING-SUSPENSION THERAPY

Sling-suspension therapy has been available to the physical therapist since the 1940s when Guthrie-Smith developed a program of remedial exercises in England. In this approach, part or all of the body is suspended in the air by ropes and slings attached to fixed points on a frame. Once the body part is suspended, the patient is free to move without the influence of gravity and friction. The therapist can adjust the points of fixation to obtain horizontal or pendular motions and to increase or decrease resistance to specific motions. Springs are added to the suspension setups to add resistance to specific muscle groups. Thus, sling-suspension therapy may be used to strengthen muscles, increase range of motion, or improve coordination. General principles of therapeutic exercise are adhered to, including anatomical and neurophysiological factors.

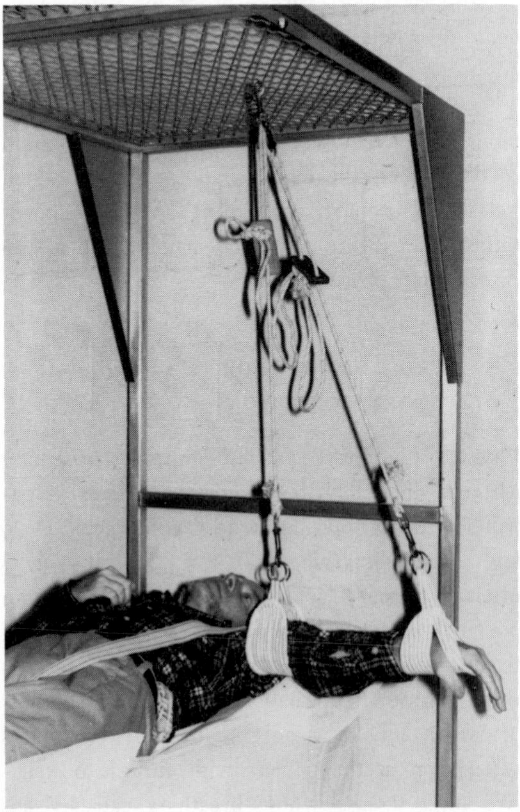

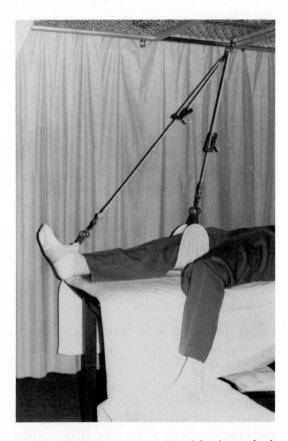

FIG. 79. Patient performing abduction and adduction of shoulder. Note webbing strap to prevent shoulder-girdle elevation during movement.

FIG. 80. Patient performing hip abduction and adduction: uninvolved limb is fully abducted flexed over edge of plinth, minimizing lateral trunk flexion and stabilizing pelvis.

This type of therapy has specific advantages for use with the geriatric or chronically ill patient. It provides an independent means of exercising in which the patient must actively cooperate if he is to improve. When the body part is supported, the patient is often more relaxed than if a therapist were attempting to move the part. Conversely, the therapist is also free to observe the patient more closely or to engage in facilitatory techniques. It also lessens general body fatigue, because the movement occurs on a localized level. Finally, it offers versatility to an exercise program because of the numerous ways in which an exercise can be varied. See Figures 79 and 80.

ADVANCED APPROACHES TO THERAPEUTIC EXERCISE

Bobath's Neurodevelopmental Approach

Chronically ill patients with brain dysfunction involving the motor system may benefit from a neurodevelopmental approach to treatment developed by Dr. and Mrs. Karl Bobath. The Bobaths have organized their treatment rationale around the concept that these patients suffer from a disorder of the higher coordinating system, which forms, sets in operation, and controls patterns of movement. Thus, their approach is directed toward influencing these higher centers. Specific goals of treatment include the improvement of postural tone, the normalizing of the postural reflex mechanism, and the promotion of selective and functional movement patterns. Abnormal reflexive postures are definitely avoided. Thus, the Bobaths are concerned with total body reactions, tone, and movement patterns rather than with specific, localized problems.

Accurate assessment of the patient is stressed as the basis of a successful treatment. This assessment determines which normal postural and movement patterns the patient has and which he lacks. The Bobaths define the normal postural reflex mechanism as the integrated activity of the righting, protective, and equilibrium reactions, which serve to coordinate movements and control postures with respect to the physical environment. These reactions bring with them a normal distribution of muscle or postural tone. Assessment also includes the investigation of abnormal patterns which are usually governed by the presence of tonic reflexes. The ease and extent to which these abnormal patterns can be modified are noted along with the effects of activity in one part of the body upon other parts. Thus, the evaluation of abnormal muscle tone receives careful attention. Finally, the Bobaths stress complete evaluation of the sensory system, for normal postural control and balance are dependent upon unimpaired sensations.

The Bobaths have developed many procedures and techniques for changing the incoordinated motor behavior found in these patients. Most require an intensive training session with the Bobaths or their instructors. Many of these techniques have been misinterpreted or misused. The Bobaths stress the need to tailor treatment techniques to each patient. These techniques include the use of dynamic reflex-inhibiting patterns, handling key or proximal points of control, tapping, and doing activities in the basic developmental postures. All may be used at one time or another in the course of treatment.

While the Bobaths have worked mostly with cerebral palsy and adult hemiplegia, their basic concepts and techniques are applicable to treatment of other disorders of the motor system. A program based upon their approach might well include the following goals and suggestions. In the spastic hemiplegic, reflex-inhibiting patterns are used very early to break up the spastic synergies of the arm and leg. Postural control and movement are first sought at the proximal joints. Associated reactions and tonic reflexes are avoided while balance and postural support responses are facilitated. Weight-bearing activities on all extremities are stressed. See Figure 81.

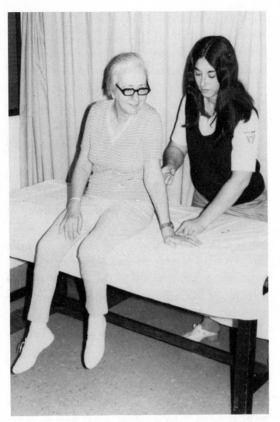

FIG. 81. Weight bearing on heel of affected hand of hemiplegic patient facilitates extension of affected elbow and postural support.

BRUNNSTROM'S MOVEMENT THERAPY

The many peculiarities of the motor behavior of the adult hemiplegic led Miss Signe Brunnstrom to develop principles and techniques of movement therapy. Her years of research into the sensorimotor problems common to these patients have yielded many practical therapeutic suggestions which have had increasingly widespread use in recent years.

One of her major contributions to physical therapy has been her comprehensive analysis of the motor behavior of the hemiplegic. After an initial period of flaccidity, these patients characteristically show basic limb synergies in both the upper and lower extremities. These synergies are stereotyped, mass-movement patterns which may occur either as a reflex response or voluntarily.

In either case, at this stage of recovery, the patient is unable to recruit these muscles for different movement combinations. These characteristic synergies are defined below. The typical resting posture of the hemiplegic is usually comprised of the strongest components of each synergy. Attitudinal or postural reflexes also directly influence motor behavior. Thus, a knowledge of the tonic neck reflexes (symmetrical and asymmetrical), tonic labyrinthine reflexes, the tonic lumbar reflexes, and associated reactions is a basic requirement in understanding the treatment techniques of this approach.

COMPONENTS OF THE MOTION SYNERGIES IN THE HEMIPLEGIC

Flexion synergy—upper (a) retraction or elevation of the shoulder girdle; (b) abduction and external rotation of the shoulder (hyperextension may appear instead); (c) flexion of the elbow and supination of the forearm.

Extension synergy—upper (a) protraction or fixation of the shoulder girdle; (b) adduction and internal rotation of the shoulder; (c) extension of the elbow and pronation of the forearm.

Flexion synergy—lower (a) abduction, flexion, and external rotation of the hip; (b) flexion of the knee; (c) dorsiflexion and inversion of the foot; (d) dorsiflexion of the toes.

Extension synergy—lower (a) adduction, internal rotation, and extension of the hip; (b) extension of the knee; (c) plantar flexion and inversion of the foot; (d) plantar flexion of the toes.

Evaluation and treatment are based upon the typical recovery stages which have been described by Miss Brunnstrom. Immediately following the acute episode, flaccidity is present and no movement can be elicited (stage 1). As recovery begins, minimal movement in the basic limb synergies may be possible; spasticity begins to develop (stage 2). Thereafter, the patient gains voluntary control to move in these synergies while spasticity becomes its strongest (stage 3). Next, the patient can begin to perform movements not common to these synergies, under the effects of decreasing spasticity (stage 4). If progress continues, more difficult movements are learned (stage 5). Spasticity disappears while individual coordinated joint movements become possible (stage 6). Not all patients proceed through these stages to normal recovery, however, for patients can plateau at any stage.

Evaluation thus includes the patient's movement patterns and the degree of spasticity and synergy dominance. Gross testing for sensory loss is also included. Training procedures begin in bed and are carried out in a number of positions as the patient improves. Specific aims of treatment are to reinforce recovery at any stage and to promote recovery in the higher stages. The same sequence which occurs in spontaneous recovery is followed. In the early stages, movements are encouraged in synergies and can be initially elicited and then reinforced through the use of tonic reflexes or associated reactions. Once voluntary control in synergy is achieved (stage 3), movement combinations which deviate from these patterns are facilitated. During this phase of training, reflex reactions are no longer used and facilitatory techniques are gradually reduced. Specific exercises for the lower extremity promote the movement combinations needed for normal walking. Upper-extremity training usually stresses the alleviation of a painful shoulder and functional movements (see Fig. 82). Progression in treatment and functional carry-over occurs over a period of weeks or even months. Most stroke patients achieve some recovery spontaneously. This approach attempts to capitalize on these strengths and to promote further recovery through an orderly sequence.

ROOD APPROACH

A third approach to the treatment of patients with neuromuscular dysfunction is that of Miss Margaret Rood. This approach represents a philosophy of treatment concerned with the interaction of somatic, autonomic, and psychic factors and their role in the regulation of motor behavior. The aim is always to obtain as normal a response as possible by applying the appropriate stimuli to produce movement or postural reactions. These are sought in the same automatic

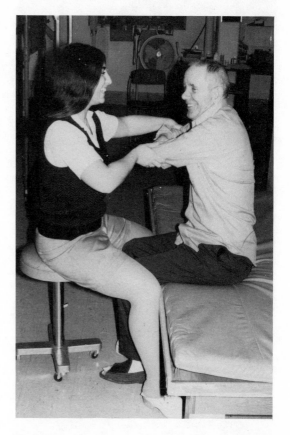

FIG. 82. Actively assisted mobilization of shoulder girdle is facilitated by asymmetrical tonic neck and lumbar reflexes.

manner as they occur in the normal, without the need for conscious attention to the response itself.

A knowledge of the development of the human nervous system during the first five years of life and its functions is essential to an understanding of this approach. Miss Rood suggests that all functions and structures of the neuromuscular system can be related to one of two purposes. Man responds either for protection and mobility or to gain control of his environment through stability. Unless mobility and stability are achieved first, the more complex skills cannot occur. Thus, Miss Rood stresses normal development and adheres closely to its sequence of events, a procedure which develops first mobility, then stability, then movement with stability, and finally, skill. The main stages in this sequence are shown in Figures 83A–H.

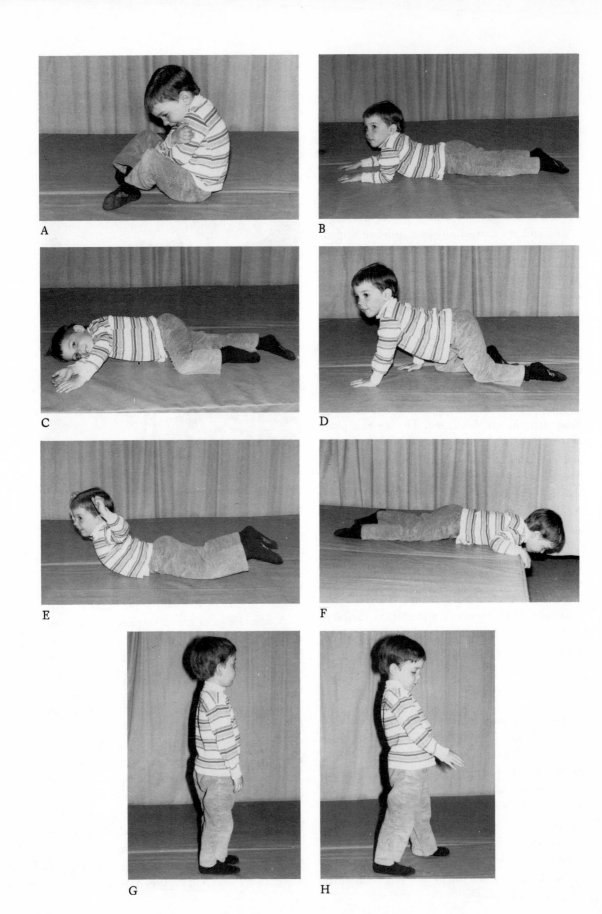

A

B

C

D

E

F

G

H

Sensory factors and their relationship to motor functions assume a position of major importance in this approach. Both the somatic and autonomic systems are employed to activate, facilitate, or inhibit motor behavior. Some types of sensory stimulation techniques commonly used in this approach are listed below. Miss Rood stresses the need to choose appropriate stimuli in order to obtain the desired responses. These responses are sought in the developmental positions in which they are first developed in the normal infant. In addition to a skeletal function sequence, Miss Rood also identifies a vital function sequence in which respiratory, sucking, and eating patterns are developed. Treatment suggestions for problems in this area are also included in this approach which is based upon normal sensorimotor learning. It employs sensory stimulation techniques applied to muscles acting in movement patterns which follow an orderly sequence of development.

In adult hemiplegia, for example, treatment is dependent upon the presence of spasticity. If the patient is spastic, the program begins with fast brushing to the skin area over the stabilizing shoulder muscles. Stretch and joint approximation are also used to facilitate these muscles. Weight-bearing positions, on elbows (see Fig. 84) or all fours, are used until cocontraction of the shoulder muscles is achieved. Then, mobility of the distal muscles is sought in functional movement patterns. Voluntary initiation of movement is thus preceded by the development of stability through appropriate sensory stimulation.

SENSORY STIMULATION TECHNIQUES

Stimulus	Response
Proprioceptive	
stretch	
quick	Facilitates muscle stretched; inhibits antagonist
sustained	Facilitates flexors, adductors, and multiarthrodial muscles; inhibits extensors and abductors
contraction	Inhibits muscle contracting; facilitates antagonist
contraction with resistance	Facilitates muscle holding
pressure	
joint	Facilitates postural muscles; inhibits flexors
muscle	Facilitates if applied to belly; inhibits if applied to insertion
Exteroceptive	
touch	
fast brushing	Facilitates tonic response of muscle brushed; inhibits antagonist
slow brushing	Facilitates phasic responses
stroking	Of posterior spine has a central inhibitory response
icing	
slow icing	Immediate inhibition, then maintained facilitation of muscle iced, inhibition of antagonist
quick icing	Inhibits muscle iced; facilitates antagonist

PROPRIOCEPTIVE NEUROMUSCULAR FACILITATION

An improvement in motor control in the elderly or chronically ill patient can also be achieved through the use of proprioceptive neuromuscular facilitation (PNF). This technique, based upon

FIGS. 83 A through G. Rood's main stages in ontogenic sequence of motor development.
A. Withdrawal—supine—total flexion response—develops mobility.
B. On elbows—develops stability, movement with stability and skill—arms, eyes, speech.
C. Roll over—flexion arm and leg—one side—develops mobility.
D. All fours—develops stability, movement with stability and skill—creeping.
E. Pivot prone—total extension—develops mobility and stability.
F. Neck cocontraction—develops stability and movement with stability.
G. Standing and walking—develops stability. H. shows movement with stability and skill while walking.

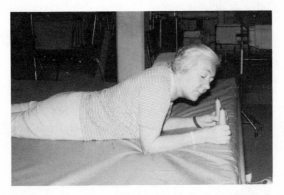

FIG. 84. The on-elbows position in developmental series of exercises is ideal for improvement of stability in scapular region. As patient gradually shifts his weight to one side, he increases stabilization through joint approximation; by squeezing a cone with its larger part on ulnar side of his hand at the same time, he stretches ulnar intrinsic muscles, thus facilitating further shoulder cocontraction.

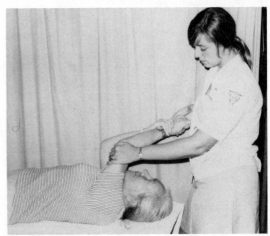

FIG. 85. Patient brings up left upper extremity in flexion, adduction, and external rotation against the therapist's resistance; bilateral asymmetrical use of both upper extremities promotes interaction of both sides of body. As the shortened range is approached, techniques of approximation and repeated contraction are applied to improve strength and stabilization.

the techniques of Dr. Henry Kabat, was developed by two physical therapists, Miss Margaret Knott and Miss Dorothy Voss. They define PNF techniques as methods of promoting or hastening the response of the neuromuscular mechanism through the stimulation of the proprioceptors. A knowledge of normal motor development and the neuromuscular mechanism is also basic to this approach.

In this method, total patterns of movement are performed in oblique or diagonal directions. These movements are rhythmic and reversing in character and are performed optimally in goal-directed activities. Normal sequences of motor development are followed. This approach aims to promote balanced reciprocal relationships between antagonistic groups of muscles. Thus, weakness in a specific muscle group is strengthened in total patterns of movement designed to correct imbalances. Since lasting improvement is dependent upon motor learning, several basic procedures are utilized to promote this learning. These procedures include positioning for maximum postural support, commands, manual contacts, stretch, maximal resistance, joint approxi-

mation and traction, and normal timing. See Figure 85.

Specific techniques which are largely dependent upon the patient's cooperation and voluntary effort are employed to stimulate or facilitate and to relax or inhibit certain muscle groups. These techniques require intensive study and practice in order for one to become proficient at them. Techniques directed primarily toward the agonist include rhythmic initiation and repeated contractions. Those directed toward the antagonist include reversal of antagonists, slow reversal, and rhythmic stabilization. The final group, aimed at promoting relaxation and inhibition, are the relaxation techniques of contract-relax and hold-relax. This approach utilizes specific procedures and techniques aimed at improving strength, coordination, and timed sequence of antagonistic groups of muscles. Spiral or diagonal patterns of movement which can be performed in developmental patterns are utilized.

Specific aims of this approach in the treatment

of the adult hemiplegic might include the promotion of voluntary movement with balance between antagonistic groups of muscles and between the two sides of the body. Patterns would use the reversal-of-antagonists technique and would include head rotation, scapular motions, and elbow extension. Lower-extremity patterns would emphasize balanced interaction of antagonists. Basic procedures to hasten motor learning would also be employed.

COMMON DENOMINATORS

These advanced approaches to therapeutic exercise have many common denominators which enable the experienced therapist to select and use certain procedures from each in the treatment of a specific problem. All recognize that sensation and motion are intimately related in the normal functioning of the human nervous system. Each method utilizes sensory input to some degree to facilitate or inhibit movement. Each method also stresses the importance of understanding the sequence of normal human motor development. All recognize that early motor behavior is largely reflexive and use these reflex mechanisms to facilitate or inhibit movement. Concepts of motor learning, such as repetition of activity, frequency of stimulation, and employment of sensory cues, are also common to these approaches. Finally, they focus on the "total patient" and the interaction of the body segments as a whole. Perhaps these denominators best summarize the directions in which physical therapy is proceeding. They indicate changes which have occurred in therapeutic exercise out of a need to incorporate recent advances in our understanding of neuromuscular physiology, motor development, and motor learning. Physical therapy itself is changing, growing, and expanding to better meet the needs of the patient.

REFERENCES

BOBATH, BERTA. *Abnormal Postural Reflex Activity Caused by Brain Lesions*. London: Heinemann, 1970.

BOBATH, BERTA. Observations on adult hemiplegia and suggestions for treatment. *Physiotherapy* 45: 279–289, 1959; 46:5–14, 1960.

BONNER, C. D. *The Team Approach to Hemiplegia*. Springfield, Ill.: Thomas, 1968.

BRUNNSTROM, SIGNE. *Movement Therapy in Hemiplegia*. New York: Harper & Row, 1970.

BUCHWALD, E. *Physical Rehabilitation for Daily Living*. New York: McGraw-Hill, 1952.

BUCHWALD, JENNIFER. Proprioceptive reflexes and posture. *Am. J. Phys. Med.* 46:104–113, 1967.

BUCHWALD, JENNIFER. Exteroceptive reflexes and movement. *Am. J. Phys. Med.* 46:121–128, 1967.

DANIELS, L., WILLIAMS, M., and WORTHINGHAM, C. *Muscle Testing, Techniques of Manual Examination*. Philadelphia: Saunders, 1956.

ELDRED, EARL. Peripheral receptors: their excitation and relation to reflex patterns. *Am. J. Phys. Med.* 46:69–87, 1967.

FLANAGAN, ELEANOR. Methods for facilitation and inhibition on motor activity. *Am. J. Phys. Med.* 46:1006–1011, 1967.

HOLLIS, M., and ROPER, M. *Suspension Therapy in Rehabilitation*. London: Baillière, Tindall & Cox, 1958.

KENDALL, H., and KENDALL, F. *Muscles: Testing and Function*. Baltimore: Williams & Wilkins, 1949.

KNOTT, M., and VOSS, D. *Proprioceptive Neuromuscular Facilitation*. New York: Harper & Row, 1969.

KOLB, MARY. The challenge of success. *Phys. Ther.* 46:1157–1164, 1966.

LICHT, SIDNEY. *Therapeutic Exercises*. New Haven: Elizabeth Licht, 1965.

METCALF, V., and YEAKEL, MARY. Documentation of hand function with the use of office copying equipment. *Phys. Ther.* 52:935–943, 1972.

PERRY, CATHERINE. Principles and techniques of the Brunnstrom approach to the treatment of hemiplegia. *Am. J. Phys. Med.* 46:789–812, 1967.

PINKSTON, DOROTHY (Ed.). Analysis of traditional

regimes of therapeutic exercise. *Am. J. Phys. Med.* 46:713–731, 1967.

Scott, Pauline (Ed.). *Clayton's Electrotherapy and Actinotherapy*. London: Baillière, Tindall and Cassell, 1965.

Semans, Sarah. The Bobath concept in treatment of neurological disorders. *Am. J. Phys. Med.* 46: 732–785, 1967.

Stockmeyer, Shirley. An interpretation of the approach of Rood to the treatment of neuromuscular dysfunction. *Am. J. Phys. Med.* 46:900–954, 1967.

Thacker, Winifred. *Postural Drainage and Respiratory Control*. London: Lloyd-Luke, 1968.

Voss, Dorothy. Proprioceptive neuromuscular facilitation. *Am. J. Phys. Med.* 46:838–898, 1967.

12
Occupational Therapy

Occupational therapy can best be discussed after first reviewing the following definition and functions of occupational therapy, as prepared and distributed by a special task force sponsored by the American Occupational Therapy Association in February, 1972:

Occupational therapy is the art and science of directing man's participation in selected tasks to restore, reinforce, and enhance performance, facilitate learning of those skills and functions essential for adaptation and productivity, diminish or correct pathology, and to promote and maintain health. Its fundamental concern is the development and maintenance of the capacity, throughout the life-span, to perform with satisfaction to self and others those tasks and roles essential to productive living and to the mastery of self and the environment.

Since the primary focus of occupational therapy is the development of adaptive skills and performance capacity, its concern is with the factors which serve as barriers or impediments to the individual's ability to function, as well as those factors which promote, influence, or enhance performance.

Occupational therapy provides service to individuals whose abilities to cope with the tasks of living are threatened or impaired by developmental deficits, the aging process, poverty, cultural differences, physical injury or illness, or psychologic and social disability.

Reference to occupation in the title is in the context of man's goal-directed use of time, energy, interest, and attention.

The practice of occupational therapy is based upon concepts which acknowledge these factors:

1. Activities are primary agents for learning and development and an essential source of satisfaction;

2. In engaging in activities, the individual explores the nature of his interests, needs, capacities, and limitations; he develops motor, perceptual, and cognitive skills, learns a range of interpersonal and social attitudes and behaviors, sufficient for coping with life tasks and mastering elements of his environment;

3. Task occupation is an integral part of human development; it represents or reflects life-work situations and is thus a vehicle for acquiring or redeveloping those skills essential to the fulfillment of life roles;

4. When activities match or are related to the developmental needs and interests of the individual, these activities not only afford the necessary learning for development or restoration but also provide intrinsic gratification which promotes and sustains health and evokes a strong investment in the restorative process;

5. The end product inherent in a task or an activity provides concrete evidence of the ability to be productive and to have an influence on one's environment;

6. Activities are *doing*, and such focus upon productivity and participation teaches a sense of self as a contributing participant rather than recipient.

These principles are applied in practice through programs reflecting the profession's commitment to comprehensive health care. These programs are:

DISABILITY-PREVENTION AND HEALTH-MAINTENANCE PROGRAMS

The fostering of normal development, sustaining and protecting existing functions and abilities, preventing disability, and/or supporting levels of restoration or change make up the disability-prevention and health-maintenance programs. The central concern is provision of activity experiences which enable the individual to use productively his existing skills, capacities, and strengths: those which provide personal gratification and meet the basic human needs for acceptance, achievement, creativity, decision-making, autonomy, self-assertion, and social relationships; those which provide opportunities to pursue and develop interests, explore potential, develop capacities, and learn to recognize the resources within himself and within his external world.

REMEDIAL PROGRAMS

Remedial programs focus on the reduction of pathology or specific disability, providing task and activity experiences which may diminish the particular impairment and restore or develop the individual's capacity to function. In this context, the tasks or activities selected will be those whose characteristics and properties will, for example, provide specific exercise and motor learning, offer appropriate sensory stimuli, and improve response. They will also promote muscle strength, endurance, and coordination, alter disorders in thinking and/or feeling, teach and enhance interpersonal skills, offer the necessary psychological gratification, correct faulty concepts of self and identity, and develop attitudes and skills basic to the pursuit of independent functioning.

DAILY-LIFE TASKS AND VOCATIONAL-ADJUSTMENT PROGRAMS

These are primarily concerned with work adaptation and work-role adjustment. The tasks chosen are those which promote and teach independent functioning, develop and enhance the ability to work, and/or fulfill age-specific life tasks and roles. This focus involves the identification and examination of those roles and skills essential for the individual's adaptation to his community, assessment of the nature and level of his work capacities, attitudes, and self-care skills, identification of what learning needs do occur and in what sequence, and provision of graded task experiences which teach the necessary skills and attitudes.

These programs are not mutually exclusive but often occur simultaneously. Thus, for example, the child with a developmental deficit may be helped to achieve the necessary learning and growth through involvement in a game, by working a puzzle, or learning spatial relationships by painting a picture. The physically impaired person may regain necessary muscle control through the grasping exercise in a personally gratifying game of checkers or in a woodworking project; or perhaps he may be taught to compensate for his loss through a competitive sport, by learning to sculpture or to operate a calculator. Normal growth and development of the disadvantaged child may be supported and encouraged through participation in a storytelling group, by building an airplane model, or working with colored blocks. His parents may be helped to develop a sense of being able to influence his environment by involvement in a homemaking-skills group, a housing project, discussion group, or by developing relevant marketable job skills. The socially maladapted or emotionally disturbed person may be helped to develop more realistic responses to failure and success, more flexibility in responding to the demands of his world through participation in gardening or other group projects, to perfect job-related skills, or to learn to manage his feelings and test his adequacy through creative painting, writing, or drama.

The task or activity experiences within each frame of reference may be offered in the context of a group setting, where the dynamics of the group are used to facilitate participation and goal achievement, or on an individual basis wherein the one-to-one relationship is used as a motivational and supportive force.

The overall service functions of the occupational therapist are to: (1) evaluate the individual client's or patient's performance capacities and deficits; (2) select tasks or activity experiences appropriate to the defined needs and goals; (3) facilitate and influence client or patient participation and investment; (4) evaluate response, assess and measure change and development; and (5) validate assessments, share findings, and make appropriate recommendations.

Occupational therapy provides service to a wide population in a variety of settings, such as hospitals and clinics, rehabilitation facilities, sheltered workshops, schools and camps, extended-care facilities, private homes, housing projects, and community agencies and centers. Occupational therapists both receive from and make referrals to the appropriate health, education, or medical specialists. The teacher, the public-health nurse, physician, physical therapist, psychologist, speech pathologist, social worker, and recreation leader are some of the professionals with whom the responsibility for comprehensive care is shared.

Delivery of occupational-therapy services involves several levels of personnel. The basic entrance level qualifications, roles, and functions of each may be broadly defined and differentiated. A copy of these qualifications, roles, and functions for the registered occupational therapist, certified occupational therapy assistant, and the occupational therapy aide may be requested from the American Occupational Therapy Association, 251 Park Avenue South, New York, New York, 10010.

Patient Evaluation, Goal Setting, and Treatment

For the purposes of this publication, the theories and rationales expressed are confined to the context of occupational therapy responsibilities in remedial programs for the physically disabled. Patient evaluation, goal setting, and treatment techniques cannot be defined as separate entities because of their essential interrelationships and the practical necessity that they be constant ongoing and overlapping processes. To clarify the role of the therapist in this process, a systematic strategy for gathering and utilizing basic patient data is illustrated.

It must be assumed that it is the quality of the occupational therapist's understanding of the patient's mental processes, physical deficiencies and abilities, and emotional stability which influences the setting and actual achievement of appropriate goals. In order to set these goals, certain evaluatory processes must take place. Each evaluation must provide information which, when integrated, can satisfy a series of questions encompassing as much of the totality of human behavior as present skills and theories allow. Four major areas form the basis of the occupational therapist's focus: (1) cognitive functioning; (2) social functioning; (3) physical functioning; and (4) activities-of-daily-living functioning.

Cognitive functioning involves the assessment of: the patient's insight into his own disability, his orientation to time and place, his concentration or attention span, the quality of his recent memory, his ability to follow directions, and what type and level of directions are most easily understood. Also, within this area of cognitive functioning, the therapist must evaluate whether the patient can initiate purposeful activity or whether he must await outside direction; whether he can utilize old habit skills and patterns, such as self-feeding, which do not require any adaptation to be carried out. The next area of critical importance is the assessment of whether he retains new-learning skills, such as the technique for one-handed wheeling of his wheelchair, which involves the mental processes of problem solving and motor planning. Can the patient accurately use his body in a new and unfamiliar way? Without this new learning capacity, adaptation is extremely difficult, and regaining independence demands this capacity for adaptation.

In assessing the areas of *social functioning*, the therapist is most interested in observing whether the patient is aware of himself, his own importance, his right to be involved in decisions related to him; whether he is aware of others and can interact with them or whether his actions are perhaps totally self-centered. What does his behavior suggest in terms of his emotional balance? Is he appropriately depressed? Does he withdraw from any involvement with his disability? Does he have a sense of humor? Can he comfortably ask for help or express his concerns without fear of rejection? These areas cannot be measured or tested, but without an impression of the patient's level of self-esteem, treatment approaches could very well be not only inappropriate, but ineffective.

The third broad area of focus is the area of *physical functioning*. The occupational therapist shares a similar approach and concern in this area as does the physical therapist, and these two specialists work quite naturally in close conjunction and cooperation. The occupational therapist will observe, test, and measure specific physical capacities in the context of their importance to total body functioning in basic tasks, i.e., feeding, dressing, reading, writing, etc. He (or she) will evaluate sitting and standing balance and endurance, upper-extremity strength and coordination, sensory integrity of the upper extremity in terms of touch and position in space, and sensory integrity of the visual fields, hearing, and the physical mechanisms for verbal and nonverbal communication. The limiting factors in both active and passive joint range of motion would also be noted. Upon completing the initial assessments, the physical history and prognostic course of the neuromuscular systems involved in the presenting diagnosis would be reviewed. Adaptive equipment, such as hand splints, arm supports, walking slings, or other mechanically assistive devices might be indicated either to prevent contractures, edema, or pain, or to promote endurance, facilitate or replace weakened mobility for specific functions, or to place the weakened part in the optimal posi-

tion for gaining specific strength. The occupational therapist assumes the responsibility either to design, construct, or supervise the construction and appropriate application of any of these remedial devices.

The fourth general area for investigation is the status of the patient's activities-of-daily-living (ADL) skills. What is his capacity to accomplish self-care, such as washing, dressing, grooming, and toilet activities? What is his capacity to move around and accomplish basic household tasks, such as answering and/or dialing the phone, transporting objects from room to room, getting items in and out of the refrigerator, handling the stove, or putting out the garbage? Also, what is his capacity to resume special interests, to return to work, or to enjoy his weekly poker game? Cognitively, socially, and physically, can he resume at least some aspects of those activities which were particularly meaningful, important, or just enjoyable before the onset of his present disability? What ready talents and unexplored human potentials are available to him to be realized as valid and self-satisfying capacities and responsible contributions within society? Again, the occupational therapist will assume the responsibility for constructing or locating any one of a number of commercial self-help devices, such as: one-handed rocker knives for cutting and preparing foods, special elastic or zipper shoelace replacements, long-handled combs and shoehorns, special grasping devices to extend reach, adapted typewriters and handwriting devices, raised toilet seats, adapted telephones, alarm devices, labor-saving kitchen appliances, or totally redesigned kitchens, bathrooms, or office areas. Whenever natural function cannot be improved, the occupational therapist will work with the patient to redesign the environment or the tools with which to accomplish the task. He will provide relevant experiences, so that the patient may learn and assess the usefulness of this equipment as well as explore his own potentials for solving the problem satisfactorily.

The data collected in these four areas soon become complex, since the therapist is dealing with a variety of intricately connected factors. Some of these factors are measurable, as is the assessment of physical power and sensory integration. Some are theoretical, as are perception and other components of the cognitive learning processes. Still others are subjective, as in estimates of emotional investments and needs, those areas which act as the major catalysts in allowing reintegration processes to take place.

It is essential to discard the assumption that a simplistic approach and generalized or routine treatment can be applied to a presumed common diagnosis. No diagnosis is simple or common, and treatment can be effective only when devised and individualized in relation to the specific factors observed in these myriad, yet potentially understandable, interlocking systems.

The following ten steps demonstrate the manner in which the therapist organizes the necessary information into an individual treatment program that not only assures relevance in goal setting and actual patient achievement but also provides sufficient information to educate and orient the patient and his family to the exact nature of the limitations imposed by the disability and the nature of the remaining potentials.

Step one is the development of rapport with the patient initially to reassure him of his acceptability as he is and to reduce the emotional anxiety which normally follows any catastrophe, such as severe physical dysfunction. Rapport and some degree of trust are essential in order to gain his cooperation to make valid observations and evaluations of basic physiologic and psychologic functioning.

Step two is to evaluate clinically the patient's musculature and sensory integrity, coordination, and functional performance, either self-initiated or available to command.

Step three is to test clinically as well as to observe, in functional performance, the integrity of the patient's cognitive and learning processes which allow information to be processed and adaptation to take place.

Step four is an overall evaluation of the preceding information to establish a baseline of present function, an assessment of the degree of dysfunction, and an appreciation of the focus of the patient's physical and emotional needs at this time. This information directs the development of a primary and tentative goal.

Step five is an analysis by the therapist of the physiological, cognitive, and psychological demands of the tasks necessary to achieve the initial goal. What sequence and type of preliminary physical tasks can be graded to strengthen effectively the essential muscle groups preparatory to attempting the goal tasks? What are the critical clues to which the patient need be alerted? Can the patient be oriented to attend to these clues? What minimal and general abilities must the patient have for the task to be successful? To what level of competence must this task be learned in order to be effective? Will the demand for intensive cognition confuse the learning of the task (because of the interference of brain damage), and can the task be learned instead on a lower brain, reflex, or rote basis? How much time can be given in the training process to achieve this goal? Will the eventual learning emotionally and physically enhance future performance? Does the task demand the understanding of an abstract concept, or is it composed of more easily learned, concrete steps? The therapist must answer not only these questions but must know the approach and the quality of response expected in order to teach any task requiring a new type of integration.

Step six is an orientation (if a cognitive approach is required) to how the task will meet the patient's needs. This should assist him in focusing his attention, directing his purpose, and thereby eliciting his motivation to sustain his effort.

Step seven is the actual teaching and learning process in an environment where distractions can be controlled, the patient's dignity preserved, and normal self-consciousness respected.

Step eight is the gradual withdrawal of the therapist's direction, in order to determine the effectiveness of the patient's self-direction.

Step nine is a reassessment of the practical use

of the new function in more distracting and thus more normal environments.

Step ten is the combined therapist-patient setting of the next goal, with a repetition of the same steps already described, until either a plateau of function and capacity has been realized, or until the patient knows the method and can realistically assess his own needs and reintegrate solutions entirely on his own.

This strategy by no means implies a system for achieving total independence and normal functioning. It is merely a system for assessing multiple functions, setting *achievable* goals, and defining the most probable means for retraining. Ultimately, the patient is utilizing his own fullest capacities and potentials with some genuine satisfaction and the dignity that self-determination implies.

OCCUPATIONAL THERAPY MEDIA

Based upon the foregoing evaluation, goal, treatment theories and rationales, an infinite variety of treatment media is available in occupational therapy to provide the means for achieving mutual goals. Whether the activities are the traditional and popular crafts and manual arts, such as woodworking, weaving, claywork, tile setting, and drawing and painting, or games such as checkers, cards, pool, shuffleboard, or prevocational tasks such as typing, using business machines, electronic assembly, filing or collating, or basic functional activities, such as washing, dressing, grooming, feeding, cooking, housework, or direct strength and coordination exercises, such as lifting weights or pulling springs, each activity will be selected because of the type of experience it can provide. The activity is never an end in itself. Although the role of any activity as a tool to gain therapeutic results is obvious, even more important is the therapist's personality and his capacity to develop trusting relationships and sensitivity in the timing, approach, and relevance of each activity choice.

To demonstrate the tremendous adaptability that a single activity could have in therapeutic

use, the example of a simple wooden breadboard project can be viewed from the four major occupational therapy focal areas previously discussed, i.e., cognitive function, social function, physical function, and activities-of-daily-living function.

Cognitive processes are brought into play because of the concrete nature of the breadboard project. The task is defined and the directions can be as simple as "sand that edge until it is smooth," or "paint that side red." Initially, decisions are not required and distractions are controlled, so that the patient has both reason and opportunity to focus and increase his attention span. Each direction provides a tangible goal which the patient can see being accomplished, and the amount of time and effort expended can be controlled by the therapist to maintain a successful experience. The repetitious nature of the tasks of sanding and painting allow for simple learning or old-habit skills to be utilized and also provide something tangible and nonthreatening to be remembered from day to day. Problem-solving experiences can also be provided by more complicated directions, or no directions at all. A different woodworking project, however, of multiple parts, requiring finishing and assembly, would obviously provide a higher level of trial and error and problem-solving experiences.

In the area of social function, it is more often the atmosphere surrounding the breadboard task that becomes therapeutic. A highly anxious and withdrawn patient can be eased into focusing his attention and realizing, symbolically, the availability of his existing capacity by following simple directions, not demands, in the finishing requirements of a precut breadboard. He can be in an atmosphere where he sees others using their available skills despite their obvious disability. He can have opportunity to accept and provide assistance to others in a natural give-and-take manner. If he chooses to give his finished project to a family member, he can influence the normalizing of their attitudes toward him. The activity can also channel destructive, compulsive, or hostile feelings and can allow outlets for control and masculine or feminine identification. As mentioned earlier, the sensitivity of the therapist's approach will turn the emphasis of the experience toward whatever social and emotional areas require the most support.

Physical functioning is more tangibly observed in the physical activity demonstrated in completing the project. Strength and endurance can be increased either by the position of the project, the position of the patient, or by the weight of the tools used. The breadboard placed on an increasingly inclined and raised plane will exercise shoulder and back musculature. The breadboard placed at table height and sanded with a special weighted sanding block will strengthen elbow flexors and extensors. The sanding tool can be designed to be used bilaterally or unilaterally, and special, gravity-eliminating suspension slings can support a weakened extremity yet allow for successful and coordinated bilateral activity. Again, the repetitive nature of sanding, sawing, or painting provides the benefits of any repetitive exercise, and the adaptability of the tools and equipment allows the therapist to isolate the muscle groups requiring attention. The friction and resistance experienced in performing the task facilitate normal physiological sensory-motor integration and promote the recovery of coordinated patterns of motion. A patient who has lost the total function of his dominant arm can gain dexterity in his remaining arm through tasks which gradually put finer and finer demand on the coordinated use of this arm. If increased standing balance is the goal, the steps of the breadboard activity can be done from a standing position. If a visual-field loss is interfering with external activities, the breadboard project or written directions concerning it can be gradually positioned into the blind area

so that the patient has reason to compensate for the blindness by exaggerated head positioning, which will eventually be refined into a useful habit.

Activities-of-daily-living skills are increased as a secondary gain of involvement in the breadboard project. Daily tasks require the cognitive capacity to be goal-directed; to focus attention; they require the social and emotional capacity to risk and maintain the motivation to relearn mundane, taken-for-granted, and highly personal tasks; and they require also the physical capacity to maintain balance and sustain physical strength to complete the task. The breadboard project could provide the necessary preliminary experiences which would indicate the physical and psychological moment when relearning of activities-of-daily-living skills could be effective. For the housewife who will be preparing food with only one hand, the breadboard can serve as a self-made assistive device, if three long nails are grouped so they protrude through the top of the board to act as a stabilizer for peeling potatoes or other vegetables. For the patient who must learn again to write, but with his nondominant hand, the dexterity required for wielding a paintbrush in finishing the breadboard is a good and necessary prewriting, coordination exercise.

Any activity, whether a craft or the operation of an adding machine, can be similarly analyzed to determine whether or not it can be adapted to meet the therapist's and especially the patient's needs. The creativity and ingenuity required to provide therapeutic and relevant activity experiences make the role of occupational therapy a unique one in its contribution to the total rehabilitation process.

REFERENCES

LaQue, K.   Unpublished Data.

Luria, A. R.   *Higher Cortical Functions in Man.* New York: Basic Books, 1966.

Special Task Force.   Occupational therapy: its definition and functions. *Am. J. Occup. Ther.* 26: 204, 1972.

13
The Speech Therapist

The ability to communicate is one of man's most precious possessions. Loss of this ability affects not only the patient, but also all those with whom he comes in contact. It is not only the spoken word that may be involved, but the whole system of language.

Interpersonal communication may be brought about by verbal and nonverbal or gesture language. It is this exchange of thoughts and/or opinions which enables human beings to interact with and socialize in their environments. Communication takes place through a system of arbitrary signs: oral language, written language, and everyday gestures, to name a few. Loss of this communicative skill, both verbal and/or nonverbal, results in feelings of frustration, anxiety, depression, and withdrawal. In some instances, the emotional trauma supersedes the language loss. This feeling of desperation is dramatically illustrated in the book *The Bells of Bicetre*, by Georges Simenon:

At half-past nine, Rene Maugras was still unaware that it was half-past nine, and he woke up again more sharply and dramatically, as though after a nightmare, as if he had dreamed that he must, at all costs, cling to something solid. Only his strength had left him. His limbs were moving aimlessly, at random, uncontrolled. Then he tried to call out, to shout for help. His mouth opened. He was practically sure that he opened his mouth wide, but no sound came out of it.

This chapter will be concerned with the process of communication, both expressive and receptive, with emphasis on the etiology, associated physical and psychosocial sequelae, and treatment of communication disorders frequently found within a geriatric population.

APHASIA

Frequently the geriatric stroke patient finds himself with a breakdown in symbolic-language communicative skills. This disorder in language processing is referred to as *aphasia*. More specifically, aphasia is a disruption of and/or reduction in the abilities to use and/or comprehend the conventional linguistic elements of a language that has been previously acquired. It is usually due to a left cerebral vascular accident, which interferes in some way with the blood supply from the left internal carotid artery and its tributaries, which in turn supply arterial blood to that part of the brain responsible for language functioning. Aphasia may also be caused by any type of trauma, i.e., a fall, an auto or motorcycle accident which injures the language center located in the left cerebral hemisphere.

Expressive and Receptive Modalities

As stated, aphasia is a disruption of and/or reduction in a patient's ability to express himself in and/or to comprehend the conventional linguistic elements of a language system. Expression within a language system involves talking, writing, and the usage of gesture language. Reception or comprehension within this system involves reading and understanding the spoken word.

185

Thus, in aphasia, there is a breakdown in these language modalities.

In addition, the system of calculation and numerical ability, also a symbolic process, may be impaired. This involves the computation of arithmetical tasks, such as telling time, handling money, reading calendars and instruments; e.g., reading a thermometer requires numerical ability.

LANGUAGE AND CONVENTIONAL LINGUISTIC ELEMENTS

To better understand the language disorder, the terms *language* and *conventional linguistic elements* need to be clearly defined. Language is a system of symbolization and rules whereby each referent has a given written and spoken symbol and the grammar is a given set of rules. The process of symbolization enables one to associate an object with a symbol and gain meaning.

A language system consists of expressive and receptive modalities and four major subdivisions which are: (1) the phonological or sound system; (2) the lexicon or vocabulary system; (3) the syntactical or grammatical system; and (4) the semantic or meaning system. In aphasia, there is a breakdown in the usage and/or comprehension of these subdivisions. That is, the patient may have difficulty recalling how sounds are made and thus may have difficulty in producing and sequencing sounds to form words; in naming objects, because he has become unable to associate the referent object with its spoken symbol; in understanding the spoken or written word symbol, because he has become unable to associate it with the correct referent object. He may have lost all or only some of the rules of grammar, i.e., plurality, possessiveness, verb-subject agreement, proper word order, and formulation of passive and/or question structures. He may make word-choice errors and not be able to use words with the correct meaning. In most instances, words will be used concretely with an absence of the abstract attitude.

It may be observed that the geriatric aphasic patient has social automatic phrases, i.e., "How are you?," "Thank you very much." In addition, he is able to perform some automatic oral tasks, e.g., singing words to familiar songs, counting, and reciting the days of the week. Since the aphasic is often frustrated at this inability to communicate and express his thoughts, he may revert to the use of profanity and swearing as an emotional release. He may not be aware of his swearing or be able to inhibit it.

DYSARTHRIA: A DISORDER OF SPEECH

In some cases, the speech of the aphasic patient may be impaired by a superimposed problem of dysarthria. This is a motor-speech problem.

It is important to realize the differentiation between speech and language. Speech is an overlaid function. The organs involved are primarily designed for eating and breathing. Speech is a motor process involving the intricate coordination among several neuromuscular mechanisms, including the respiratory, phonatory, resonatory, and articulation systems. In addition, it involves the auditory pathways concerned with perception. The primary components of speech are: auditory perception, articulation, voice (quality, pitch, tone, and loudness). These three components work in an integrated fashion to receive and produce words.

The vital function sequence is comprised of functions involved in food intake and respiration and the combining of these functions in speech. The sequence involves inspiration, expiration, sucking, swallowing, phonation, and chewing. Speech articulation is the skill level of the sequence. Clear speech is not possible if steps in the sequence are defective.

Dysarthria may exist by itself or in combination with aphasia. More specifically, dysarthria is a disorder of the oral peripheral speech mechanism which may interfere with the patient's functional speech intelligibility, thus impairing his phonation, pitch, loudness, rate, vocal quality, intonation, articulation, and/or respiration for speech. Dysarthria is caused by impairment of the central nervous system, which directly controls the muscles of articulation. Therefore, the patient's speech may be quite slurred or completely unintelligible because of paralysis or paresis of the tongue, soft palate, lips, and/or jaw. In addition, dysarthric patients often have difficulty with reflexive oral functioning, such as swallowing, sucking, chewing, and coughing. A dysarthric type of speech pattern is found with patients who have suffered a right cerebral vascular accident.

ORAL APRAXIA: A DISORDER IN COORDINATION OF ORAL MOVEMENTS

A second motor problem which may impair an aphasic's speech is apraxia, the inability of a patient to use his articulators to produce purposeful oral movements, and/or sounds, or to sequence sounds into syllables, words, and/or sentences in the absence of a paralysis or paresis of the musculature. This is due rather to a loss of the normal pattern of motion and the ability to guide the muscle groups necessary for the coordination of oral movements and speech. In severe cases of motor apraxia, the patient is unable to protrude or lateralize the tongue or imitate isolated vowel sounds.

CLASSIFICATION SYSTEM

The issue of classification of aphasic patients remains controversial with the field of aphasiology, as the factors on which to base a system have not met with universal agreement. One recent system is based upon the neurological site of lesion, linguistic analysis of the patient's language content, patient's fluency rate, patient's repetitive and naming abilities, and his auditory verbal comprehension. There are four divisions within this system: Broca's aphasia, Wernicke's aphasia, conduction aphasia, and anomic aphasia.

BROCA'S APHASIA
Patients with Broca's aphasia have a suspected lesion in the posterior inferior portion of the

frontal lobe in the motor-association cortex. Their oral production is characterized by non-fluent, telegraphic speech, consisting of nouns and verbs and the omission of endings and small grammatical words such as prepositions, adverbs, and adjectives. Their speech is produced with great effort and poor articulation and lacks normal rhythmic features. These patients exhibit a similar disorder in their written output but may comprehend spoken and written language with minimal difficulty. In addition, their melodic ability to sing familiar songs may be intact.

WERNICKE'S APHASIA
Patients with Wernicke's aphasia have a suspected lesion in the posterior superior region of the temporal lobe. They exhibit fluent, effortless speech. The prosodic and rhythmic features of their speech are normal; the content of their language, however, consists of filler words, circumlocutions, neologisms (nonreal words), and paraphasia. Literal paraphasias occur when sounds are substituted within a word, i.e., sleep/sleet. Verbal paraphasias occur when in-class word substitutions are made, i.e., car/bus. The language of Wernicke's aphasics reflects intact grammar but lacks nouns and verbs (content words). Their written language is similar to their oral deficits; that is, they produce well-formed letters, words which are misspelled, and incoherent sequence letters, i.e., "leatter" for letter. They have considerable difficulty understanding spoken and written language. Psychologically, these patients may exhibit paranoid tendencies but are not to be confused with true cases of paranoia. Rather, they exhibit a severe auditory verbal-comprehension problem.

CONDUCTION APHASIA
Patients with conduction aphasia typically have a suspected lesion in the lower parietal lobe, disconnecting Wernicke's area from Broca's area. Thus, they exhibit a gross defect in repetition. Their oral production is characterized by fluent,

paraphasic language. The comprehension of both the written and spoken word in these patients appears to be intact.

ANOMIC APHASIA

Patients with anomic aphasia have a suspected lesion in the parietal area. Their spontaneous speech is fluent and their comprehension of the spoken word and repetitive ability are unimpaired. Their major difficulty is a severe naming problem.

AUDITORY AGNOSIA

In some instances, patients may be unable to perceive the spoken word or written word in the absence of auditory or visual acuity loss. Pure word deafness or auditory agnosia exists when the patient is unable to understand the spoken word and yet has normal hearing acuity. He displays normal oral and written language expression as well as comprehension of the written language. Damage in this instance is usually deep in the left temporal lobe, destroying the direct auditory pathway to the left hemisphere and the callosal connections from the opposite auditory region.

ALEXIA

Pure alexia exists when the patient is unable to read the printed word yet has normal visual acuity. The patient may be able to copy words and to write spontaneously but later is not able to read what he has copied or written. All aspects of his language are normal with the exception of his inability to read. Probable damage in this instance may be to the left visual field and posterior portion of the corpus callosum connecting the visual areas of the two hemispheres.

APHASIA: A SYMPTOM COMPLEX

As one works with the geriatric aphasic patient, one must take into consideration his emotional adjustment to his communication, perceptual, and physical deficits. The patient must be seen in his entirety, and one must try to understand how he feels. His premorbid personality should be considered and changes which may have occurred since the stroke. It should be emphasized that a patient's language performance does not relate to his previous intellectual functioning. Rather, his language performance and behavior depend upon the site and severity of neurological insult. Aphasia is a symptom complex consisting of the language disturbance or inability to retrieve the previously learned language code caused by brain injury with physical and psychological sequelae.

PSYCHOLOGICAL SEQUELAE

The psychological sequelae of brain damage may further modify the geriatric aphasic patient's behavior and personality. Behavioral changes may occur in the form of perseveration, concrete attitude, distractibility, and lability. Some patients may exhibit perseveration, or the inability to shift to new acts and thoughts; they maintain a response which is no longer appropriate since the stimulus has been removed. Most patients exhibit the inability to deal with and use abstract concepts and are said to have a *concrete attitude*. Some have a reduction in attention span and are easily distracted. At times, some patients may exhibit inappropriate emotional responses—either laughter or crying—which they cannot inhibit, and they are said to be labile.

Geriatric aphasic patients often exhibit personality changes. Most patients develop increased dependency needs and require a great deal of understanding and support from those who care for them. They may exhibit defense mechanisms in the form of withdrawal and denial. Many aphasics, having lost the ability to communicate with others in their environment, shut themselves off and prefer to be alone. Other patients deny the language deficit because they are unable to work through the reality of the situation. It should be remembered that the geriatric aphasic has normal reactions of fear, anxiety, depression, and shame, which should be dealt with by those who care for and treat him.

A period of spontaneous recovery may occur within the first three months to a year after the onset of injury. If this occurs, a patient has fairly good prognosis of language return. During spontaneous recovery, patients improve steadily and do tasks each day that they could not do the day before.

PROGNOSIS: FACTORS DETERMINING RECOVERY

A geriatric aphasic patient's prognosis in terms of improvement in language skills is contingent upon several factors. If it is observed upon initial evaluation that the patient exhibits a severe motor apraxia and is unable to imitate speech sounds or oral movements, he is believed to have poor prognosis for speech return. Some of the contributing factors which enable one to prognosticate a geriatric aphasic patient's prognosis are as follows:

One of the most important factors in determining the nature and severity of aphasic symptoms and response to treatment is the locus and extent of damage in the brain. A second significant element is his general response pattern to therapy. If the patient exhibits lethargy and/or verbal perseveration, his ability to learn will be considerably inhibited. Motivation for improvement is needed if he is to make significant therapeutic gains. A third factor is the patient's level of functioning in each language modality, including oral expression, writing, reading, auditory verbal comprehension, and calculation ability. A severe reduction in auditory comprehension will make therapeutic and functional gains minimal, unless spontaneous recovery contributes favorably to the patient's understanding of the spoken word. Therefore, the aphasic's level of intactness in each language area will determine his prognosis and therapeutic goals. A fourth factor influencing his extent and rate of progress is error-awareness and self-corrective ability. The more aware he is of his inability to communicate accurately and to correct his errors, the better his chance of progress and language return. Lastly, a psychological estimate of the patient's emotional functioning will contribute to the rate and extent of expected language recovery. A patient who exhibits a severe depressed, frustrated, or anxious attitude is less likely to make significant clinical and/or functional gains than a patient who appears well-adjusted to his communication deficit.

EVALUATION PROCEDURES

Language impairment is assessed by a speech pathologist through informal functional and formalized testing procedures. In this way, the speech pathologist becomes aware of the patient's functional performance as well as his abilities in a formalized situation. A functional assessment may be performed to see how the aphasic meets his daily communication needs, to judge the severity of his handicap, and to obtain a profile of his language, which will describe his residual language in terms of activities of daily living (ADL). In such an assessment, the therapist wants to know if the patient can make his needs known verbally or through gesture, if he is aware of and can identify environmental sounds, if he knows the names of family members and common objects, can understand conversation or television, and if he can read street signs, letters, magazines and/or books. Formalized clinical assessment, on the other hand, is done to obtain an estimate of the degree of his disorder, his present level of functioning, and to measure the progress he has made.

TREATMENT: SETTING OF GOALS

There is no prescription for aphasia therapy, rather, each aphasic patient requires a unique treatment program based on his personality and language needs. There do exist criteria for the selection of long- and short-term goals. In a majority of instances, the long-term therapeutic goal deals with the improvement of the patient's expressive and receptive linguistic skills, enabling him functionally to communicate his daily needs. Short-term goals are determined by the level of functioning the patient exhibits in each language modality.

GROUP VS. INDIVIDUAL THERAPY

Therapy may be either individual or group. In the individual setting, the therapist is able to work directly with the patient and to focus his energies on the patient's emotional needs and responses. Individual treatment enables the therapist to provide immediate reinforcement to the patient's answers. Initially, most patients require a one-to-one relationship. Group therapy provides him with an opportunity to socialize with other aphasic patients. It enables him to release commonly shared emotions and to realize that he is not alone in his communication loss; there are others who can speak less or more fluently than he.

SUBSTANTIATION FOR APHASIA TREATMENT

Few valid conclusions on the efficacy of treatment are permissible today, because very little is known about the pathophysiology of aphasia and less about the recovery process. One is not able to explain the observed losses in the absence of a thorough understanding of normal language processes. A contended issue is, on the one hand, that the involved brain cells are destroyed and the functions are irretrievably lost; on the other hand, there is the multipotentiality of brain tissue and a concept of language organization not wholly dependent on anatomical factors.

One should perhaps question whether or not the effort to teach the aphasic and plan a treatment program has substantiation for success. An effort to teach necessarily implies that there is a residual communication system in the aphasic's brain which can increase in capacity. In all likelihood, the aphasic's communication centers have been damaged and cannot function spontaneously or be trained to function as they did prior to the insult.

THE RECOVERY PROCESS: STIMULATION, FACILITATION, AND MOTIVATION

According to J. M. Wepman, if aphasics are left untreated, they plateau and develop secondary reactions with anxiety, depression, a sense of worthlessness, feelings of futility, and an overall attitude of insecurity.

If their environment is sheltered, they may become overly dependent, invalidized, and infantilized. Instructive, supportive therapy is needed to help patients regain a wholesome self-concept. Stimulation is important to promote action. Both internal and external persuasion should be utilized.

Therapy is a form of stimulation based on the patient's needs, drives, and motivation. Aphasia therapy is a process by which the therapist provides stimulating materials in the area of the patient's greatest need, at the time when his nervous system is capable of utilizing it for the facilitation of cortical integrations leading to language performance. Facilitation is the physiological ease and strength of the drive to motivate action. Motivation is the amount of goal-directed behavior the patient has. The operation of these three concepts at maximal level increases the probability of successful therapy.

AUDITORY STIMULATION

Clinical findings indicate that improvement of articulation, word finding, reading, and writing often results from the use of a single therapeutic principle: intensive auditory stimulation. There are six important principles involved in the use of effective auditory stimulation:

1. The material used should be meaningful to the patient and relevant to the context in which it is used. The therapist names objects in the patient's immediate environment.

2. The length of each auditory unit must be carefully controlled. One must use language units short enough for the patient to grasp. The length of the unit varies from patient to patient and increases as therapy progresses. An effective device for controlling the auditory unit is the

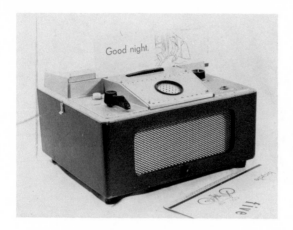

FIG. 86. Language Master auditory unit.

Language Master (see Fig. 86). This machine was developed by Bell and Howell and consists of a dial for patient and instructor to play back. The patient is able to record his response and play it back. The Language Master cards may be blank or printed and contain a strip of recording tape on the bottom. The prepared printed cards may contain short, one-word units, i.e., nouns, present-tense action verbs, and the corresponding picture, also phrases or sentences of increasing complexity.

3. The patient should make a specific response to each language unit presented. The therapist must wait for this response and reinforce it with repetition of the stimulus, timing this repetition to coincide with the patient's response. If the patient has no available oral response, the required response may be pointing to an object or picture named by the therapist. The clinician gives the direction and repeats it as the patient performs. Most patients begin to verbalize spontaneously with the clinician during this step.

Two variations which help the patient advance from talking with the clinician to more voluntary speech are as follows: (1) ask the patient to repeat what he has just said; (2) before a set of stimuli are presented, the patient is instructed casually, "Say it if you can. If it doesn't come, listen, think it, say it with me."

The patient is given an opportunity to do so if he can. If the word does not come, the therapist pronounces it; if it does, additional stimulation is given by using the word in short, common phrases: lock the door, open the door, close the door.

In more progressive stages of therapy, patients are asked to repeat words, phrases, and sentences of controlled length and to write these units from dictation. The Language Master is helpful in this procedure. The patient's ability to form sentences (oral and written) improves with his ability to retain language patterns.

The transition from repeating and writing from dictation to independent formation may be accomplished by giving the patient a few additional easier words each session. Materials change from pictures of familiar objects to single-activity pictures and then to complex situational pictures in which the patient describes what is happening, adding more details as language increases. See Figures 87A–F.

4. Abundant and varied materials should be used during each clinical period. The basis for this is that the patient *has* words, even though they are not readily available to him. The process of therapy is not teaching words but stimulating damaged processes to function again. It is also based on the observation that giving the patient a great deal of auditory stimulation in controlled units and giving him time to respond to each unit produces a good deal of language in a short time.

5. A maximal number of verbal attempts should be made by the patient during each clinical period, allowing him to speak during each clinical period to provide him with confidence in his ability to talk. Because of this experience, he is more apt to try to talk when he goes back to the ward.

6. Defective responses usually should not be corrected. Early correction is frustrating, but errors tend to decrease and disappear as more language becomes available. Correction should be provided when the patient begins to monitor his own speech and asks for help.

Techniques for Auditory Stimulation. Many

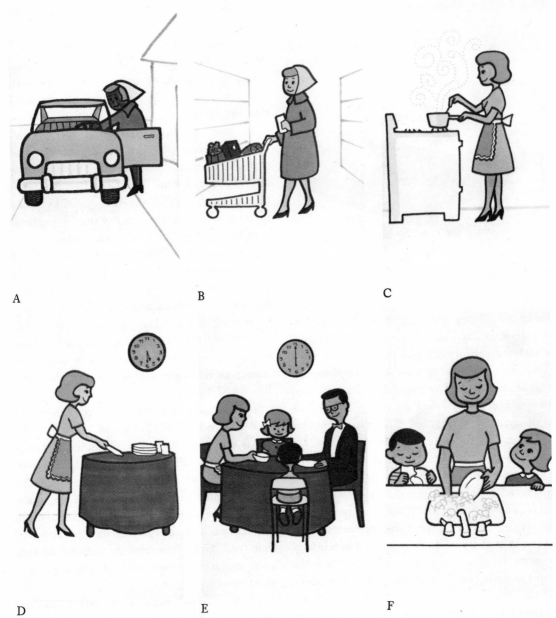

A   B   C

D   E   F

FIGS. 87 A through F. Sequential picture cards that progress from single activities to more complex situations which patient must attempt to describe.

methods for auditory stimulation involve reading and writing. This is recommended because one language modality serves to reinforce another. It should be stressed that the techniques must always be adapted to the patient's interests, his level of performance, and his pattern of impairment:

1. Present objects or pictures. Ask patient to point to stimulus named and attempt to say it with therapist, who repeats it as patient identifies it correctly.

2. Ask patient to carry out simple directions; the patient verbalizes actions with the therapist as he performs them.

3. Have patient count, say days of the week, months, and alphabet with therapist.

4. Ask patient to point to objects, using phrases.

5. Present phrases and sentences, using common associations, and ask patient to complete phrase, e.g., A cup of _____, or I go to bed at _____.

Techniques for Increasing Vocabulary and Language Usage. The methods for auditory stimulation also increase the patient's vocabulary. As the patient acquires more language, he should acquire an increasing responsibility for his speech. The following activities are useful in stimulating language and vocabulary expansion:

1. Carry on simple conversation, involving greetings, patient's name and address, names of members of his family, and his daily activities.

2. Have patient name objects and describe pictures.

3. Word association. Therapist speaks a word and asks patient to name as many things as he can that the given word makes him think of.

4. Have patient define words.

5. Ask patient to explain techniques or processes with which he is familiar, e.g., how to fix a tire.

SENSORIMOTOR TECHNIQUES

Sensorimotor techniques are used when aphasia is complicated by sensorimotor involvement of dysarthria or oral apraxia. These methods are usually required when the following conditions exist: (1) when the patient has difficulty imitating gross movements, such as opening and closing the mouth, protruding the tongue, blowing out a match, or initiating phonation; (2) when alternating movements, such as protruding and retracting the tongue or moving the tongue laterally and vertically, are markedly hesitant and uncertain, and when speech is unintelligible.

Sensorimotor techniques may be divided into three parts: for general facilitation of movement patterns, for obtaining specific sounds, and for reinforcing and facilitating learned patterns.

TECHNIQUES FOR FACILITATION OF MOVEMENT PATTERNS

Observed in some stroke patients is impairment of the ability to alter pitch voluntarily, irregular pitch intervals, impairment of the ability to sustain phonation, decrease in volume, and impairment of the ability to initiate phonation.

The therapist may ask the patient to:

1. Say "ah" with prolonged phonation. (Timing phonation obtained may increase the patient's interest level.)

2. Vocalize up and down the scale.

3. Open and close jaw on rhythmic count.

4. Protrude and retract tongue on command.

5. Blow out a match.

6. Sing a familiar song.

7. Blow in a spirometer.

TECHNIQUES FOR OBTAINING SPECIFIC SOUNDS

One of the most effective ways to produce specific sounds with the aphasic patient is to use minimal placement clues combined with visual and auditory ones. The patient's observation of the therapist and of himself in a mirror helps. As sensorimotor processes begin to function, new sounds tend to emerge. The following minimal placement cues are effective:

(*m*) Close lips. Hum.

(*b*) Press lips together.

(*p*) Press lips. Whisper.

(*l*) Press tongue up. Sing.

(*d*) Press tongue up. Say sound.

(*t*) Press tongue up. Whisper.

(*g*) Press with back of tongue.

(*k*) Press with back of tongue.

(*r*) Say *ah*. Raise tongue gradually to say sound of *r*.

(*th* voiced) Bite tongue. Say sound of *th*.

(*th* unvoiced) Bite tongue. Whisper.

(*z*) Close teeth. Say sound of *z*.

(*s*) Close teeth. Say sound of *s*.

(*sh*) Close teeth. Blow. Like *s* but make it bigger.

(*w*) Lips round. Say sound of *w*.

(*j*) Press tongue down. Say sound of *j*.

(*ch*) Close teeth. Press tongue up. Whisper to make sound of *ch*.

TECHNIQUES FOR REINFORCING SOUNDS AND FACILITATING SPEECH MOVEMENTS

The following methods are needed for reinforcing speech sounds:

1. Combine consonant immediately with "ah." Repeat with increasing rate.
2. Combine consonant with other vowels the patient can make.
3. Repeat short familiar words beginning with the desired consonant.
4. Associate the learned sound with the printed symbol. Write and say.
5. Place cards with learned sound on table. Ask patient to indicate sound produced by the therapist.
6. Have patient imitate learned sounds daily with only auditory stimulation.
7. Present learned sounds on individual cards; give patient opportunity to initiate sound on presentation of symbol. Give patient

set of cards with learned sound for practice.

TECHNIQUES FOR VISUAL INVOLVEMENT

Aphasic patients who need special techniques for reading and writing impairment have the following difficulties:

1. Confusion of letters with similar visual configurations, e.g., EF, CG, PBR, and WM.
2. Confusion of words which look alike, e.g., WATCH, MATCH, and BARK, PARK.
3. Special difficulty with ends of words.
4. Slowness of word recognition.
5. Confusion of upper- and lower-case letters in writing.
6. Reversals of letter sequences in words.
7. Special difficulty with double letters in spelling.
8. Tendency to spell phonetically.
9. Difficulty in keeping place and in following a line.

The following devices may be helpful in improving the patient's reading and writing skills:

1. Writing and naming individual symbol simultaneously.
2. Writing and saying letters in alphabetical order in groups of 5 or 6.
3. Pointing to letter named by the therapist.
4. Naming letters presented in random order.
5. Writing letters from dictation.
6. Writing words from dictation.
7. Reading single words.
8. Reading phrases.
9. Writing sentences to dictation and reading back.

ROLE OF FAMILY MEMBERS

Treatment of the aphasic patient goes beyond the patient to his family members. They are an integral part of his overall language rehabilitation. It is important that they understand the nature of his communication loss and how best to deal with him to minimize frustration. Their understanding of the medical and neurological aspects of the stroke and resulting aphasia may be initiated by the practitioner. Relative or family counseling is often performed by the speech pathologist in conjunction with social service.

During counseling it is stressed that the family members try to provide an understanding and stimulating companionship with the patient. This may be accomplished in several ways. The first is by spending time with the patient when he is most responsive and alert. The length of time may gradually increase as he progresses in his recovery. The family is also advised that it is important that the patient have some time to himself to develop a sense of freedom.

Second, it is recommended that the family make a list of the patient's interests and use material from it when visiting with him. Although the patient may be unable to express what his preferences are, it is up to the family to find out what stimulates and interests him.

The relatives are advised to accept the patient as he is at the moment. They should try to be relaxed and casual about oddities in his behavior. They should give him sufficient time to respond and perform simple tasks, as he may be extremely slow in responding. They should try to remain relaxed about his future and reassure him during his course of recovery. It is important that the family praise and reward the patient for his accomplishments rather than indicate that he should do better.

It is recommended that family members increase the patient's independence as much as possible. He should be encouraged to do as much on his own as possible within the limits of his abilities. Any advance in self-help should be acknowledged.

The relatives are told to include the patient in family affairs. It is important that he be treated in a manner similar to the way he was treated before his illness. This will help the patient to maintain his status and dignity in the family. He should be encouraged to join in meals and other family events. It is relevant that the family understand that the overall goal of recovery is socialization and that language is only one means of achieving this goal.

A significant portion of family counseling is devoted to assisting the relatives in better communication with their aphasic relative. They are told to talk to him simply and naturally and to keep instructions and explanations simple. They are urged to encourage him to respond in whatever way he can. For patients who have difficulty expressing themselves, family members should ask questions requiring a simple yes or no response, indicated by a head nod or oral response. The use of gestures may also be encouraged whereby the patient can show what he means by pointing. If a patient responds slowly, he should be given time to search for the word he desires. If he is unsuccessful after several attempts, the word should be provided for him, in order to eliminate frustration. The aphasic person should be encouraged to use greetings and social exchanges, i.e., "Hello," "Thank you," and "Good-bye," since these are automatic phrases which should be easy for him. Relatives are told that if they are unable to understand what the patient is trying to say, they should try to change the subject or return to the issue later.

ROLE OF THE PHYSICIAN

The physician has certain responsibilities to the geriatric aphasic patient and his family. It is he who initally informs the patient that he has had a stroke and then describes what has happened. An explanation should be provided to the aphasic patient if his auditory verbal comprehension appears intact, despite a severe deficit in speech and language expression. The physician's explanations and instructions should be kept as simple as possible and should be accompanied by gesture to make sure the patient understands. This type of communication with the patient should exist in subsequent meetings, until the aphasic demonstrates significant gains in his auditory verbal comprehension for more complex conversations.

It is the physician who explains the patient's

medical and neurological condition to the family and informs them of the patient's apparent communication loss. He must not assume that because the patient is not speaking he does not understand. Therefore, confidential medical information should not be stated in the patient's presence. The physician may be the person to explain the aphasia initially to the relatives and to make referral to a speech pathologist for a language evaluation. It is important, then, that the physician have a great enough understanding of the nature of aphasia to enable him to relate to the aphasic patient and his relatives and to know when a speech referral is needed.

LARYNGEAL CARCINOMA

Carcinoma of the larynx occurs most frequently in middle and old age and is more prevalent in males than in females.

Since there are no lymphatic vessels in the vocal folds, lymphatic metastasis will occur only when considerable invasion of the larynx has occurred.

Direct extension of the tumor in the early stages is confined to the membranous and muscular tissues of the larynx and limited by its cartilaginous structures and is of low malignancy. A tumor usually is not painful in its initial stages and gives no danger signal of its existence. Laryngeal tumor produces immediate symptoms of hoarseness followed by discomfort, obstruction, and an irritating cough if allowed to progress. Early diagnosis will promote a prolonged lifespan and, in some instances, a permanent cure.

TREATMENT OF LARYNGEAL CARCINOMA

Treatment of carcinoma may be by surgical intervention or radiotherapy. Surgery tries to cure the cancer by total excision of the growth. Radiotherapy attempts to destroy or arrest active growth and stimulate fibrous tissue formation. Radiotherapy may be alternative to surgery or ancillary to it at any stage of treatment. It is prescribed for: (1) cases who refuse operation, (2) people who are too ill to undergo operation hazard, (3) cases in which the tumor is not well encapsulated, so that isolated particles may remain after removal of main mass and recurrence is a danger.

A more extensive penetration of the pharynx will necessitate partial pharyngectomy with a laryngectomy. The total procedure is called a *pharyngolaryngectomy.*

PARTIAL LARYNGECTOMY

Partial laryngectomy is performed only in cases of well-localized tumor situated on the extreme outer edge of the fold.

Usually both vocal fold and verticular band and the thyroid ala of the affected side are removed together. Eventually, in the place of the thyroarytenoid muscle a substitute vocal fold forms. The healthy fold passes over the midline to meet the adventitious fold and a serviceable voice is acquired.

TOTAL LARYNGECTOMY

Excision of the entire larynx is necessitated if the carcinoma has penetrated the surface tissues of the larynx, involving the muscles. Surgical technique is not related directly to speech proficiency; it is related, however, to the final form of the reconstructed pharyngeal tube.

PATIENT'S POSTOPERATIVE PROGRESS

The patient is usually well and cheerful 10 to 14 days after the operation, if no complication arises.

The most common postoperative complication is bronchitis, caused by the aspiration of secretion into the bronchi during operation. The patient has notable difficulty breathing and is fatigued in his effort to cough up mucus. To alleviate the patient's distress a Moure's cannula is inserted in the tracheal opening, at first. This cannula consists of two tubes which fit one within the other. Usually the outer tube is left in position until the wound has healed, but the inner tube may be removed, cleaned, and sterilized. Suction apparatus may be used to extract mucus from the cannula.

The laryngectomized patient is able to cough efficiently by using abdominal muscles and diaphragm for increasing intrathoracic pressure.

Persistent postlaryngectomy bronchial catarrh may hold up the patient's recovery for several weeks. Treatment may consist of breathing exercises and postural draining of the lungs undertaken by the physical therapist. The speech pathologist and physical therapist should consult to avoid possible conflict of exercises and instructions.

PSYCHOLOGICAL SEQUELAE TO LARYNGECTOMY

An initial consideration in the treatment of a laryngectomized patient is his psychological state before and after the operative procedure. One must realize the importance of the larynx in communication and of the voice as a vehicle for the expression of feeling and of personality. Thus, excision of the larynx may produce profound emotional reactions in the patient.

The initial emotional reaction of the patient may be a reactive depression upon learning that the larynx is cancerous and must be removed. The patient has a gamut of feelings which may include fright, anxiety, insomnia, confusion, self-pity, fear of death, and suicidal impulses.

The patient will have anxieties about eating, breathing, speaking, and cohabitation. He will wonder how he will be able to cough or to blow his nose. Generally, he will be concerned about his ability to return to work and his/her loss of attractiveness and desirability.

Both the surgeon and the speech pathologist should try to allay the patient's fears and those of family members. The patient may be greatly comforted if preoperating arrangements can be made for him to meet and speak with a proficient esophageal speaker. The laryngectomized rehabilitated person is thus able to describe from actual experience what laryngectomy means in

terms of physical discomfort and personal, social, and economic difficulties.

SPEECH REHABILITATION
AFTER LARYNGECTOMY

The laryngectomized patient may acquire a functional means of oral communication. In place of vocal folds, he learns to use the esophageal sphincter as a vibratory reed or pseudoglottis, and the upper portion of the esophagus serves as an air reservoir. Both the sphincter and upper portion of the esophagus consist of striated muscle. Voluntary relaxation of the sphincter must be acquired in pseudo-voice production. According to Stetson, the valvular lips of the esophageal sphincter separate as air bursts through and vibrates them. Closure of the lips is automatic as the air pressure below decreases. Air intake and expulsion is somewhat dependent upon changes in intrathoracic pressure which coincides with normal respiration for speech.

The air content in the esophagus is constantly replenished during esophageal speech in two ways: (1) air is aspirated into the esophagus at the same time as lung inspiration; (2) small quantities of air are injected into the esophagus by muscular compression of air in the oral cavity. Injection is accomplished by closing the lips and elevating the soft palate with slight tensing of the cheeks and tongue, causing air to be compressed in the oral cavity, pressed backward into the pharynx, and injected into the esophagus.

SPEECH THERAPY PROCEDURE

It is suggested that preoperatively the patient engage in preliminary relaxation techniques and intercostal diaphragmatic breathing. Postoperatively, the patient should be encouraged to experiment when he feels inclined and may spontaneously produce voice. Once voice has been mastered, the patient is able to speak using his articulatory mechanism which remains intact. Speech is slower than normal, allowing time for more emphatic articulation. A majority of laryngectomized patients have difficulty mastering the basic elements of esophageal voice and single-vowel sounds. The first goal in teaching is the production of a sound, regardless of the manner in which it is achieved.

It is important to remember that the therapist should not insist upon acquisition of esophageal voice when it is not possible. The ultimate decision should be arrived at in collaboration with the laryngologist who can assess the surgical result. The patient's esophopharyngeal structure, its size, shape, and dilatability should be examined by cineradiographic filming.

The following factors may make the acquisition of esophageal voice difficult:

1. A poor postoperative result with formation of scar tissue which restricts facile dilation of the hypopharynx and cricapharyngeal sphincter.

2. Damage to the nerve supply to the pharynx and tongue by surgery, producing paralysis.

3. Old age and frailty accompanied by lack of drive to learn.

4. Deafness and inability to monitor speech.

5. Low intelligence and inability to master the necessary new muscular coordination.

6. Distaste for esophageal speech.

VOCAL METHODS

Three major vocal methods exist for teaching esophageal speech. The methods include: air swallowing, injection method, and aspiration method.

AIR SWALLOWING

Air swallowing consists of the eructation of air from the esophagus or belching. This requires control over the relaxation and dilation of the esophageal sphincter. Some patients, especially females, develop an aversion to this method due to psychological inhibitions and social taboos against burping.

INJECTION METHOD

Air injection is preferable to air swallowing. Small quantities of air may be injected into the esophagus by muscular compression of air in the oral cavity. Injection is accomplished by closing the lips and elevating the soft palate with slight tensing of the cheeks and tongue causing air to be compressed in the oral cavity, pressed backward into the pharynx, and injected into the esophagus.

ASPIRATION METHOD

The aspiration method is recommended if the laryngectomized patient is tense and breathing is shallow. This method entails proper instruction in relaxation and central breathing. Breathing exercises need not be taught in relation to phonation exercises. Rather, the patient may learn to produce voice by the injection method independently, and then attention may be focused upon connection between voice and respiration. In most laryngectomized patients breathing exercises are advisable early in treatment, to increase the air reservoir and thus to enable the patient to obtain longer phrasing and greater volume of voice.

GROUP THERAPY

Group therapy is the most satisfactory medium to work with for laryngectomized patients. The beginner feels extreme self-consciousness over his voice, which he thinks is conspicuous and socially unacceptable. Thus, working with a group in a warm, sympathetic atmosphere breeds confidence and gives the patient the courage to speak freely at home and eventually in the outside world.

TREATMENT PROCEDURES

1. Experiment with vocalizing syllables with initial consonants p, t, and k.
2. Practice a syllable once it is voiced until achieved easily.
3. Practice different syllables beginning and ending with voiced and voiceless plosives and containing different vowels.

4. Practice polysyllabic words.
5. Extend to sentences, omitting difficult consonants and words beginning with vowels.
6. Practice phrasing, whereby breathing technique is integrated with speech.
7. Try whistling and blowing a mouth organ in staccato blasts from the esophagus by diaphragmatic and thoracic movements.
8. Practice increase of vocal volume.
9. Extend to improvement of tone and pitch.

ARTIFICIAL VOCAL AIDS

Some patients may be unable to acquire esophageal speech or they may have a personal preference for using an aid rather than esophageal voice. They should be helped to obtain the most suitable aid and instructed in how best to use it.

Old age and poor health provide further conditions for using a vocal aid. The aged have difficulty in managing the aid and synchronizing the artificial voice with articulatory movements. The electric vibrator has to be switched on and off and speech has to be adjusted to the noise generated. The best speakers are those who switch on and off for each word or short phrases.

Deafness renders use of the vocal aid impossible. Many patients with a high-frequency loss are unable to understand their own speech. They are literally deafened by the vibrator.

Two recommended available vocal aids are the Cooper-Rand electronic speech aid, which is manufactured by the Rand Development Corporation. It is recommended for the aged and consists of a hand-operated oscillator, generated by a transistor battery. Western Electric Company and Bell Telephone Laboratories manufacture a Bell electronic larynx, consisting of an electric vibrator contained in a cylinder, over the end of which a flexible diaphragm is stretched. The vibrator is operated by a press button and a continuous buzzing is produced. When the pulsating diaphragm is placed firmly against the pharynx, the sound of the vibrator is transferred to the pharyngeal cavity and is converted into speech by ordinary movements of articulation.

HEARING IMPAIRMENT

Effective communication for speech involves the auditory pathways concerned with perception. Speech is the process by which oral symbols are perceived and produced. Focus will now be placed on these auditory pathways and hearing loss will be discussed. This difficulty is a frequent communication impairment in geriatric patients.

HEARING LOSS

By the term *hearing loss* one means the symptom of partial impairment of auditory sensitivity or the medical condition that underlies it. By *deafness* one means peripheral impairment with a severe loss of sensitivity, so that sustained communication by the unaided, unamplified voice is impossible or very nearly so. The hearing level for speech is at least 82 dB.

There are three major types of hearing loss which have diagnostic significance: conductive, sensory-neural, and mixed.

CONDUCTIVE HEARING LOSS

This type of loss may be defined as a hearing impairment caused by interference with the acoustic transmission of sound to the sense organ, usually in the outer or middle ear. In pure conductive hearing loss, the hearing threshold levels measured by bone conduction are usually near normal and the air-bone gaps are large.

Conductive loss may be caused by plugging of the external canal, damping the free movement of the drum, or restricting the movements of the ossicles. Any of these conditions will reduce the intensity of the air-borne sound that finally reaches the inner ear. Among the etiological conditions resulting in a conductive impairment are: congenital malformation, impacted wax, external otitis, otitis media, chloesteatoma, and otosclerosis.

CONGENITAL MALFORMATIONS

Congenital malformation or absence of the external ear may be associated with aberrant formation of other structures. Atresia, or closure of the external ear canal, is such a malformation.

IMPACTED WAX

The most common cause of hearing loss from the external canal is wax or cerumen, which may harden in the canal and become impacted so that it prevents sound waves from reaching the drum and middle ear.

EXTERNAL OTITIS

Changes may occur in the skin of the external canal which permit the growth of bacteria and fungi. Infection of the skin and inflammatory changes involving other structures produce external otitis. This occurs most frequently in hot, wet climates. The most prominent symptom of this condition is pain on manipulation of the auricle.

OTITIS MEDIA

The middle ear is a chamber which contains the mechanism that conducts sound from the air in the external ear to the fluid in the inner ear. The components of this mechanism are: the eardrum, the ossicles (malleus, incus, and stapes) and their ligaments. Diseases of the middle ear, when they produce a hearing loss, involve one or more of these structures, and the loss is conductive in nature.

Inflammation in the middle ear is the most common cause of conductive hearing loss. The inflammation is called *otitis media*; and usually develops from a cold in the head. Nasal secretions infect the eustachian tube. The infection travels along the tube until the middle ear is reached. If the tube is inflamed, air pressure in the middle ear cannot be equalized. Thus, oxygen in the middle ear is absorbed by the blood and a partial vacuum is formed, forcing the eardrum inward and fixating the ossicles. A clear fluid exudes from the mucous lining. This is called *nonsuppurative otitis media*. As the disease progresses, the watery serous secretion thickens into a pus. When material in the middle

ear becomes infected, the disease is in the suppurative or purulent stage.

CHOLESTEATOMA

Cholesteatoma is a cyst lined internally with skin. It grows from the upper part of the drumhead. It originates from chronic wetting of the deep parts of the external canal or from inflammation of the middle ear. The cyst enlarges and may erode the ossicles or other bony structures and cause symptoms. The patient usually complains of intermittent discharge from the ear. The hearing level may be within normal limits or within 15 or 20 dB of a normal threshold.

OTOSCLEROSIS

This is a unique bony disease that affects the bony capsule surrounding the inner ear. This bone becomes invaded by a softer bone which grows intermittently and then becomes hard again, i.e., sclerotic. The most common site of this growth is in front of and below the oval window. The growth tends to fixate the footplate of the stapes in the oval window and hence impedes the stapes movement. Therefore, vibrations carried to it from the eardrum through the incus and malleus are not transmitted to the fluid of the inner ear.

Otosclerosis is a hereditary disease. It is a disease of youth and its associated hearing loss is usually first observed in adolescence or the early twenties. In its initial stages the loss is purely conductive with loss of lower tones. As loss for high tones increases, tinnitus (ringing in the ears) becomes severe. The hearing may remain the same for a long period of time, with gradual additional loss occurring when sensory-neural hearing loss of old age compounds the conductive loss.

SENSORY-NEURAL HEARING LOSS

Sensory-neural hearing loss means a hearing impairment due to abnormality of the sense organ, the auditory nerve, or both. Some or all of the hearing levels by bone conduction are abnormal but the air-bone gaps are small or absent. Contributing etiological factors include: advancing age, drugs, and prolonged exposure to loud noises.

DYSACUSIS

Dysacusis is an inclusive term indicating hearing losses which are not simple losses of sensitivity of hearing. They are due to malfunction of the sense organ or abnormal function of the brain. Included within this category may be: diplacusis, presbycusis, discrimination loss, hysterical loss, block, agnosia, and phonemic regression.

Central Dysacusis. By *central dysacusis* one means impairment of hearing which is unexplainable by abnormality of the sense organ or auditory nerve. Rather, the etiology is localized in the central nervous system. The term *central* implies that the impairment is more than a faulty function of the ear. *Dysacusis* implies that the condition is a sensory rather than a motor difficulty.

Any type of general disease of the brain, such as brain tumors, arteriosclerosis, cerebral hemorrhage, plugging of the cerebral blood vessels via thrombosis or embolism, multiple sclerosis, or brain abscess, may affect the auditory pathways from the auditory nerve through the brain stem and up to outer layers of the temporal lobe.

Psychogenic Dysacusis. Psychological changes in a patient's personality may result in auditory difficulties. There may be a partial or total inability to hear, with no structural change in the auditory apparatus. Nerve impulses reach the brain but are not consciously heard. Such deafness is called *psychogenic dysacusis*.

PRESBYCUSIS

The most common cause of sensory-neural hearing loss, and probably of all hearing loss, is advancing age. Partial atrophy of the organ of Corti and of the auditory nerve is common after the age of forty. The development of a certain amount of high-tone sensory-neural hearing loss seems to be part of the natural course of growing older. This type of loss is known as *presbycusis*.

The structured change responsible for this loss involves the degeneration of the sensory cells in the part of the organ of Corti toward the base of the cochlea.

DRUGS

Some drugs have been thought to produce tinnitus and sensory-neural hearing loss. Ototoxicity has been attributed to quinine, salicylates, dihydrostreptomycin, and kanamycin. The hearing loss from dihydrostreptomycin often does not appear for two or more months after the medication has been taken.

NOISE: TEMPORARY HEARING LOSS

Auditory fatigue, or temporary hearing loss, is produced by long exposure to loud sounds. Recovery from this loss is so complete that the hearing loss may be considered a fatigue rather than an injury, and thus it is referred to as a temporary threshold shift. For most noises the temporary effect is usually a partial high-tone loss, most severe for frequencies above the range essential for speech.

NOISE: PERMANENT HEARING LOSS

The intensity required to cause real disintegration depends in part on how long the noise lasts. *Acoustic trauma* is a term used to refer to injury to the ear by a single brief exposure to sound. In acoustic trauma it is easy to identify the actual incident, the time that it happened, and the responsibility for it.

MENIÈRE'S DISEASE

This condition is typified by vertigo (dizziness), tinnitus, and sensory-neural deafness. The sensory-neural loss may be greater for low tones than for high tones.

Often associated with this condition is distention of the membranous labyrinth. Etiological theories have been proposed indicating causative factors in this disease process. The most popular theory is that it is caused by a kind of spasm or intermittent partial blocking of the circulation of the inner ear. Some have postulated that a psychosomatic element underlies the disease process.

PHONEMIC REGRESSION AND OLD AGE

Phonemic regression is a condition found in the aged, which is loss of the ability to comprehend all the words in a sentence or even single words, spoken at normal tempo, in spite of relatively good sensitivity for pure tones or slow speech.

Patients who exhibit phonemic regression have a diminished attention span. They have more difficulty with complicated acoustic patterns of speech than with simple pure tones. These patients have the high-tone sensory-neural hearing loss of presbycusis, but their failure to understand words is greater than can be explained by the loss alone.

The cause of phonemic regression is in the brain. Generalized cerebral arteriosclerosis is the most common cause.

A hearing aid is not helpful in improving phonemic regression, because amplification will not assist the patient's comprehension of speech. It is more important to speak clearly, simply, and slowly for these people.

HYSTERICAL DEAFNESS

The most common type of psychogenic deafness is called *hysterical deafness*. Deep emotional conflicts within the personality structure involve the sense of hearing and manifest themselves in a total loss of hearing. Unconscious conflicts are the cause of hearing loss. The disturbing emotional problem is converted into an impairment of hearing. Such substitution for the emotional problem is called conversion, and the resulting deafness is termed *conversion hysteria*. The patient is unaware of the conflict, which has found a substitute solution, or he does not understand its true nature.

MALINGERING

Psychogenic dysacusis should not be confused with malingering. The patient who exhibits malingering knows that he can hear but pretends that he is deaf to escape unpleasant duties and responsibilities. The possibility of malingering must be considered in the military situation and in medicolegal circumstances whenever the patient being tested may gain financially if he has a sufficient impairment in hearing.

CONSERVATION OF HEARING IN ELDERLY PEOPLE

For the geriatric population, the problem of hazardous noise-exposure becomes less important, and the maintenance of reasonable hygiene of the ear becomes more routine. There are fewer risks, as people grow older, from dirt and water or from the common cold. The characteristic hearing loss of old age is neural in etiology, and there is no effective precautionary measure to guard against it.

Something can be done, however, to protect communication by speech. As hearing begins to deteriorate in elderly persons, they can begin to use hearing aids. They can take lessons in speech reading, and if their hearing losses become severe, they can learn how to keep their own voices pleasant and intelligible.

The problem is to begin soon enough while the geriatric patient is still adaptable, able to learn, and willing to make the necessary effort.

REFERENCES

American Heart Association. *Aphasia and the Family*, pp. 17–22 (1969).

CARROLL, V., SCHUELL, H., STREET, B. S. Clinical treatment of aphasia. *J. Speech Hearing Dis.* 20: 43, 1955.

N. GESHWIND. The organization of language and the brain. *Science* 170:940, 1970.

GREENE, M. C. L. *The Voice and Its Disorders.* Philadelphia and Toronto: Lippincott, 1964.

SIMENON, GEORGES. *The Bells of Bicetre.* New York: Harcourt, Brace and World, 1963.

STETSON, R. H. Esophageal speech for any laryngectomized patient. *Arch. Otolaryng.* 26:132, 1937.

WEPMAN, JOSEPH M. A conceptual model for the processes involved in recovery from aphasia. *J. Speech Hearing Dis.* 18:4, 4–13, 1953.

14

The Social Worker

The aged and the chronically ill face many changes in their relationships to society and in the reactions of society toward them. Some of these effects of increasing age or disability are summarized as follows:*

Increasing social isolation brought about through:

1. Death of contemporaries—either family or friends.

2. Physical limitations on ability to get about.

3. Physical limitations on communication—failing sight, impaired hearing, etc.

4. Retirement from daily contact with fellow employees.

5. Children growing up and moving away.

Growth in problems of daily living:

1. Inability to perform at the same level of physical competence as in younger days. Caring for the house, shopping, getting on and off the bus, etc., all become more difficult.

2. Having to assume new duties that were formerly performed by husband or wife.

3. Housing arrangements suitable during younger days become a burden to manage; there may be too many rooms to care for, steep stairs, a difficult furnace, a large yard.

4. Limitations on ability to plan activities ahead because of the difficulty of predicting how one will feel at a given time, weather conditions, etc.

Limitation of personal choice:

1. In addition to the limitations imposed by financial need and physical infirmity, there are

limitations imposed by lack of community resources.

2. No services may be available which will enable the person needing some help in daily living to remain in his own home, so the only alternative may be permanent removal to a nursing home.

3. The kind of nursing-home care available may offer little choice to the individual either in quality of medical care or in the type of personal treatment.

4. There may be denial of employment opportunities or other types of arbitrary exclusions solely on the basis of chronological age.

Decreased sense of present value as a person because of:

1. Increasing social isolation.

2. Limitations on personal choice.

3. Lack of interesting ways to occupy one's time.

4. Lack of things to do that are useful to others.

5. A feeling of being a burden to others, especially to children with whom one must live or upon whom one must depend for financial support.

6. The tendency of younger people to equate lack of physical competence with lack of mental competence or to equate transitory periods of confusion with permanent and complete incompetence.

7. Self-awareness of memory loss, of periods of confusion and worry about what the future holds.

Increased physical infirmities:

1. Tendency to poor dietary habits of those living alone (tea and toast).

* After Foster, H. B. *The Role of the Caseworker.* Bureau of Public Assistance, Public Assistance Report No. 30. Department of Health, Education and Welfare, 1958.

2. Cumulative effect of chronic conditions developed during one's lifetime.

3. Increased susceptibility to severely disabling illness and worry about future ability to care for oneself.

4. Need for regular medical care which ameliorates effects of or retards advance of chronic illness.

To help the aged and chronically ill cope with these altered social relationships and their many related problems and to deal with such a wide variety of personalities, preferences, and socioeconomic backgrounds of patients, the social worker requires a range of understanding and skill which can only be acquired through professional training. The term *social worker* is defined as the professional person whose education, preparation, and practice qualify him, or her, for membership in the National Association of Social Workers (NASW). Currently, there are seventy-five schools of social work in the United States and Canada accredited by the Council of Social Work Education, with student enrollment amounting to 12,000 and yearly graduating over 5,000 with MSW (Master of Social Work) degrees. There are also more than two hundred colleges which have undergraduate programs in Social Welfare that offer a baccalaureate degree and train social workers to perform work requiring lesser skills. The National Association of Social Workers, with its 50,000 members, sets the standards for the profession. The Social Security Administration, in 1965, specified that the provider of medical care and nursing care to be covered under Medicare must identify medically related social needs of the patient and provide services to meet them while the patient is undergoing treatment and care.

Illness must be viewed as a disturbance in a person's life. Inasmuch as it can cause changes in a person's life-style and goal, one must not focus upon it to the point that the total person is overlooked. Aging is a normal phase in the life process rather than a time of crisis. The need for psychological and social support should,

therefore, be expected as a natural and appropriate course. Hospital administrators, having considered emotional and social components of illness and the normal needs of the aged in patient care, have enlarged the function of the hospital from merely treating diseased individuals to treating patients as persons. By attending to the psychosocial needs in addition to physical needs, medical service is thus humanized.

Today the hospital has a responsibility which extends beyond its doors. In Massachusetts, recent legislation requiring hospitals to implement continuity of care and to establish continuing-care services, supervised by nursing and social-service personnel, is an attempt to ensure that the total person is being served. A good continuing-care plan begins even before the patient enters the hospital. To ensure appropriate admission, selective preadmission screening is encouraged. Regularly held staff meetings focused on continuing care to establish treatment goals for each patient, to review plans periodically, to recommend discharge goals, to evaluate progress of continuing-care activities, and to report on follow-up findings of discharged patients, are essential when the patient's psychosocial needs are regarded.

Traditionally, social service workers in hospitals worked with referrals from physicians, nurses, patients, or families, and outside agencies. Priority was usually given to crises or noted discharge problems. Recognizing that illness, disability, and hospitalization represent crises to most aged and chronically ill patients and their families, and that the degree of anxiety associated with them generally weakens existing adaptive mechanisms and defenses, social service has become an integral part of comprehensive medical care. It is geared to cope with all problems of aged and chronically ill patients and is not limited to handling only concrete details, such as financial matters or discharge planning.

A recent study done at the Mt. Sinai Hospital, New York, where 165 social-service case records for patients 65 years or older, selected at random, were analyzed, identified twelve categories of social needs requiring social service. They are: (1) anxiety reactions to hospitalization, (2) anxiety as a hindrance to discharge, (3) chronic institutional care, (4) complaints, (5) concrete aids, (6) convalescent care, (7) home help, (8) housing, (9) finances, (10) potential discharge against medical advice, (11) problem patients, and (12) transition in role relationships. Experience has shown that these needs are also typical of those found in a rehabilitation and chronic-disease hospital.

The admission interview is a good point of entry for forming a relationship necessary to attend to the social needs. It serves to identify the patients and families who may need short- or long-term social service and to uncover soluble problems before they become critical. It relieves much of their stressful experience, particularly upon learning of diagnosis, prognosis, prescribed medical care, and changes in social situation. A psychosocial summary on the medical chart, alerting the staff to the patient's specific needs, helps to form an effective comprehensive treatment plan and increases the staff's ability to deal with the patient and family. Progressive medical care begins not only with the patient and family understanding what services are available, but with their comfort in knowing someone cares about the patient's psychosocial needs.

The American Hospital Association, in 1961, defined, as follows, the functions of social workers in their cooperation with physicians, nurses, and other paramedical personnel in providing services for the sick:

1. To give the entire health team a better understanding of the patient and his social and emotional environment.

2. To help the patient and his family accept the illness and residual physical disability.

3. To assist the patient and his family with problems precipitated by the illness.

4. To encourage optimum utilization of medical care.

5. To help the individual achieve his fullest capacities.

6. To encourage more effective use of hospital beds for the acutely ill through the utilization of other community resources for the chronically ill when hospital care is no longer needed.

7. To encourage development of new resources for unmet social-service needs.

8. To participate in studies which will contribute toward improved patient care and improved health programs in the community.

Recent emphasis on an effective delivery system of health care has been of major concern, and the social worker's role has, therefore, expanded. In 1971, the same organization recommended that a hospital social-work program be divided into three categories of services, here summarized in part:

1. Services to the patients and their families:
   a) Casefinding: the staff is expected to seek out patients who need help, not just wait for referrals.
   b) Direct service—through casework or group work which includes continuity of care as a hospital responsibility.
   c) Consultation—as an indirect service to or on behalf of the patients or their families.
   d) Collaboration—using team approach within the hospital or community on behalf of the patients.

2. Service to the hospital:
   a) Involvement in hospital committees, e.g., in program planning and policy and procedure development.
   b) Education of staff and students.
   c) Research and demonstration to help the hospital provide better patient care and develop future social-work programs or total-care programs.

3. Service to the community:
   a) Participation in community action to advocate social changes.
   b) Keeping the community informed about the hospital in order to give the public a better understanding of health-

care needs and programs and to stimulate them to effective action.

Generally speaking, the social worker, who is trained to recognize the psychosocial difficulties and needs of disabled people and their families, can perform either one of the following roles when serving the patient. He can be a change agent in a health setting promoting a better health-care system, an enabler in an individual therapeutic situation using social casework or group-work methods; or he can be an advocate participating in community or legislative reform to achieve better services of a wider scale and of permanent nature. In 1967, it was estimated that 20,000 social workers were employed in the United States in health-related programs.

The major function of the social workers in most health settings, which are concerned with comprehensive health care, is direct service to the patients and families, since psychosocial stresses that interfere with the effective use of preventive, rehabilitative, and follow-up services must be alleviated in order to make efficient use of health manpower and resources.

To achieve this objective, social workers use various treatment modalities, such as social casework, group work, and family conference. Social casework helps the patient find a satisfactory solution or adjustment to physical, social, emotional, and economic problems. Mary E. Davis wrote that social casework begins with the establishment of a relationship with an individual, in which the individual feels accepted as a person and at ease during the purposeful interviews with the social worker. She stated also that this method, itself, is based upon the same principle of management as those used by administrators (planning, organizing, staffing, directing, and controlling).

Ann Hartman wrote that in the practice of crisis intervention, the client, with the help of the worker and the utilization of personal and environmental resources, is enabled to turn a threatening, and possibly debilitating, life experience into an opportunity to grow, to develop new coping mechanisms, and even to work through old, unresolved losses or conflicts that emerge as a result of the current crisis.

Through the use of interviewing skills, the social worker explores those elements in the patient's situation, both current and past, that directly affect his health problem. Exploration may include the patient's ideas, feelings about illness, his relationship with members of his family and with others, his religious beliefs, and his occupational goals. On the basis of the information obtained, a social diagnosis is made by evaluating how these factors may be affecting the patient's illness, treatment, recovery, and maintenance of health. Social treatment includes a plan of action to help the patient and his family either to resolve the problem or to adjust to the situation. In short, the social worker endeavors to achieve some of the things that practitioners in the past accomplished by intuition, and which today's specialized and busy physician can no longer handle adequately.

Social group-work programs can be used for various purposes in hospital or health settings. Louise A. Frey said, "The hospital is an authoritarian setting usually characterized by a great gap between the patient system and the staff system, and it can be a bridge between them when the social worker becomes involved in the patient system by working with spontaneous natural groups." It can serve as a medium for healthy group interactions, allowing members with the same disability to assemble regularly and purposefully to help them assume responsibility for themselves and handle their emotional responses to illness and hospitalization. It can also serve as a means to help the patients to clarify their misunderstandings about matters relating to illness and to increase their receptivity of information, such as diagnosis and prognosis, through group process.

The family conference is used to increase understanding of realities in the patient's situation and, very often, can lead to attitudinal changes of relatives toward the patient and his disability. It is a very important tool when used to set therapeutic goals with the cooperation of the relatives, particularly in a rehabilitation program. In multichildren families, the share of responsibility toward a patient's care to be taken by each person can be worked out in a family conference where the social worker plays an objective role. The patient's participation is sometimes necessary to effect a sound decision regarding his care.

Old-age and chronic illness cause more severe and extended disruptions of social relationships and create more serious economic problems than most acute illnesses. In these situations, the support offered to patients and their families by social workers is important and leads to better adjustment of both the patient and the relatives. The social worker's responsibility in a rehabilitation plan includes helping identify the direction and potential strength of the patient's motivation for recovery or work. It is the social worker who is most concerned with helping the patient to recognize his potential and work toward reaching it. Needless to say, work toward change and growth in the patient is done with an understanding and acceptance of the limitations of both the social worker and the patient.

The role of the social worker is important, not only during a patient's hospitalization and rehabilitation, but also during confinement to a nursing home. Social workers are often the only link with the outside world for nursing-home inmates, because they alone assume the role which ordinarily is the family's function, namely, to give these lonely patients a sense of someone still caring. Even though some families take good care of their aged and chronically ill, keeping them in their homes or visiting them often in institutions, such families may still benefit from consulting a social worker who is familiar with social agencies and community services, which may stand ready to assist with their problems. The prevention of social deterioration or breakdown by the use of accurate multidisciplinary assessment is always the social worker's objective.

Just as to neighborhood health facilities and visiting nurses serving the aged at home, the patient's accessibility to social service help is important. Often times, the local public-assistance social worker is the only one available.

Helping an elderly person to review his past or to reminisce enables him to increase his understanding of himself which may lead to a sense of fulfillment and direction and self-esteem. Dealing with death and dying, which are natural phenomena, has also been included as a social-work responsibility in many facilities caring for the aged and chronically ill. Depression among the aged relating to loss or reduced physical ability is very common and many are mentally not ready to accept dying. Social workers are aware of the psychological process that takes place after learning of a poor prognosis, and their objective should be to help the patient live out the remaining days with minimal emotional stress.

"*Team work* is a necessity in any public health or medical setting in order to coordinate the services of many specialists," wrote Margaret Bourg. An understanding of the various functions of team members and a respect for their judgment are essential in team work. In caring for the aged and chronically ill, the social worker brings to the team her knowledge of social and community resources as well as her understanding of the psychosocial needs of the patients. She must be at all times aware of the patient's medical situation in which the physician makes the decision.

Social service is known to have a dual role of helping the patient and collaborating with the team to make patient-care decisions. Harriet Bartlett wrote that she is not only concerned with the interplay of medical and social factors and their bearing on the patient, she is continuously concerned with all the significant working relationships that are involved in the care of the patient. These include the worker-patient relationship, the patient's relationship with all the team members who are closest to him, and the worker's own relationship with them in turn. The role of the social worker differs from that of physician and nurse in that her permissive approach is in contrast to the authoritative approach of the medical staff. Essentially, it is with the permissive approach that she can help reduce psychosocial stress and conflict and enable the patient to increase social functioning. Successful team work depends on the staff's conviction about its value and its benefit to the patient as well as understanding the role of each member.

REFERENCES

BARTLETT, H. M. *Social Work Practice in the Health Field*. New York: National Association of Social Workers, 1961.

BERKMAN, BARBARA GORDON, and REHR, HELEN. Social needs of the hospitalized elderly: A classification. *Social Work Journal* 17:4, pp. 80–88, 1972.

BOURG, MARGARET S. The medical social worker's role in the clinical team. *Med. Soc. Work* 1,3, pp. 33–37, 1952.

DAVIS, MARY E. The practice of social work in hospitals. *Hosp. Prog.* 52, pp. 60–62, January, 1971.

Encyclopedia of Social Work. New York: National Association of Social Workers, 1971.

Essentials of Social Service Department in Hospitals and Related Institutions. Chicago: American Hospital Assoc., 1961.

Essentials of Social Work Programs in Hospitals. Chicago: American Hospital Assoc., 1971.

FOSTER, H. B. *The Role of the Caseworker*. Public Assistance Report #30. Washington, D.C.: Bureau of Public Assistance, 1958.

FREY, LOUISE A. (Ed.). *Use of Group in the Health Field*. New York: National Association of Social Workers, 1966.

HARTMAN, ANN. But what is social casework? *Social Casework* 52:7, pp. 411–419, July, 1971.

Health Resources Statistics, 1968. Washington, D.C.: National Center of Health Statistics, Public Health Services, U.S. Department of Health, Education and Welfare, 1968.

LURIE, HARRY L. (Ed.). Preface. In *Encyclopedia of Social Work*. New York: National Association of Social Workers, 1965.

15
The Dietitian

When one looks at elderly persons and considers all the ramifications of their nutrition, one comes to the conclusion that the majority of the aged have everything going against them. For example, at least eight million of the nineteen million persons over age 65 are edentulous, and about 23 percent of these have dentures which are ill fitting or unsatisfactory in one way or another. This usually leads to increased intake of improper foods which are low in bulk.

A sharp decrease in financial income frequently limits the choice of foods which the elderly can purchase. Less expensive high-carbohydrate foods are mainly available as the geriatric individual finds himself able to buy less meat and dairy products, fewer fresh vegetables and fresh fruits.

Many senior citizens are infirm, have residual physical disabilities, are poorly motivated, and by habit seem to seek out convenience foods which require little or no preparation. These are usually higher in carbohydrates and fats. Loneliness, anxiety, and depression may also reduce their appetites.

Basically, the older citizens' nutritional requirements are the same as they were at age 25, except for the calories. By the time sunset years have arrived, however, dietary patterns have been set, and these people continue to eat as many calories as they did when young, which often leads to obesity. In general, the National Research Council states that an intake of 2,200 calories per day is adequate for the average older person. To offset this tendency and to decrease caloric intake, a reduction of the foods high in carbohydrates and fats should be instituted. This

is not easy and more time has to be spent adjusting the meal pattern. One may emphasize that eating is a social event. Thus when an elderly person lives alone, it might help to invite a guest to dinner, thus making the meal a special event. A glass of wine or a bottle of beer adds zest, provided, of course, the people involved are allowed to drink. Food patterns and eating habits are frequently influenced by long-standing cultural backgrounds, religious beliefs, and socioeconomic factors. Most people have formed very definite ideas about their food likes and dislikes and, unfortunately, sometimes even about their own dietary needs.

When counseling people about dietary modifications, it is important to individualize each plan. If one does not seriously consider the individual factors, any chance of the patient's success in adhering to the diet will be limited. It is necessary to know about previous eating patterns (take a nutrition history), economic status, home conditions, and physical abilities or limitations. Then all persons involved in the care of the patient should be included in the final instructions. This may include family and/or the visiting nurse, as well as a homemaker, friend, and/or the patient himself, if mentally competent. The dietitian should include her work telephone number on the instruction sheet so that further consultation may be made.

DIETARY NEEDS

Some of the dietary problems encountered in the care of the chronically ill are greater when the effect of illness on eating is considered. As stated previously, eating is a social function, a time to join with family and friends. In the hospital, especially at first, the patient becomes tense because he is away from his family and friends, and in some cases, he is also depressed and frustrated because he can no longer care for himself. The illness itself may have an effect on the eating habits of the patient, for example, physical handicaps resulting in poor motor skills and limited range of motion; or paralysis of the face or throat muscles may make eating messy and cause the patient to feel thwarted and even to seek isolation from the rest of the patients. If this occurs, it may, in turn, cause a reduction in food intake. As he improves, he should be encouraged to join others for a more sociable mealtime relationship. To help him become more self-sufficient the food should be cut into bite size or put into sandwiches for easy handling. More and more demand is being made for medical institutions to provide group dining areas.

Medical Problems of Diet

Long-term immobilization may cause nutritional problems, such as nitrogen and mineral loss, which can lead to decalcification of bone, gastrointestinal malfunction caused by poor functioning of the biliary tract, formation of decubiti, and even obesity. Chronic illness can also lead to malnutrition, which in turn can complicate the underlying disease. Since many immobilized patients have poor appetites, a great deal of ingenuity is necessary to stimulate the increase of food intake. The tray must look appetizing; the food must taste good and must be served hot. In some cases, caloric and/or protein supplements must be added. For those patients with nitrogen loss or decubiti, higher protein diets as well as a lowered intake of calcium may be beneficial.

A common complication for paraplegics is urinary infection, and an insufficient fluid intake may contribute to the cause. Stroke patients also very often become dehydrated, so in both cases, a close supervision of their fluid intake is neces-

sary. At least 5 quarts of water or other beverages should be taken each day.

In paraplegics, a high incidence of decubiti may be decreased by increasing the daily protein to 100 to 150 grams a day.

During a rehabilitation program, patients will be using muscles in a more strenuous manner. Muscle strengthening is necessary, and protein is the main body-building source. The body stores proteins in different areas, such as muscle, skin, bone, lungs, and brains, but there is a greater turnover in the liver, pancreas, blood plasma, kidneys, and intestinal wall. Because of this, protein may be transferred from muscle to other areas needing protein, thus causing wasted muscles and general weakness. Along with this, the patient may become more susceptible to infection. Approximately 25 grams of protein daily are needed for maintenance, and since not all the protein ingested is utilized, larger amounts of protein may be necessary daily for long periods of time.

In addition to the above, other disorders such as atherosclerosis, hypertension, and diabetes occur. All three are aggravated by obesity, which can be a real problem for this type of patient. Because of their lack of activity and constant thought of food, weight control can become very difficult for everyone involved. Families must be informed of what, if any, foods can be brought in to the patient. The patient, also, should be instructed so that he will understand why all those rich or highly salted foods he likes are excluded from the diet.

Following onset of a stroke, patients may have to be fed very soft or strained foods. Diets of this type can be very depressing, as they make patients feel even less independent. Whenever possible, give whole vegetables or fruits which can be mashed. Also, if patients have aphasia, they may have difficulty communicating their preferences, thus leading to apathy and discouragement with loss of appetite and decreased food consumption. When this occurs, a periodic evaluation of their intake should be made to prevent further weight loss and weakness. Body weights should be followed weekly. Much patience and understanding is necessary when working with this group.

The most popular and basic diet recommended for the sick is the normal, regular, or so-called house diet. This diet is prescribed for the majority of ill patients, and the proper nutrition provided may aid in faster recovery. Then too, therapeutic diets are usually modifications of the normal diet.

When planning a basic menu, include the following foods:

MILK GROUP

Two or more glasses of milk (fat free, regular, or powdered instant milk reconstituted). Cheese, ice cream, and other milk-made foods may be substituted.

MEAT GROUP

Two or more servings of meat, fish, or poultry a day. Eggs are another possibility but should not be eaten more than twice per week. Dry beans, peas, lentils, nuts, and peanut butter may be used as alternates.

VEGETABLES AND FRUITS

Four or more servings. Include one serving of citrus fruit for vitamin C and one serving of a dark-green vegetable or a dark-yellow vegetable at least every other day for vitamin A.

BREADS AND CEREALS

Four or more servings (enriched, whole-grain, or restored).

FATS, OILS, AND SUGARS

These are not included in the basic four groups since these foods are used more to enhance the flavor of the above foods. Fats and oils are the most concentrated sources of calories, also the most satisfying, because they take longer to digest. As a means of preventive medicine, a good rule is to use polyunsaturated fats in the form of vegetable oils and spreads made from vegetable oils. Meat should also be served lean.

Sugars provide empty calories—meaning that they are foods which are low in nutrients but high in calories. Often, too, these foods taken in large quantity may promote tooth decay.

WATER

At least 10 large glasses of water or other liquid should be taken.

Without the fats and sugars, the four main food groups provide approximately 1300 calories. The fats and sweets will add about 500 to 1000 calories, bringing the total daily intake up to 1800 to 2300 calories.

SAMPLE MENU

Breakfast
½ cup of orange juice
1 hard cooked egg
1 slice of buttered toast
1 glass of milk
Coffee with cream and sugar
Lunch
Fruit-salad plate with cottage cheese
1 roll
1 pat of margarine or butter
1 serving of tapioca pudding
Tea with milk and sugar
Supper
½ cup of soup
1 serving of roast beef
1 baked potato with margarine or butter
1 serving of cooked carrots
Lettuce and tomato salad with vegetable-oil
    dressing
Ice cream
Coffee with cream and sugar
Snack
Small glass of fruit juice
Sugar cookies

To increase the protein, add more meat, fish, poultry, milk, eggs, and cheese. Powdered milk may be added to whole milk, soup, gravies, or cakes. Occasionally, concentrated protein supplements may be necessary, especially for patients with poor appetites. These can be difficult to mix but may be used as directed by adding to water or milk. Even in the powdered form they may be added to applesauce or fruit juice. To increase the calories, the following foods may be added to the basic diet: cream, cakes, cookies, pastries, puddings, custards, jams, jellies, and nuts.

To reduce calories, do not use most of the above high-caloric foods and substitute fruits for high-caloric desserts, and if acceptable, use skim milk instead of regular milk. Food portions may also need decreasing.

To help the physician choose the proper caloric level, refer to the table on Recommended Dietary Allowances (see Table 5).

LIQUID DIETS AND TUBE FEEDINGS

Patients with throat cancer or those who have difficulty swallowing may require a liquid diet for an extended period. This may be taken either orally in the form of strained fruit juices, strained soups, thinned-out cooked cereals, jellos, puddings, and milk, or they may be taken through a tube utilizing blenderized meals. To increase calories and protein in a liquid diet, add creams, soups, milk shakes, eggnogs, and ice cream.

In the case of tube feeding, a blender is very useful. A diet consisting of bread, milk, fruit juice, strained meat, and vegetables is blended, liquefied, and strained through a fine-meshed strainer. There are also special commercial mixtures which meet the basic nutrient requirements that may be more convenient. The levels of nutrient intake can be controlled more accurately by tube feeding than by any other diet. But in all cases, physicians should be aware of the vitamin content since a vitamin supplement may have to be prescribed.

Diarrhea is a complication of tube feedings and may sometimes be avoided by giving small, frequent feedings with proper refrigeration and short-term storage.

When the patient has left the hospital, there are further resources to utilize if necessary. Some communities, aware of certain problems, have set up services such as Meals on Wheels. Hot meals are prepared and delivered to those unable to shop or prepare foods for themselves. The price usually depends upon what each person can afford. The meals are usually planned by a dietitian so that special diets may be included. One hot meal, usually the noon meal, is sent out; but cold meals, such as a sandwich or dessert, may be included to be used later in the day.

Another service is the Homemaker or Home Health Aide Service. A trained Homemaker goes into the home and helps the family maintain a regular routine when the patient first returns. Help in planning, preparing, and even purchasing the food necessary for meals is included in this service.

In the past few years, a new service has been instituted in many large cities called *Dial-A-Dietitian*. This is a free telephone service offered to the community by the State Dietetic Association. There are trained dietitians and nutritionists who have volunteered their services to provide information on normal nutrition, nutrient content of food, special diet recipes, food additives, food preparation and purchasing. Diets may not be prescribed and medical advice is not given, but the client may be referred to a family physician or appropriate agencies. This is an answering service, the question is recorded and sent to the dietitian who has volunteered for that day. She returns the call with the answer within 48 hours.

Another unique service is called *Eldecare Services, Inc.* For $59.00 a week, this service delivers three meals a day to an elderly person's home, cleans the house once per week, does whatever shopping is needed, takes the person to the doctor, dentist, or hospital for appointments, and even empties the trash. For extra cost, they can also provide nursing or live-in help. Phone service is maintained over a 24-hour period for emergencies.

Embellishments such as a lily at Easter time,

TABLE 5. RECOMMENDED DIETARY ALLOWANCES

	Age in Years	Weight (kg)	Weight (lbs)	Height (cm)	Height (in)	K Cal	Protein (gms)	Vitamin A I.U.	Vitamin D I.U.	Vitamin E I.U.	Ascorbic Acid (mg)	Folacin (mg)	Niacin (mg) Equiv.	Riboflavin (mg)	Thiamin (mg)	Vitamin Bb (mg)	Vitamin B₁₂ (mg)	Calcium (gms)	Phosphorus (gms)	Iodine (mg)	Iron (mg)	Magnesium (mg)
											Water Soluble Vitamins							Minerals				
Males	10–12	35	77	140	55	2500	45	4500	400	20	40	0.4	17	1.3	1.3	1.4	5	1.2	1.2	125	10	300
	12–14	43	95	151	59	2700	50	5000	400	20	45	0.4	18	1.4	1.4	1.6	5	1.4	1.4	135	18	350
	14–18	59	130	170	67	3000	60	5000	400	25	55	0.4	20	1.5	1.5	1.8	5	1.4	1.4	150	18	400
	18–22	67	147	175	69	2800	60	5000	400	30	60	0.4	18	1.6	1.4	2.0	5	0.8	0.8	140	10	400
	22–35	70	154	175	69	2800	65	5000	—	30	60	0.4	18	1.7	1.4	2.0	5	0.8	0.8	140	10	350
	35–55	70	154	173	68	2600	65	5000	—	30	60	0.4	17	1.7	1.3	2.0	5	0.8	0.8	125	10	350
	55–75+	70	154	171	67	2400	65	5000	—	30	60	0.4	14	1.7	1.2	2.0	6	0.8	0.8	110	10	350
Females	10–12	35	77	142	56	2250	50	4500	400	20	40	0.4	15	1.3	1.1	1.4	5	1.2	1.2	110	18	300
	12–14	44	97	154	61	2300	50	5000	400	20	45	0.4	15	1.4	1.2	1.6	5	1.3	1.3	115	18	350
	14–16	52	114	157	62	2400	55	5000	400	25	50	0.4	16	1.4	1.2	1.8	5	1.3	1.3	120	18	350
	16–18	54	119	160	63	2300	55	5000	400	25	50	0.4	15	1.5	1.2	2.0	5	1.3	1.3	115	18	350
	18–22	58	128	163	64	2000	55	5000	400	25	55	0.4	13	1.5	1.0	2.0	5	0.8	0.8	100	18	350
	22–35	58	128	163	64	2000	55	5000	—	25	55	0.4	13	1.5	1.0	2.0	5	0.8	0.8	100	18	300
	35–55	58	128	160	63	1850	55	5000	—	25	55	0.4	13	1.5	1.0	2.0	5	0.8	0.8	90	18	300
	55–75+	58	128	157	62	1700	55	5000	—	25	55	0.4	13	1.5	1.0	2.0	6	0.8	0.8	80	10	300

Recommended Dietary Allowances. (7th ed.). Food Nutrition Board National Academy of Sciences National Research Council, Pub. No. 1694, 1962.

a St. Patrick's Day carnation, or a little gift on a birthday add the human touch.

HELPFUL REFERENCES FOR THOSE ON SPECIAL DIETS

DIABETES MELLITUS

Behrman, Deaconess Maude. *A Cookbook for Diabetics*. Available from the American Diabetes Association, Inc., 18 East 48th Street, New York, New York—10017. $1.00.

Forecast. A bimonthly magazine for diabetics, published by the Diabetic Association, offers recipes which give the exchange values.

SODIUM RESTRICTED DIET

Payne, A. S., and Cablahan, D. *The Fat and Sodium Control Cookbook* (3rd ed.). Boston: Little, Brown, 1965. This may be purchased in a bookstore.

Materials from the American Heart Association Inc., 44 East 23rd Street, New York, New York—10010, or your local Heart Association. Patient copies require physician's prescription, but there is no charge.

Booklets:
Your 500 Milligram Sodium Diet
Your 100 Milligram Sodium Diet
Your Mild Sodium-Restricted Diet
The Cook Book for Low Sodium Diets

FAT-CONTROLLED, DECREASED SATURATED FAT, LOW-CHOLESTEROL DIETS

Dobbin, V., et al. *Low Fat, Low Cholesterol Diet*. Garden City, N.Y.: Doubleday, 1970.

Materials from the American Heart Association, Inc., 44 East 23rd Street, New York, New York—10010, or your local Heart Association. Patient copies require physician's prescription, but there is no charge.

Booklets:
Planning Fat-Controlled Meals for 1200 and 1800 Calories.
Planning Fat-Controlled Meals for 2000–2600 Calories.

Leaflets:
The Way to a Man's Heart
Recipes for Fat-Controlled, Low-Cholesterol Diets.

16
The Psychiatrist

The state of well-being is at once a physical sensation and an emotional experience. Familiar phrases such as "feeling hale and hearty" or "relaxed and happy" illustrate our common association of the states of physical and mental health.

On the other hand, when we feel tense and anxious or tired and depressed, such combinations of physical and emotional discomfort suggest dysfunction in either or in both the bodily and the mental spheres. The effect of even minor illnesses, such as a common cold, on our ability and willingness to perform unpleasant tasks, while they actually affect very little our capacity to engage in rewarding and absorbing activities, is an example from everyday life of the myriad ways in which the soma and the psyche mutually influence each other and are indelibly bonded together.

In patients who have suffered a major physical trauma, a stroke, a serious brain injury, or a mutilating operation, the interplay between body and soul, between physical and emotional states is sometimes dramatically, at other times more subtly, reflected in the vicissitudes of their rehabilitative course. Depressive reactions, attempts to deny the seriousness of their condition, or regressive demandingness and excessive complaining, all are anticipated signs of a painful readjustment process. One or more of these reactions will, without fail, occur at some time with varying intensity in all these patients during their recovery period.

Hospital personnel, who devote their lives to the rehabilitation and care of such sick persons, may either fail to notice these reactions or consider them so much part and parcel of the expected so-called "normal" course of events that they take them for granted. As long as these adjustment reactions do not noticeably protract the patient's rehabilitative course and do not cause serious management problems, the daily hospital routine can absorb a considerable amount of fluctuation in mood and behavior of patients and personnel alike.

When a patient's depression does not lift, however, but increases in severity, when he refuses to get out of bed or to cooperate with the prescribed rehabilitative program, the helping staff often experiences increasing frustration and mounting resentment against him, which can paralyze their efforts and so jeopardize his treatment even further. Mrs. H. is a good example of a patient who, because she had great difficulty in coming to terms with her physical impairments, presented initially a considerable problem to a rehabilitation-center staff.

A 64-year-old widow, Mrs. H. had been in good health until her stroke, which occurred four months prior to her hospitalization at the rehabilitation center. According to the reports of her married daughter, Mrs. H. had always been a hard-working, proud, and energetic woman who believed that hard work could cure anything. Widowed early in her marriage, she took pride in supporting herself and her only child by working as a cleaning woman. Now, following her stroke, Mrs. H.'s right arm was paralyzed.

Upon arrival, Mrs. H. seemed full of good cheer and "expecting a miracle," but after a month at the center, she became completely disillusioned. She saw her disability as a sign of personal failure, because, as she and her daughter told us, illness and disability are conditions "not to be given in to." The patient was unwilling to learn to use her left arm more skillfully, because she could not accept the paralysis of the right and could not tolerate "doing something in thirty minutes which used to take her ten." Empathy, reassurance, and appeal to reason had, if any, only an adverse effect upon this patient; she had become more and more stubbornly resistive, outraged, and fractious.

Over and over again, we see that knowledge of a patient's earlier life experience, style, and premorbid personality traits are extremely important in determining how he can best be motivated to cooperate with some type of rehabilitative regime. Mrs. H., an energetic, no-nonsense person before her cerebrovascular accident, could not tolerate explicit expressions of sympathy and concern for her illness, because she could not empathize with herself as a handicapped person. Sympathy with and attention to these handicaps only served to reinforce her self-depreciation and self-condemnation. When it dawned on Mrs. H. that despite her most fervent desires, she would not be able to return home as good as new, she slumped into an angry, resistive, and reproachful attitude. She succeeded in making the physical-therapy staff feel guilty for not fulfilling her magical expectations, but as they redoubled their efforts to help her, Mrs. H. felt worse.

As soon as the psychiatrist's recommendation for a more matter of fact, no-nonsense approach to Mrs. H. was adopted, however, her reproaches toward herself and others diminished considerably. A sensible routine was established, and Mrs. H. was kept busy with a full range of regularly scheduled, precisely defined, and prescribed tasks, activities, and exercises, which she was expected to accomplish and which left her little time to derogate herself and others. This regime capitalized on this patient's need to be active and doing. It provided her with some of her own medicine, which had carried her along successfully and happily for so many years. She was minimally fussed over, treated matter-of-factly, and kept constructively busy.

When the staff was able to take a more realistic attitude toward this patient's handicap, Mrs. H. herself could let go of her magical expectations. This made her more appreciative of what she could accomplish with help from others and relieved her own as well as their feelings of obligation and guilt that the impossible could not be achieved. Very soon thereafter, Mrs. H. began to make substantial progress, regained some of her lost self-esteem, and was able to perform simple household tasks sufficiently well to be able to return to her home much improved.

Unfortunately, the story of Mr. F., who was also a source of serious concern, had a less favorable ending.

Mr. F., a 45-year-old patient with severe diabetes, was admitted for rehabilitation following an amputation above his right knee. The amputation had become unavoidable when he developed gangrene in his right foot. From his history, it seemed likely that the severity of his diabetes was in part due to Mr. F.'s own unwillingness to adhere to a diet and also to bouts of excessive drinking. His wife described him as a moody and frequently depressed man with a low tolerance for frustration and disappointment, who was very dependent upon her.

The staff was extremely upset at Mr. F.'s unwillingness to stay on a diet, his total refusal at times to eat, his withdrawal from other patients, his despondency, utter passivity, and his increasingly demanding and regressive behavior. Upon several occasions Mr. F. had wet his bed. When his wife and children came to visit him, he turned away from them.

The description of this patient's behavior, his total apathy and increasing withdrawal, impressed the psychiatric consultant as suicidal in nature, and a review of Mr. F.'s earlier history helped him to understand this patient's emotional fragility.

The victim of a very deprived childhood, he was orphaned at an early age and shifted from pillar to post all during his childhood. Relatives would take him into their home for periods of time, but either Mr. F. could not stand them or they became tired of him. He married a woman several years his senior who ran the house and him. She kept both financially afloat during periods when Mr. F., who was a short-order cook, was out of work or unable to work because of ill health.

Mrs. F. made no bones about her exasperation with her sick husband, whom nobody could effectively help because he refused to be helped. She dreaded his return home as a total invalid, who would require 24-hour attendance and force her to give up a job which was bringing her both financial security and a great deal of satisfaction. Mr. F.'s low incentive for living was not helped by his awareness of his wife's reluctance to take him back into their home in his dependent and regressed condition. Not to be accepted by her on his own terms increased his resentment even more.

Our inability to motivate certain patients like Mr. F., who have severe emotional as well as serious physical problems, was most difficult for a devoted, energetic young rehabilitation-center staff to accept. Such patients cannot muster the energy and will to live, especially if their severe chronic and debilitating disease requires repeated and grossly mutilating surgical interventions.

For Mr. F., the loss of his leg was like the proverbial straw that broke the camel's back. A very dependent, emotionally labile, and insecure person, he had found it increasingly difficult to bear the continuous stress of a strict diet and the need for regularity and moderation in his eating and drinking habits. After repeated hospitalizations to regulate his medication and diet, he had finally had to undergo the amputation which left him severely debilitated and which shattered his already low self-esteem.

Self-neglect is often the hallmark of depression or lack of self-esteem and incentive to live, especially in chronically ill patients who develop secondary complications of their disease accelerated by that self-neglect. As their physical condition deteriorates, their depression, apathy, and despondency increase, which often precipitates further abrasion of their self-esteem.

Despite massive and valiant efforts by the staff to instill in Mr. F. a will to struggle and fight for his life, the patient was unable to do so. When, at the suggestion of the psychiatric consultant, he was no longer subjected to further attempts at physical rehabilitation, his extreme withdrawal and regressive behavior let up considerably. He seemed satisfied when allowed to stay in the hospital without strings attached until his death approximately six months later.

Fortunately, patients like Mr. F. are in the minority. His case, however, illustrates in stark relief how the combination of an emotionally deprived childhood, low self-esteem, a tenuous emotional investment in others, and a debilitating physical illness can conspire to precipitate an early death—despite excellent medical care and valiant attempts to rescue such a patient from his self-destructive bent.

Many patients whose rehabilitative course is unsatisfactory or atypical turn out to be lonely people who have led rather isolated lives and do not have the resilience needed to make the new adaptations their ailments require, because they have nothing and nobody to live for. Excessive demandingness, chronic complaining, and lack of progress are often their ways of expressing their resentment and frustration, their limited coping ability, and their anxiety about the future. Examples of such patients are Mr. A. and Miss C.

A consultation was requested for Mr. A. because his treatment had reached an impasse. Mr. A. had been referred to the rehabilitation center at his own specific request. Three years prior to admission, he had fallen backward down a flight of stairs and, because he complained of continuous intractable pain, a laminectomy was performed one year later. He subsequently sustained a mild stroke and was sent to a nursing home. There, he became dissatisfied with his care and requested referral to a rehabilitation center, where he wished to be readied to live by himself again as he had been doing prior to his accident.

Mr. A. complained of extreme weakness in

his arms and legs which made it impossible for him to stand up straight, to maintain his balance, or to perform a transfer using his arms. Muscle examinations did not show any abnormalities, and he had no observable sequelae of any kind, although he reported having had two strokes.

Because of the inconsistencies between the physical findings and his performance, because of the contrast between Mr. A.'s strongly expressed desire for independence and his inability to make substantial progress in that direction, an impasse had developed which led his physical therapist to request a psychiatric consultation.

Mr. A., a tall, handsome 42-year-old man, was seated in his wheelchair when the consultant came to see him. He made no spontaneous effort to wheel himself down the corridor to the interviewer's room, clearly expecting her to push him there. In a mild-mannered fashion, he complained about his fate, his ineffective medical treatment, the poor care he had received in the nursing home, the weakness of his arms and legs, and his overriding desire to return to the rooming house where he had previously lived by himself.

Members of the Social Service Department knew that Mr. A. had had a long history of physical disability beginning in childhood, namely, a weak leg that tended to buckle whenever he was surprised by a sudden noise or appearance of a person. He had indicated to them that this condition had prevented him from participating in sports and had led to a youth of isolation and loneliness. He did not remember what treatment had been prescribed for the knee, nor had this condition ever been satisfactorily diagnosed. He ascribed his lack of friends and paucity of social contacts to his physical handicap which he considered to be the cause also of his dropping out of school in the eighth grade. His father was an alcoholic who had abused the patient's mother. After his father deserted the family, Mr. A. continued to live with his mother until her death; thereafter he lived by himself until the accident of his fall down the cellar stairs.

At no time during the interview did Mr. A. seem open to reason. He reiterated repeatedly that he had come to the rehabilitation center because he wanted to live by himself and in order to do so, he had to learn to walk; having not yet mastered this skill, he was compelled to stay in the hospital, much against his own wishes. When the psychiatrist pointed out that his physical therapist seriously doubted whether he could make further progress, in which case he could not remain in the hospital, Mr. A. stated that he would, under no circumstances, return to a nursing home but must find a room for himself instead. Asked how he could manage to live by himself if he were not able to stand up, let alone walk, he reverted to his former statement that he would stay in the hospital until able to walk and live by himself.

The psychiatrist suggested to Mr. A. and his physical therapist that he be given two weeks' time to find out if he could make any substantial progress. If not, he would be discharged to a nursing home. Were he able to make major gains during this period, his stay at the hospital would be extended for another defined period of rehabilitation.

This recommendation was accepted by the patient and staff. For several days following the interview, Mr. A. found himself unable to get out of bed in the morning to attend his therapy sessions. This behavior convinced the staff that this was Mr. A.'s way of telling them that he felt unable to cope with life independently. He was discharged from the rehabilitation center in a wheelchair to a nursing home at the agreed time.

The case of Mr. A. illustrates the discrepancy which can exist between a patient's verbally expressed desires for independence and his covert wishes to be taken care of and dependent. Here the discrepancy was manifested in this patient's lack of progress and inability to perform tasks for which he had sufficient physical equipment. If realistic goals and alternatives are presented to such patients and flexible but well-defined time limits are set to accomplish what must be accomplished if they are to resume independent living upon discharge from the hospital, the rehabilitative course, without fail, points out which solution is preferable under the circumstances.

Mr. A., a passive, lonely, and schizoid man, was not able to muster the energy and motivation needed to continue living alone. Even though he resented being dependent on nursing-home personnel and would have wanted both his dependent and independent longings to be gratified at the same time, his regressive reaction following reality confrontation by the psychiatrist made clear to the staff what course of action had to be followed.

The startling contrast between word and action understandably creates a good deal of confusion in the minds of therapists and relatives alike. Their feelings of guilt, of mounting frustration and bewilderment can foster an atmosphere of hostility and impatience which, unless clarified, can in time result in long, fruitless periods of hospitalization culminating in angry separations and absent or poor after-care planning.

A psychiatric consultation was requested for Miss C. about whom the rehabilitation staff had also become quite concerned.

Miss C., a 62-year-old spinster, had been referred for rehabilitation following a hip fracture. Despite satisfactory repair as shown on the x-rays, the patient continued to complain about intractable pain in her leg. She was uncooperative with her physical therapist, and in general, very slow moving. She demanded a great deal of attention and made minimal effort to regain her independence. Very agreeable to the idea of seeing a psychiatrist, Miss C., during the interview, was mainly concerned with money matters and very well informed about her available financial resources. Rather quickly, she made it clear that she felt completely boxed in. Because of her age and because of reorganization at her place of work, she had been dismissed from her job as bank clerk. She could not take another job because, were she again able to work, her disability insurance would be taken

away from her. She might be rehired by her former company but could not accept a job offer because it would require a great deal of walking, which was impossible for her because of the pain in her leg. Too young for social security benefits, Miss C. pointed out that she could not live on that amount of money either.

Not only had Miss C. broken her leg, but she had also sustained other minor accidents over the last three years. These accidents followed closely upon the loss of her friendly and supportive supervisor at her place of work, increasing alienation from her only brother, and other losses because of age or geographic moves. Miss C. mentioned these and the recent loss of her apartment and landlady because of the hip fracture, all without any show of emotion. When the psychiatrist commented that her mental distress might be expressed in physical pain, Miss C. politely acknowledged this possibility but denied any awareness of sad feelings now or in the past. She quickly dropped any further discussion of her emotional state and returned to complaints about her painful leg and her insoluble problems.

Miss C., a rather withdrawn, rigid, and uncompromising person, had begun to lose interest in her work when her supervisor left the job. She apparently was unable to adapt to a new person and, lacking the previous supportive relationship, she could not maintain her work performance at the old level; her self-confidence diminished and she became discouraged and depressed. Miss C. could not admit to these feelings and ascribed several minor car accidents, breaking her wrist and finally her hip in the course of three years, to bad luck. Unable to bear depression, faced with old age and loneliness, now in addition handicapped by her hip fracture, she was doomed to lead the life of an invalid. Although unwilling to go to a nursing home, she could not muster enough energy and strength to face a more independent but very lonely and isolated existence.

Had we been able to provide Miss C. with partial financial support, enough to permit her to take a half-time job and thereby provide her with sufficient funds to maintain her own living quarters, the outcome of her rehabilitation program might have been more successful. It would also have given us a leverage to help her modify her rigid standards.

Unfortunately, disability and insurance policies confirmed Miss C.'s perfectionistic views that one is either all well or all sick and that there is no room for relative health and infirmity or for relative dependence and independence.

After a long stay in the hospital, during which she made little progress, she was finally discharged to a nursing home, still totally incapacitated by pain.

Although it is impossible to tell whether their depressed state was the cause for or the result of their accidents, both Mr. A. and Miss C. achieved limited gains from their rehabilitative programs; and their subsequent chronic physical and emotional invalidism becomes more understandable viewed in the light of their prior history.

To understand how Mrs. H. ticked did much to help the staff remove the emotional roadblocks which interfered with this patient's ability to use the treatment to her best advantage. Awareness of the depth of Mr. F.'s depression and sense of defeat made it ultimately possible for the hospital to resign themselves to the irrevocable outcome of his hospital course. An appreciation of Mr. A.'s and Miss C.'s predicaments helped their physical therapists to lower their expectations of these patients and to be satisfied with limited achievements.

Mrs. B.'s case is another illustration of the extreme importance of understanding a patient's personality, his coping modes, and the contingencies of his life situation.

Mrs. B., an extremely obese 38-year-old school teacher, was admitted to the rehabilitation center following a laparotomy necessitated by circulatory complications resulting from her obesity. Immediately, Mrs. B. was put on a strict diet; because physical therapy was not very effective as long as the patient was so much overweight, she was enrolled only in the occupational therapy program.

Mrs. B. came to the consultant's attention because her behavior had given rise to a great deal of anger on the part of the staff. She did not adhere to her diet: friends and relatives conspired in bringing her candy and other forbidden foods, much to the nurses' and doctors' annoyance. Mrs. B. complained bitterly about the hospital food and the occupational-therapy program. She was extremely demanding of attention and, at times, verbally abusive to the staff. As she became more difficult to please, the staff tended to become more restrictive and punitive with her. By the time the consultant was called in, Mrs. B. had been threatened with dismissal from the hospital, with dire predictions of a return of her former condition, of strokes due to high blood pressure, and of a life of chronic hospitalization, invalidism, and a fatally downhill course, unless she religiously followed her prescribed regime. As a last resort, she had been threatened with a visit from the psychiatrist and, needless to say, from all accounts, she vociferously objected to this encounter!

Mrs. B. had been a gregarious, much beloved, and very competent kindergarten teacher. A great many visitors and a large number of get-well cards testified to her popularity. In listening to the reports, the consultant surmised that the rather extensive operative procedure and subsequent enforced inactivity, coupled with oral deprivation, had conspired to increase Mrs. B.'s anxiety and frustration enormously. Her already shaky self-esteem was further eroded by the constant critical attention paid to her weight. A teacher herself, she rightly found the simple tasks presented to her in occupational therapy, tasks suited for severely handicapped people, beneath her dignity. The restrictive and authoritarian ways in which her doctor and some of the nurses forbade her certain foods evoked a strong obstreperous and rebellious reaction in her. If she were being treated like a child, she would indeed behave like one!

It was only after the psychiatrist had been

able to clarify for the staff what psychological forces were mobilized by their attitudes and ways of dealing with Mrs. B. that a drastic change in the management of and approach to this patient could take place. The perfectionistic standards for Mrs. B.'s weight were modified to meet more realistic goals. Medication suited to counteract depression and at the same time suppress the patient's appetite was prescribed, and her diet was less strictly enforced. Mrs. B. was asked to assist the occupational therapy staff in helping other patients and definite plans for discharge from the hospital as soon as possible were set into motion. Mrs. B. rightly had become increasingly anxious about her job and her financial future.

The enforced inactivity had served only to heighten her anxiety and to promote a regressive infantile reaction in her. After discharge, Mrs. B. resumed her teaching and continued to come for her physical-therapy treatments as an outpatient; she regained her former sunny disposition and was able to maintain her weight at a far from ideal, but for this patient, manageable, level.

Therapeutic goals and management need to be tailored to a patient's personality structure and character style. While Mr. A. and Miss C. will have to be taken care of, Mrs. B. will no doubt continue to fight fiercely for independence and achieve it as long as possible.

Although it is important to encourage the handicapped patient and necessary to keep him motivated to strive for optimal rehabilitative results, overzealous or inexperienced ward and rehabilitative personnel tend, at times, to underestimate the emotional after effects of physical traumata which severely interfere with a person's ability to function independently. This is especially so when a patient does show no visible sadness or despair but his depression takes on an atypical form, as in Mr. A.'s and Miss C.'s case, or is expressed in recalcitrance as in Mrs. B.'s case.

The management of such patients tends to become contaminated by feelings of anger, guilt, and resentment on everybody's part.

The necessity to grieve the loss of a body part or its function before a person can become genuinely intent upon trying to compensate for its loss or to retrieve its function cannot be overstressed.

Angry rebellion, excessive demandingness, withdrawal, and apathy are normal forms of posttraumatic reactions. They are attempts to deal with depressive feelings and likely to subside relatively quickly if met with empathetic understanding. Often a period of visible sadness and crying spells follow in which the patient consciously mourns his loss. If sustained by mature understanding on the part of ward personnel and visiting relatives, and if supported by a consistent, carefully devised therapeutic regime, the behavior of most patients does not create any major management problems. Neither does the period of sadness necessarily interfere with their ability to cooperate successfully in a rehabilitative program.

In a small number of patients, difficulties do arise which are apt to stem from specific personality problems or to rejection by relatives. If such a patient feels that there is nothing or no one who makes life worth living, he has little resilience to invest in strenuous regimes for his rehabilitation. Premature pressures for top performance or overindulgence and infantilization by hospital personnel or relatives complicate their course still further. Most often, major impasses occur through a combination of these three most common factors.

Timely consultation and judicious interaction by psychiatrically trained social-service staff and psychiatric consultants can do much to improve the understanding of the patient and his reality situation. Relatives can often be effectively helped with their feelings of distress and despair by a competent social worker.

Special problems arise at times with a patient suffering from progressively debilitating diseases, such as multiple sclerosis or rheumatoid arthritis. These diseases lead to increasing physical restriction, helplessness, and, in some instances, chronic pain.

For these illnesses, there is, at present, no cure and their origins are insufficiently known. Patients suffering from such diseases have usually been subjected to long periods of observation, to multiple diagnostic procedures, some of which are quite painful, without any benefit other than a confirmed diagnosis, an uncertain prognosis, and no prospect of cure. Referral to a rehabilitation center is often experienced by them as a rejection by the original hospital or clinic which made the diagnosis, or as a personal failure, or a punishment for true or imagined sins. Some react to their new environment with suspicion; they compare the new one unfavorably with the old and blame the nursing staff for true, partially true, or imagined oversight. Such direct attacks are hard to take but often are attempts on the part of these patients to relieve themselves of inner despair and impotent rage regarding their plight. Engrossed in a struggle between their reasonable thinking and unreasonable feeling values, they attempt to externalize this most painful inner conflict. They create dissent between and within the various professional groups in charge of their therapeutic regime, play one against the other, and attempt to manipulate their relatives into battles with the hospital staff on their behalf. Only an understanding for the intensity of their emotional conflict, for their anxiety about their future, and their helplessness in the face of an incurable, crippling disease can protect their caretakers from angry rejection and retaliation or from a hopeless embroilment in numerous controversies.

These patients need a consistent, secure, and disciplined approach to their illness. They cannot be allowed to rule the ward or to create dissent between family and the hospital staff or between the various specialists within the rehabilitation center upon whose efforts and assistance they are dependent, often for many years to come.

Different but equally pressing problems often occur in the course of rehabilitating adolescent patients who have been severely injured in a car or athletic accident.

Mr. D., for instance, was a 17-year-old boy who sustained a severe head injury in a car accident. He had been in a coma for several weeks and upon return of consciousness was hemiparetic and unable to speak. In the course of several months, his speech returned, he became able to move his at first paralyzed arm, and though ataxic, he could take some steps with support.

A consultation was requested by the nursing staff because Mr. D. was becoming a problem. This was the more puzzling to them because, according to everyone concerned, the patient was making excellent progress and his negativism, irritability, and gloomy outlook on life made little sense to the ward personnel, who felt increasingly annoyed with him.

In a psychiatric interview, Mr. D., a typical adolescent, complained bitterly about the many old people on the ward and the lack of peer companionship. He worried about his future: would he regain his physical strength and be able to participate in sports again? He felt pushed around, imposed upon, and lacking in privacy.

To the consultant, Mr. D. seemed a typical normal adolescent. The serious car accident, followed by long loss of consciousness, loss of memory of the event, loss of speech, and partial loss of motor function had been a major traumatic event, not only in the physical, but also in the emotional sense. Coming at a time when developmentally he was struggling with age-appropriate concerns about his future and his ability to succeed in life, his strivings for independence and self-sufficiency had been seriously jeopardized by the helplessness inflicted upon him by a car accident for which he had no personal responsibility. His concerns about his future and complaints about his present situation made sense to the consultant.

Following the consultation, the hospital staff made a concerted and successful effort to move Mr. D. into a room with patients closer to his age. He was treated less authoritatively and with greater flexibility. When occasionally depressed and withdrawn, his wish to be left alone was respected. The social-service staff provided a tutor for him as soon as he was ready to turn to school learning. The volunteer group was alerted to this patient's need for male companionship and for opportunities to "rap" with peers. His family assumed responsibility for encouraging and organizing friends and schoolmates to visit their son in the hospital.

Subsequently, Mr. D.'s progress picked up considerably, and he was discharged from the rehabilitation service with very good results and sooner than anyone had expected. He maintained contact with the hospital after discharge and has made excellent use of a number of rehabilitative and training opportunities in his community.

The ravages inflicted upon young people by injuries they sustain in car accidents or sports events often have consequences which confront them, the hospital personnel, and their parents with an agonizing reality. Due to the present-day excellence of medical care, many of these young victims survive, who would formerly have died of severe brain or spinal injuries. Often for days or weeks in coma, they find when they regain consciousness that their arms and legs are paralyzed, their face and bodies disfigured, or that they are unable to speak or make themselves understood. Irreparable loss or lasting severe impairment of motor function, speech, eyesight, memory, or comprehension can create monumental problems for the patient who is doomed to a life of invalidism and for his family and relatives burdened with the life-long responsibility for his care. Feelings of anger, guilt, and remorse can seriously interfere with the patient's progress and optimal recovery. Overindulgence or attempts by the family at cheerful denial of the extent of his handicap can create a severe strain for the patient and his environment. Fits of impotent rage, bouts of gloom and despair are common reactions. They have to be understood, tolerated, endured, and judiciously dealt with if the patient and his family are to resume a relatively satisfying life together in a stable,

mutually supportive, and, for the patient, growth-promoting atmosphere upon his discharge from the hospital.

Fortunately, rehabilitative efforts may pay off in unexpectedly favorable ways because of the young person's physical and emotional resilience. On the other hand, the strength of his resentment, the vehemence of his anger, and the depth of his despair are often greater than those of the older patient. Severe management problems, persistent resistiveness to the rehabilitation program, and strong suicidal urges can complicate and prolong the rehabilitation course of the adolescent patient. At such times psychiatric intervention can be most helpful. Commonly, a steadfast empathetic attitude toward this group of patients, flexible and purposeful ward management, a varied rehabilitative program which pays special attention to an individual adolescent's needs, skills, and areas of competence are needed to achieve optimal results. Family counseling can be extremely useful in planning for the patient's return home. The combination of his infirmity, which makes him dependent upon his parents and others, and his natural adolescent strivings for independence and self-sufficiency creates serious conflicts for him and his environment in everyday living.

Equally important as helping the young person to live as productive a life as he is capable of is one's willingness to respect and accept in the old or incurably ill person the wish to die with dignity and some sense of autonomy.

Late one evening, the psychiatric consultant was called in great distress because Mr. P., a 68-year-old man, suffering from advanced cancer, insisted on leaving the hospital that very night. According to the nurse, he was totally unwilling to listen to reason, had refused to take his pain-killing medicine, tranquilizer, and sleeping pills, and had tried to bully his wife and children into taking him home that very minute.

His wife, a rather nervous and justifiably helpless person, felt completely incapable of taking responsibility for the care of her severely ill husband. His daughters agreed that their father should remain in the hospital, but nobody was able to quiet Mr. P. down. He was hollering and screaming at the doctor and nurses, who, with soothing words, tried to persuade him to take his pills so they would not have to resort to more drastic means of quieting him down. When the psychiatrist entered upon the scene, it was clear to her that everyone was in a state of panic and helplessness. Only too glad to leave her alone with the patient, relatives, nurses, and the doctor in charge all rapidly cleared the room as Mr. P. was struggling to get out of bed and yelling that he was going to go home never mind what it took.

When the psychiatrist inquired what had caused Mr. P. to become so upset, it became clear to her that he was afraid of dying and that leaving the hospital was his way of trying to escape death.

He was also resentful at having to take a large variety of pills which, so he said, left him feeling doped and unable to think clearly. The acute upset was triggered off by the night nurse's insistence that he take his sleeping pill, because at 10 p.m. he was supposed to go to sleep. Mr. P. wondered why he could not stay awake if he wanted to. In the old days at home, he never used to go to sleep before 1 a.m. What was wrong with his staying awake now if he did not make any trouble?

When the psychiatrist agreed with Mr. P. that she too did not see any good reason why he should have to take a sleeping pill if he did not want to, Mr. P. quieted down almost immediately. Within the next half hour, Mr. P. was able to make his fears and complaints very clear to her, and she was then able to explain his behavior to his family and the ward personnel. Mr. P. did not really want to go home; he wanted to escape death. To be forced into a passive position, heavily sedated and isolated with a group of withdrawn noncommunicative roommates was like a premature death to him, which he was fighting tooth and nail.

For the next ten days, a major effort was made by the social-service staff to make sure that Mr. P. could visit other wards and play cards every day with a group of more lively and communicative patients. One of the social workers assumed the responsibility of mediating between Mr. P. and those among the nursing staff who feared that he might die en route, make for trouble, or become agitated again.

The psychiatrist tried to persuade her medical colleagues to give Mr. P. some say in what medication he was willing to take. Interestingly enough, Mr. P. never refused his pain-killing medicine, but was, at times, adamant in his refusal of tranquilizers or sleeping pills.

There were a few minor flare-ups which could be quickly resolved when the social worker was able to help Mr. P. talk with her about his awareness that his death was imminent. When allowed to remain active and to some extent master of his own fate, he was a perfectly amiable and easy-to-manage patient. He died peacefully one late afternoon in the way he had wanted, and for which he had actively fought.

The strain of having to bear with the knowledge of a patient's inevitable and impending death is particularly hard on his relatives and on the ward personnel responsible for his care.

When patients adopt a passive, resigned attitude, they are not likely to create management problems. Those, however, who fight for their lives and insist on remaining active until the bitter end by refusing medication, like Mr. P., or who insist on leaving the hospital against medical advice, are cause for a good deal of turmoil and dissent among the professional staff. They also create anxiety and guilt in their relatives who cannot honestly face in themselves or with the patient the reality of his impending death.

The majority of patients treated at a rehabilitation unit must make a new and, at times, difficult adjustment when the time of discharge approaches. Ideally, they will go back to their homes and families, having achieved an optimal return of function.

For some, however, this happy solution is not available. If their residual incapacity does not permit them to carry on independently and if there is no loving family ready to assume the responsibility for their care, admission to a nursing home becomes an unavoidable reality. Such a disposition may plunge the patient into a considerable depression, a reaction not helped by negative attitudes of relatives and friends, who although not able or willing to take him into their own homes, nevertheless strenuously object to this only feasible alternative.

Few persons can afford to return home if it means paying for continuous, 24-hour home care. Even if they have the financial means to do so, personnel willing and capable of performing such a demanding and prolonged task is rarely obtainable.

The longer a patient has been treated at the rehabilitation unit, the stronger his attachment to the institution and its personnel is likely to be. This is also true for those members of the staff who have been intimately involved in his daily care. It is painful for them to realize that, despite their concerted efforts and devotion, no further progress can be expected because of the severity of the patient's physical affliction or because a combination of physical, emotional, and environmental factors impede his optimal rehabilitation. Their disappointment and frustration may be expressed in anger at the authorities for insisting upon such a patient's discharge. Guilt reactions and doubts about their own skills and effectiveness may come to the surface. When these staff feelings are subtly, or not so subtly, conveyed to a patient, they often contribute to his difficulty in accepting his unavoidable transfer. Interprofessional tensions can arise between the social worker, who has to find a suitable placement for the patient, and members of the physical, occupational, and nursing staffs. These come to the fore in differences of opinion about the most suitable disposition for him or in growing impatience that his discharge is delayed because no place can be found on short notice.

Hospital policies governed by financial limitations or by welfare, insurance, and government restrictions tend to increase the frustration and anxiety on everybody's part, and the resulting distress often requires the intervention of the psychiatric consultant to clarify the issues and help sort out fact from fantasy. Once the staff has been able to come to terms with what, under the circumstances, is a feasible, though not necessarily the optimal, solution for their patient, they can aid him to make the change.

When a patient is to return home, social service and rehabilitative personnel play a crucial role in preparing the family for the reception of their handicapped spouse, parent, or child. Many patients may continue to come for outpatient rehabilitative work, which gives them an opportunity to maintain a relationship with the unit. This situation serves not only to consolidate and add to their further physical improvement but to provide an important source for continued emotional support. Relatives who accompany the patient on his regular visits can profit from these occasions also to review with a social-service worker, physical or occupational therapist the patient's adjustment in the home and theirs to him.

There is, at times, a vast discrepancy between the tasks a patient is objectively capable of performing and his ability to function in his family or nursing-home setting. In a climate of love and acceptance, we can see, at times, a remarkable return of physical and emotional function surpassing everyone's most optimistic expectations.

Unfortunately, the opposite is equally true. The daily care of a severely handicapped, mentally deteriorated, uncommunicative, or seemingly unresponsive spouse, elderly parent, or child can become a drain upon even the most devoted of families. To maintain a balance between caring for such a patient and protecting the household from enslavement, increasing frustration, depression, and mounting ambivalence toward such a relative is no easy task.

Most abrasive of all are those personality changes that may take place as a result of a stroke, cerebral arteriosclerosis, or other degenerative brain process. Querulousness, suspicious attitudes, sudden outbursts of accusations, and despair often tax the family's endurance to the limit and beyond. At such times, a supportive relationship with a trusted family physician, a social worker, or other professional person willing to listen to the relative's description of his plight and capable of offering sensible suggestions for the patient's management can be indispensable for sustaining the family's mental and moral equilibrium.

There is a fine line between offering such a patient life-sustaining, loving support and infantilizing indulgence. The former can enhance family unity and deepen the sense of commitment and shared responsibility for his care; the latter breeds masochistic enslavement and growing resentment. These reactions, along with the inevitable guilt, set into motion a vicious cycle of diminishing return which may cause the patient to regress physically and emotionally and may also adversely affect formerly positive interrelationships between the healthy family members as well.

Unfortunately, deterioration of the emotional climate in the family can proceed gradually and escape recognition until a major crisis occurs. Sometimes, relatives feel the need for help but do not know where or to whom to turn; shame and guilt about their growing resentment may prevent them from asking for professional assistance.

The traditional dichotomy of physical or emotional illness has adversely affected the structure and policies of many of our hospitals and aftercare settings. It also exerts a profound influence upon attitudes toward the aftercare of those patients whose mental state has been affected by their illness.

Chronic depression may go unnoticed, be interpreted as hostile resistence, as the patient's wish to be left alone, or as a sign of his physical deterioration. Patients who fight helplessness and invalidism run the risk of being considered ornery, difficult, or unmanageable, especially if they refuse to adapt themselves to the routines, rules, and regulations deemed suitable for them by their caretakers.

Caretakers may withdraw from a depressed patient, when they misinterpret outward manifestations of emotional distress, and thus increase the patient's depression. Such misunderstandings accelerate the process of mutual withdrawal so poignantly described by those who have visited large institutions offering custodial care to a vast number of wheelchair-bound, bedridden elderly patients vacantly staring into space and living to die.

Shortage of personnel and lack of psychological understanding may lead to undesirable and inappropriate prescriptions of tranquilizers and sedatives for the "obstreperous" or "agitated" patient. If these fail to tame his fighting spirits, he is threatened with expulsion from the institution or transfer to a mental hospital.

Although the difficulties of families with a handicapped member will be of a different order from those experienced by personnel of nursing homes or aftercare institutions, psychological understanding is indispensable for all persons undertaking to care for the physically handicapped, because physical handicaps do affect a person's emotional life, even if a tangible, organic mental involvement is absent.

Ideally, every rehabilitative hospital program should have the professional resources for sustained, even if only periodic, follow-up of its discharged patients.

Regular consultations with family physicians, with nursing-home and aftercare personnel, and with family members who assume the major responsibility for the patient's daily care can do much to maintain and consolidate the gains he has made during his inpatient stay and can prevent his physical and emotional regression. Needless to say, aftercare programs which can provide such continued care, guidance, consultation, and sustained support to his caretakers are few and far between. Fortunately, there is a growing awareness that rehabilitative efforts have to bridge the gap which is likely to occur when the hospitalized patient is discharged.

For the physically disabled, attention to his emotional equilibrium is as important as that given to maintaining his optimal physical functions, but a viable and optimal integration of physical and mental health care is slow in coming. Medical specialization, although necessary, also fosters organ rather than patient care.

A health model which combines prevention, intervention, and aftercare, e.g., continuous total care, has lately been emerging in the various forms of health-care centers and medical group practice. However, such total care settings are still relatively scarce. A sophisticated knowledge of intrapersonal developmental issues requires not only an appreciation and acceptance of the intrinsic indivisibility of body and soul; it also implies an understanding of the changing, dynamic relationships between physical, emotional, and intellectual factors in the course of the life-span. Disturbances, be they predominantly in the physical, emotional, or intellectual sphere, cannot fail to affect the other realms of the personality to a greater or lesser extent as well. Moreover, no individual lives in a vacuum. In his daily life he is dependent for nurture and satisfaction upon human environment. What happens to its members will, of necessity, reflect upon his state of health and well-being, and his own will affect theirs in turn.

The boundaries between health and illness are relative and fluid rather than absolute and static. Restoration of function per se is not equal to rehabilitation. In order to give his life meaning, a person has to feel needed and valued. This is possible only if he can be included as a contributing and viable member in a living environment. Only then has he been, in truth, rehabilitated. Although we cannot expect the severely afflicted person to be productive in the same way as his healthy or only slightly handicapped counterpart, his presence, in whatever setting, has to provide him with a sense of belonging, which is possible only if his presence has positive meaning to those around him.

Whenever the burdens of a disabled person's care outweigh the advantages to his surroundings, intervention is needed to reverse a potentially abrasive and malignant course. At times, rehospitalization may become unavoidable. In other instances, prolonged outpatient rehabilitative physical and mental-health services may be adequate to help particularly the chronically ill person maintain whatever function he has for as long as possible.

Relatives faced with the long-term care of an increasingly more disabled family member most likely need, at one time or another, the professional help that a family-service agency or a psychiatric or community mental-health clinic can offer. If the patient is a child or an adolescent, the services of a special school and a child-psychiatric facility may be needed, combined with those providing him with physical rehabilitation. When an institution capable of providing all necessary services under its own roof is not available, it is of major importance that sufficient contact be maintained between the various institutions and service agencies enlisted to assist the patient and his family. Only thus can optimal treatment planning take place and a comprehensive treatment regime for the total family be provided and maintained.

17

The Role
of the Family

The illness of any member of a family inevitably disrupts the pattern of family living. Acute illness will do this often for a limited period, but modern medicine, with its ability to cut short many illnesses and with its streamlined hospital organization, can adequately take care of most problems of an acute nature. People in general are quite well informed as to what to do in such emergencies, and while even short periods of disease may cause economic problems, the strains and stresses of such disease are usually within the limits of the ability of most people, and if these limits are exceeded, hopefully there are community organizations available to render assistance.

In contrast, when chronic disability strikes an older member of a family, problems emerge that, at the outset, appear insurmountable. Ignorance and well-meaning concern on the part of the family often result in poor management that, instead of helping the patient, makes him worse. Perhaps the most frequent error is the prescription of bed rest and immobilization for patients who in reality require exercise to maintain muscle strength. Although it may be easier for the family to care for these patients while they are bedridden, they will become, through this very measure of immobilization, complete cripples when, in fact, a regulated program of exercise would return them to self-sufficiency. On the other hand, there are chronically ill older patients who must remain in bed and who cannot be mobilized. How and where can they best be treated or simply cared for?

When chronic illness causes the prospect of long-term rehabilitation or immobilization, problems are posed which the average person is ill-equipped to handle and for which modern medicine and community organizations are still poorly prepared. There has been considerable progress in this field, however, and, with persistence, competent help can usually be found in most communities. We are assuming here that there is a family actually engaged in caring for the welfare of its own aged members, but, unfortunately, this is not always true. An article in *Science* has correctly depicted the plight of the aged person who must face the calamity of chronic disease alone:

In general, our 20 million people over 65 live wretched lives. Three-fourths of them have incomes averaging under $2000 a year, and half, under $1000. More than a fifth live in housing judged "substandard"—lacking private bath, toilet, or running water. Eighty out of each 100 suffer chronic ailment, yet only half have any kind of health insurance. One out of eight is on relief.

Further, the number of people living through these "sunset years" is steadily increasing: 1000 people turn 65 every day (by 1980 there will be 25 million), and there are already 10,000 Americans over 100. The proportion of age to youth is changing, too: the number of elderly people has increased six-fold since 1900, while the population as a whole has grown by a factor of $2\frac{1}{2}$.

The numbers and the miseries add up to one thing: another failure of social ingenuity to keep up with scientific change. What we have done, mainly, is to lengthen life in relation to retirement age and to curb diseases of youth without curing those of age, thereby ensuring that our aged will be not only bored and alienated but poor and ailing as well.

If the aged are victimized in general, they are also victimized in particular. Their illness, loneliness, and terrors make the aged easy prey to a growing army of charlatans in whom their vulnerability arouses instincts not of sympathy but of greed.

But families too must guard against making costly errors and against falling prey to the charlatans who stand ready to exploit the elderly sick person. The principal questions which must be answered are the following:

What is the nature of the disease? Will it require hospitalization or can it be treated adequately at home?

Is there need for long-term nursing care not feasible in the home, not requiring a hospital but rather a nursing home or extended-care facilities?

What is the proper management going to cost, and is the necessary money available?

If needed, where can one obtain outside assistance?

The family member or the individual responsible for the sick aged person should seek adequate information from a variety of sources to these questions before making his decisions. He must have some understanding of the illness, its symptoms, the residual effects on the elderly person, and the plan for the management of the problem. The aged person may need to be hospitalized briefly, to stabilize his condition or to resolve the acute problem, and then could return home if someone would provide the assistance necessary. Frequently, family members become upset and feel inadequate when an elderly person is ill and often relegate the care to others, usually to the professionals. The elderly dislike this reaction by family members and wish that they would consult with professionals but remain involved in the management of their problems and continue to care about them.

Often the sick aged can remain at home without much difficulty if there is a person available to perform the activities which prove too complex for them. The aged would prefer to remain at home in surroundings familiar to them for as long as possible, and then seek placement in an appropriate health-care facility when their care becomes burdensome to others. They should be *involved* to whatever degree it is possible in the

plans and decisions being made for their well-being. Very often, they are not included because some professionals and family members feel uncomfortable and believe that the aged person is better off not being informed. Unfortunately, the aged feel rejected and isolated by this type of action, and many become quite bitter. They have lived this long; they realize they are not as productive or as well as they once were; they know some help is necessary, and they value family affection and concern. When a lack of concern on the part of family members becomes obvious, the aged one's sense of worthlessness and loneliness is increased. Adequate resources by professionals and others should be available to any individual who has the responsibility for a sick aged person so that he can be helped to manage this complex situation to the best of his ability, and so that the aged person can know a sense of well-being and a degree of contentment.

One must begin to be concerned for the welfare of the sick aged—for all will soon reach this time in their lives. If the situation is to be corrected, the response by the people in our society to our aged must be much more vociferous and persistent. The value of life, dignity, and aging, as a right for all people, must be recognized and accepted so that the avenues by which it can be accomplished are available.

PROCUREMENT OF OUTSIDE ASSISTANCE

The answers to most of the questions posed above, although probably not to all of them, can be obtained from a competent physician. Many families may have a physician on whom they have come to rely, and he should be consulted first. If the family has no regular physician, one may be found by calling the community hospital or the county medical society, who will refer one of their staff men or members, respectively. After consultation with a physician, the needs for the proper care of the patient will become clearer. The physician may be able to refer the family to agencies which are prepared to give assistance; and if he cannot do this, he will not object to the family's consulting the local public-welfare office (county, city, or town), which will be able to provide guidance and information on all matters connected with welfare and health. The social worker in this agency can also be very helpful.

In her study, "Measuring the Home Health Needs of the Aged in Five Countries," Dr. Ethel Shanas concluded the following:

The future needs of the aged for community health services will certainly be greater than the present estimates. In part, this will result from the rapid growth of the proportions of persons over 75 years of age in the older population (U.S. Department of Commerce, 1970). Those of advanced ages are more likely to be ill than those aged 65 to 74. Further, as people become more knowledgeable about health maintenance, the demands of old people and the families of old people for services for the elderly are certain to rise.

All of the countries studied have made a start on the provision of community health services to old people. In Denmark and Britain, programs of services are already well developed. Israel, Poland, and the United States are working on the establishment of such services. The magnitude of the program is such, however, that no country studied, including those with established programs, offers services to the elderly adequate to their widespread need.

Since the enactment of Medicare in 1965, all the aged are eligible for hospital insurance benefits in Part A of Medicare, and 95 percent or more are enrolled in Part B, the supplementary medical insurance program. Chronic illness, however, usually requires care far exceeding the limited benefit periods provided by Medicare, and additional care must be covered by private sources or third-party payers, i.e., local government, public-assistance agencies, workmen's compensation agencies, rehabilitation agencies, voluntary health insurances, or prepayment plans.

Among all the third-party payers, Medicaid is the largest. In 1965, amendments to the Social Security Act also provided federally financed assistance to the states for supplying programs of comprehensive high-quality medical services to all in low-income families. The federal government pays from a low of 50 percent to a high of 83 percent. At least five basic services are required in the program: inpatient and outpatient hospital care, physician services, skilled nursing-home care for adults, laboratory services, and x-ray services.

To maintain a capacity to function at a decent level of health and well-being depends on the availability of services. The nature and number of those needing services are beyond family resources and definitely require public support. In 1970, 9.5 percent of our total population was over 65 years of age. About 96 percent of our elderly live in the community. Inasmuch as social welfare has become the inescapable obligation of government everywhere in the world to a greater or lesser extent, family responsibility toward the elderly is still the most meaningful responsibility, because it connotes the acceptance of the elderly when they are in need. Public welfare may be practical to the extent of material assistance, but the value of family interest is immeasurable. Caring for the chronically ill at home should thus be encouraged with more effort toward improving societal responsibility, establishing supportive services, and helping the family to keep the patient at home, e.g., Medicare and Medicaid with provision of home health services and the supplying of necessary equipment to make home care possible.

Local communities are becoming more aware of the needs of the chronically ill and aged and have become more responsive to the Older American Act of 1965, which authorized grants to help establish agencies and services for the elderly. These services include homemakers, friendly visiting, telephone checks, transportation, library, shopping, meals on wheels, legal aid, employment counseling, etc. There has been an increase of demonstration projects in recent years but by no means are they universally available throughout the United States. In Massachusetts, as of this writing, a master plan for delivery of home-care services to the elderly has just been put together by the Executive Office of Elder Affairs. Of all the above mentioned services, Homemaker/Home Health Aide Services are the most important and most frequently called services in assisting professional workers to meet the health and social needs of families under stress.

The term *home health aide* was officially introduced in the Title XVIII of the Social Security Act and refers to the personal-care tasks performed by the homemakers, for which special training and supervision are required. According to the National League for Nursing, home health aides are nonprofessional workers who give personal care and perform related housekeeping services in the homes of the sick, disabled, dependent, or infirm, when no family member can assume this responsibility. This service is prescribed by the physician as part of a medically directed health-care plan coordinated by a home health agency, such as the Visiting Nurse Association or a hospital-based agency.

The National Council for Homemaker and Home Health Aide Services, Inc., an organization with a membership of over three hundred agencies which provide homemaker/home-health-aide services, was cited as a national standard-setting body for such services in the United States and charged with the development of a national approval program. Their 1970 report shows that an estimate of over 18,000 agencies providing homemaker/home-health-aide services exist in the United States and that as many as 20,000 homemakers were employed; over 60 percent of these agencies were publicly operated, while the others were voluntary and proprietary. According to the Bureau of Health Insurance of the Social Security Administration, there are some 2,300 home-health agencies certified to participate in Medicare.

The role of the homemaker/home health aide can be that of helping to carry out the treatment plan, observing the patient and family relationships, reporting patient progress and any new problems to the health team. She can give personal care to the patient to provide and maintain physical and emotional comfort, to assist the patient toward independent living, and to enable the patient to remain in his own home among familiar surroundings. She can help to carry out an interim plan while the professional is assessing family and individual strengths and weaknesses, so that a long-range plan may be developed to serve the best interests of the family and the community.

She can help teach more efficient methods of household management, day-to-day living, and better methods of self-care in the presence of illness. For the family under stress, and who cannot plan their day-to-day activities, the homemaker/home health aide can help to maintain the quality of their living conditions, if a family member is also active in providing nursing care to the patient. She helps to relieve some of the demands made upon the family member and to provide an opportunity for them all to enjoy each other as a normal family group. But most importantly, she makes it possible for the chronically ill and aged to remain at home, or if hospitalized, to return home sooner.

President Nixon, at the closing session of the 1971 White House Conference on Aging, specifically stated, "We can give special emphasis to services that will help people live decent and dignified lives in their own homes, services such as Home Health Aides, Homemaker, and nutritional services, home-delivered meals, and transportation assistance." This message has stimulated and encouraged the establishment of Home Health Service Agencies to provide trained homemaker/home health aides in local areas. This service has been a tested low-cost means of keeping families together and the chronically ill at home.

The homemaker/home health aide generally works for a plan of care designated by the physician under the supervision of the Visiting Nurses Association, proprietary home health agencies, health departments, or a hospital-based coordinated home-health care program. Medicare and volunteer health insurances, such as the Massachusetts Blue Cross, furnish home-health-aide coverage for its members who hold prolonged illness coverage and Master Medical contracts. The hospital-based coordinated home-health-care type of arrangement furnishes all professional health services, equipment and supplies prescribed by private physicians to selected patients who require, and can receive, a combination of hospital type services in their homes. Regular case conferences by the team are held to evaluate the ongoing treatment and goals of the patient's plan of care at least every four weeks.

In the Greater Jackson area of Mississippi, a Home Health Agency was sponsored by a private practicing physician. It is called the Central Mississippi Home Health Agency. Other private physicians, instead of sending their patients to a hospital for care that could be furnished by the agency at home, send written orders for individually tailored care programs to the agency. The physician receives periodic reports from the agency on his patient, who must be seen by him at least every sixty days. This agency, under the supervision of a medical doctor, provides physical therapy, occupational therapy, speech therapy, and nursing services. Its nursing services include home-care instruction, management of diabetes, dietary instruction, inhalation therapy, and postoperative care with dressings, packs, catheters, tube feedings, and decubitus-ulcer prevention and management.

Other supportive services, which can also be helpful to the family, are family counseling or family service agencies, such as the Family Service Association of America. Their 335 agencies, located throughout North America, offer social casework service for any phase of personal or family life to people of all ages. Some agencies also have group-work and homemaker-service programs. This service is available also to friends and relatives of older people, who need help in planning with and for them. Fees are charged according to ability to pay.

Some churches have volunteer friendly visitors who may even act as relief for the family members for short periods of time. Local senior-citizen projects have activities which can be very

beneficial to the family and patient. Some youth groups do shopping and errands for the elderly.

Where specialized nursing care is needed, the public-health nurse may be the answer to the family's problem. These nurses are finding that more and more of their visits are made to aged and middle-aged persons with long-term illnesses. In a few cases, such service is supplied by the local health department, but, in general, this help is provided by the Visiting Nurses Association, an agency that exists mainly in urban areas. An important aspect of the visiting nurse's job is assisting and educating family members caring for the aged person.

In order for those who are working with the families of the aged and the chronically ill to be able to assess objectively the total person and his situation and to contribute toward a more realistic plan, it is necessary to update the current sociological picture. Therefore, one does not expect that every patient should or can have home care. The change of family structure has come about slowly, but its progress was accelerated by social, economic, and technological advancements. According to the United States Census 1970 report, there were relatively rapid increases in the number of individuals who live alone, which probably reflects, in part, an increasing tendency among younger persons to maintain their own apartments or houses away from their parents, and an increasing ability among older persons to maintain their own homes rather than to live with relatives or other persons.

With technological and commercial advancements which produced improvement of household appliances and mechanization of many household chores, the family and household characteristics have changed considerably during the last twenty years. Liberal thinking and social freedom of the young generation pose a different value system between the generations. Many people of the younger generation have not lived with an older person nor have they had a chance to get to know one intimately and gradually. They are less able to deal with their disabled elderly. Of the older generation now living alone, some resented the fact that they were tied down by their parents and vowed independence from their children. Social Security and other retirement benefits have helped in the process of giving them some sense of financial independence. Old-age assistance and medical assistance have further relieved the children of financial responsibility toward their parents. Divorces and separations also have added to the increased number of people living alone. Physical segregation does contribute to psychological segregation and to looser family ties; however, the majority of our elderly still enjoy affectionate relationships with their families which must be preserved.

For whatever reason, many elderly people do not choose to live with their children, and the children never plan to have them. Some have conflicts of personalities and living styles which make living together impossible. Some elderly people do not want to relinquish their own households but are not managing adequately and must have psychological and concrete support. Part-time homemaker service may enable these people to maintain dignity and independence.

For the elderly person who lives alone, the family's responsibility should be even greater to protect him from harming himself. The community should be able to guide him to better use of his own and community resources.

One assumes that persons who are ill and disabled are happier and recover better in their own familiar surroundings, and that most aged feel more dignified if allowed to maintain independent living in the community as long as possible. Following the acute phase of illness or an active rehabilitation program, the family, the hospital social worker, and the continuing-care coordinator jointly consider a continuing-care plan based on the patient's medical situation, emotional strength, social needs, family's desire and capability, and home environment, as well as availability of home-health and supportive services

in the community. The hospital physician, who has the authority to make referral for home-health care, gives approval to the plan, and the physician in the community who is taking charge of the program (if not the same as the hospital physician) must also approve. The physician who approved of a home health-care plan sees that it is a part of the continuity of care plan for the total person.

Ideally, appropriate and effective utilization of home-health-agency services should be determined by multidisciplined assessment of the total needs of the patient and planning for his care. Evaluation by physician, nurse, social worker, and other professional disciplines permits the selection of the aide best suited to give the care. Many home health agencies have social workers only as consultants, and social service is still not generally available except to a few cases.

A substantial number of our elderly people, with or without disability, do not need skilled nursing or other professional health services allowed by Medicare as a home health benefit because it is strictly a health benefit. Those who do need intermittent part-time services of a home health aide for personal care and housekeeping duties are not adequately provided for under our legislation. Families should be aware of this lag and be prepared to find other resources while working on legislative changes to formulate programs to meet the needs for in-home social services for people. Another factor is that at present, voluntary health insurances cover mainly hospital benefits, and some cover the service of a registered nurse limitedly in the home, but do not provide for a licensed practical nurse or home health aide. Many patients have no choice but to be hospitalized in order to receive medical care which could be provided by a home health agency at home.

As mentioned above, availability of community services is one very important factor determining the feasibility of home care. Experience shows that a shortage of physicians who are willing to visit patients at home is another reason why institutionalization seems to be the only way for the aging or disabled to receive medical care, or even nursing care. This institution-oriented attitude, which has developed among our professional and public servants, can very well be a result of the convenience-for-all-concerned attitude and the lack of services in the community. Unless the advantages of home health care can be widely demonstrated and proved, further development of home health services will be slow. Currently, Medicare guidelines are too restrictive, in that they limit the services of home health aides to posthospitalized referrals and cases in which the patient needs continuing medical and nursing care for the same diagnosis which caused the original hospitalization.

Regardless of how willing and devoted the family can be toward providing home care, there can be a time when the family finds it necessary to place their elderly relative in a nursing home or long-term care facility. They have usually extended themselves over a long period of time, tried alternatives, and endured severe personal, economic, and social stress in the process.

The family should be cautioned to consult with someone who has experience in nursing-home placement or continuing care in working out long-range plans. It is sometimes inadvisable to think of making temporary placement, because the elderly person can get disoriented and upset at each move. When private payment is being considered, one must have assurance that the patient can remain in the same home when his payment source changes to public assistance.

It has been pointed out that some of the common findings for the need for placement are as follows:

1. The personal and social cost to the younger generation is high.

2. Multiplicity of problems caused by middle-aged children responsible for aged parents.

3. Population grows older and more older members than younger ones need care, both financial and physical.

4. Stigma of institutionalization causes fear and guilt.

5. Professionals see institutionalization as negative and community living as positive and often are not objective enough to give good advice.

6. Lack of community-based services and intermediate facilities like day care, home health aide services, etc.

The family can play just as important a role if the patient cannot have full-time care at home. When placement in a nursing home is the wisest decision, family members can learn how to handle the patient, including transfer from bed to chair and in and out of a car, in order to take him out on weekends and holidays. The ease and familiarity of care depend on the effort of both the patient and family members. Whatever the family is willing to do, the focus must be on maintaining maximum independence of the patient. Generally, nursing-home administrators are very willing to have patients enjoy close family relationships and will encourage any positive experience from it. The patient who enjoys group living can find a nursing home a place providing socialization in addition to its meeting the nursing need.

In the recent White House Conference on Aging, strong recommendations were made that the long-term institutional care aspects of Medicaid should be completely federalized and should give patients a choice of state and location desired. It also recommended that supplementary resources need to be allocated for alternate care as well as national insurance programs to meet the needs of those who require catastrophic care, mental-health care, and social services both within and outside of institutions.

Many cities and communities are establishing neighborhood health clinics so that people of all age groups may receive health care without difficulty. The aged are a classical group of individuals who like this kind of health service. If the neighborhood clinic is located in a central area easily accessible by public transportation or car, the aged welcome the opportunity to receive professional assistance with their health problems. Most of these clinics are managed by a professional team or by professional nurses who have received additional education and supervised experience beyond their initial education.

Meals on Wheels—a specialized service offered to shut-in patients in many cities, for example, Philadelphia, Dallas, Columbus, Ohio, Chicago, Rochester, New York, and Boston—brings hot, nutritious foods to the home. Although the obvious purpose of Meals on Wheels is to feed patients who would otherwise go hungry or have to fend for themselves inadequately, the fundamental aim of the program is to increase the independence of the recipient. Services may go beyond the delivery of the meal. In Philadelphia, for instance, volunteers and the staff of the *Lighthouse*, the settlement house that runs the program, also mail letters, cash checks, call the doctor, assist with household problems, and are capable of referring patients to other resources. Applicants are evaluated as to their need for this service, and in most cases there is a nominal fee, usually based on ability to pay. Voluntary contributions cover a good part of the costs. This program is small, the average number of clients served being only 25. Although it is still in the experimental stage, those communities that have tried Meals on Wheels are most optimistic about its future.

Nearly 300 member agencies of Family Service Associations of America work with families who have problems of interpersonal relations. Most of the agencies' work is brought in by the middle-aged children of older persons. Through counseling and the provision of homemaker services, these agencies often provide the much needed help. Very often family members hesitate to seek the assistance of others until the situation becomes severe or difficult. Sometimes people are unaware of the services available to them. A most thorough public-relations program is needed so that the aged and their families can be in-formed of the local and state programs offered to assist them.

Other voluntary agencies may offer services to the chronically ill, to aged persons, and to those concerned with their care. For example, local chapters of the American National Red Cross list the provision of transportation and home visiting among the services offered; and the Junior League in many communities has initiated programs for the older members of our society, both sick and healthy. Religious groups may also offer counseling and information to their members. Moreover, activity centers for older people frequently have trained social workers and nurse specialists who are well informed on community resources and may also be able to provide counseling help.

REHABILITATION

Many patients with long-term illnesses, such as those with hemiplegia, arthritis, amputation, fractured hip, and neurological diseases, may need some form of exercise or training to restore the strength of atrophied muscles or to prevent crippling through disuse. These exercises and the methods of treating some of these specific chronic conditions are discussed in greater detail elsewhere. The United States Public Health Service and various foundations have material available upon request which describes what can be done at home for these patients.

For instance, the families of stroke victims may benefit from the description of exercises in the pamphlet *Strike Back at Stroke*, which can be obtained by writing to the local office of the American Heart Association. The American Heart Association also provides up-to-date authoritative information about the various aspects of heart disease in books and pamphlets prepared for the nonmedical public. Others recommended are: *Strokes: A Guide for the Family*, and *Heart Disease Caused By Coronary Atherosclerosis. Cerebral Vascular Disease and Strokes*, #513, a publication of the National Heart Institute (U.S. Government Printing Office, Washington, D.C., 20 cents), gives a good general picture of cardiovascular disease.

Many patients are not able to speak after a stroke, or if they can speak, their words are so badly mixed up that it is hard to understand what they are trying to say. There are many ways in which the family can help in such instances: by assuring the patient that this does not mean he is losing his mind, by making up signals so that he can describe what he wants and needs, and by exercising a great deal of understanding and patience. Methods of speech therapy are discussed in detail in Chapter 13. Additional information can be obtained from a booklet entitled *Aphasia and the Family,* published by the American Heart Association. This reference will give family members a good overview of the whole problem. The physician or nurse can help the family to work with the patient.

Other booklets published by the Public Health Service which could be helpful to patients and family members are:

If You Have Emphysema or Chronic Bronchitis, No. 367—15¢.

Diabetes and You, No. 567.

Hearing Loss, No. 207—25¢.

Multiple Sclerosis, No. 621—5¢.

Parkinson's Disease, No. 811—20¢.

The local chapter of the Arthritis and Rheumatism Foundation can tell the arthritic patient and his family what services are available in the community, and their various publications may be of help in gaining a better understanding of the different aspects of arthritic diseases— their origin, manifestations, and treatments. These can be obtained, at no cost, by writing to the local chapter of the Foundation or its national headquarters (10 Columbus Circle, New York, New York). Available are the following handbooks: *About Gout: A Handbook for Patients, Osteoarthritis: A Handbook for Patients, Diet and Your Arthritis, Home Care in Arthritis, Rheumatoid Arthritis: A Handbook for Patients,* and *Arthritis : Manual for Nurses, Physical Therapists, and Medical Social Workers.*

Many cities have rehabilitation centers with specialized equipment and well-trained specialists, where patients with fractures, hemiplegia, quadriplegia, arthritis, and other physical handicaps may be trained in the activities of daily living and where families may be able to receive practical instruction in how to care for them at home. Families should consult these centers to learn what help can be provided. In areas where there are no such centers, there are often specialists who can be called upon for help. The American Physical Therapy Association (1156 15th Street, N.W., Washington, D.C., 20005) will give the physician the name of a local chapter officer who can advise him of the newest services available.

When a person needs occupational therapy, The American Occupational Therapy Association (251 Park Avenue, South, New York, New York, 10010) can also supply the names of chapter officers who will know of services available in the particular vicinity. The American Speech and Hearing Association (9030 Old Georgetown Road, Washington, D.C., 20014) may be able to provide the names of a qualified person in the field of speech correction who lives in or near the patient's home.

GENERAL NURSING PROBLEMS IN THE HOME

Ambroise Paré wrote in 1583 that "I dressed him and God cured him." It should be added that "good nursing would have helped." Indeed, to the severely incapacitated patient, those who nurse him well do not appear merely as the handmaidens of medicine; their services may be even more important than the sporadic appearance of the physician. Some of the fundamentals of good nursing given below may seem trivial and obvious, but these often are the most important to the comfort of the patient, and inclusion here is warranted if for emphasis alone. These services should be within the ability of many families, who can make their sick loved ones comfortable at home. (For a more detailed description of general nursing procedures, see the Red Cross *Home Nursing Textbook,* available at the local chapter of the American National Red Cross for $1.50.) In many places, local chapters of the Red Cross give free courses in first aid and care of the sick and injured, which contain much information that is valuable for emergency care and accident prevention, as well as for the training of family members to give simple nursing care to the aged, ill, or handicapped person in the home. Persons interested in these training sessions should consult the chapter of the American National Red Cross serving their community.

HYGIENE

Basically this means maintaining the cleanliness and neat appearance of the patient and the provision of clean and conducive environment.

BED

The average bed, be it in the home or in the hospital, is either too soft or too hard and often misconstructed. A mattress made of foam rubber and placed on top of a hard bedboard presents an adequate surface for prolonged bed stay. Foam-rubber pillows, likewise, are more comfortable and hygienic than any other.

Except, perhaps, in the immediate postoperative period or for severely deformed patients, pajamas for those who like to wear them, or bed shirts which button in front if necessary, should be worn by men. Attractive nightgowns and bedjackets will be much appreciated by women. These garments may be chosen so that they can be opened in the front or back and in this way make it easier to handle the patient or allow the patient to be independent in this area of his daily care.

HOW TO MAKE A BED WITH THE PATIENT IN IT

The bed sheets should be changed frequently. When daily changes are not possible, a plan should be devised to change the linen twice or three times a week.

When caring for a bedridden patient in the home, it may be necessary for a member of the family to learn how to make the bed with the patient in it. The bedspread and blanket are first removed and the top sheet loosened. The new top sheet is placed on top of the old one, which may then be pulled out from under the fresh linen. The blanket may be placed on top. The patient is placed, or moves himself, to one side of the bed, and the top sheet and covers are folded over him so that the unoccupied side of the bed is exposed. The bottom sheet can then be loosened, folded, and rolled toward the center of the bed as close to the patient as possible. The mattress cover and the rubber or plastic sheet, if one is being used, are straightened, the new sheet is placed securely in position, tucked under at the corners, and rolled neatly toward the center of the bed, as far under the patient as possible. The patient can then roll over onto the freshly made side of the bed or be placed there. The used linen is drawn away on the other side of the bed, the fresh sheet now being stretched over to the unoccupied side of the bed, straightened, and tucked in. The top coverings of the bed are easily adjusted; they should not be tucked in too tightly, and the patient should be made comfortable by proper positioning and diversional activities.

The technique for changing the mattress is somewhat comparable. Three chairs are placed alongside the bed with the seats toward the bed. They must be at the height of the lower surface of the mattress. The mattress, with patient on it, is pulled out onto these chairs. Appropriately large pillows are placed on the empty side of the bed and the patient moves himself, or is lifted, onto these pillows. This frees the mattress, which may now be turned or changed. Then the patient moves back onto the new mattress, which is pulled back into place on the bed after the pillows have been removed.

BED EXERCISE

Whenever a patient is bedridden for more than one week, a regular routine of bed exercises should be carried out, unless they are contraindicated. They preserve muscle tone and prevent the formation of contractures and deformities. A list of such exercises has been published in F. H. Krusen's *Physical Medicine and Rehabilitation for the Clinician* (1961) and is reprinted as Table 6.

Other bed exercises are: sitting up from the supine position, pushing oneself up by the arms, which are placed in pronation along the body, and pushing up from the sitting position, pushing down on both palms, lifting hips and buttocks from bed. Quadriceps setting is very important to strengthen the thigh muscles. The leg is extended and by contraction of the quadriceps, the patella is moved up and down. This should be done 10 to 15 times an hour. The hip extensors can be strengthened by bending the knees, placing the soles of the feet flat on the bed, and raising the buttocks. This exercise can be done every time the bedpan has to be used, if this cannot be avoided.

THE BATH

The frequency of baths is, to some extent, determined by the severity of the illness. The majority of individuals who can walk, even with crutches, or those who are able to get around in a wheelchair, can use a shower with a chair in it or may be seated on a crossboard on top of or suspended in the bathtub and thus bathe themselves or be washed in this position. If this is impossible, complete or partial bed baths should be given daily. When bed baths are the only possible form of ablution, patients themselves should do as much of the washing as they can. This is excellent incidental exercise. After each

bathing the skin should be massaged lightly with rubbing alcohol, particularly on the back and over pressure areas, such as the heels, knees, sacrum, hip bones, and shoulder blades. This should be followed by application of lanolin or some cream preparation and by powdering. Brushing the teeth or inserting dentures and combing and brushing the hair should be part of the regular routine and should be done whenever possible by the patients themselves. Some consideration should be given by the family as to the best time to give the bath or to assist the patient with showering or bathing. Many times the person would like some flexibility in the daily schedule. Perhaps he would like partial care early in the morning and more complete care late in the afternoon or before bedtime. Since the patient is at home, there is no need to have a rigid schedule with the aged or the chronically ill unless it is specifically requested.

BED-BATH TECHNIQUE

Water in a suitable tub at a temperature from 105° to 115° F., or agreeable to the testing hand, a washcloth, soap, face towel, bath towel, rubbing alcohol, fresh bedclothes, and a soft, full-length, and light blanket are needed for giving a bed bath. The patient is first undressed and covered with the blanket. One should begin with the face and neck and work downward, washing separately the arms, chest, thighs, legs, and genitals. As each part is washed, as much of the patient as possible is kept covered with the blanket to keep him warm and give him a sense of privacy. Each part of the body is dried immediately after it is washed. A towel may be placed under each successive part of the patient during washing to protect the bed. The feet should be soaked in the tub. All parts of the body except the genitals may be rubbed with alcohol, and an emollient, such as cold cream, should be used to keep the skin soft. Talcum powder is applied, and deodorants, toilet waters, and cosmetics should be accessible, especially for women, if desired. The skin should be inspected daily and any reddened or inflamed areas must

TABLE 6. BED EXERCISES[a]

Part	Motion To Be Restored	Restoration Exercise
Fingers	Flexion and extension	"Practice" piano-playing; squeeze rubber ball, water pistol, sponge, crumple newspaper, knead bouncing putty
Wrist	Flexion and extension	Rest hand over edge of table: first passively, and later actively move it up and down; crumple newspaper, knead bouncing putty
	Abduction and adduction	Rest hand on table: carry sideways, then actively move it sideways; crumple newspaper
Forearm	Flexion and extension	Shadow-boxing; "chinning," either on rings, bar, floor, or end of bed
	Supination and pronation	Rotate poker, broom, or water pail
Arm	Abduction	Scratch head and comb hair lying down; then do same standing up
	Circumduction	Swing pail in a circle over head
	Internal and external rotation	Rotate a water pail at arm's length
Jaw	Flexion and extension	Chew gum
Neck	Flexion and extension	Toss head back and bring chin to chest
	Rotation	Look over right and then left shoulder
Clavicle	Gliding	Swing pail in a circle over head
Spine	Flexion, extension, and rotation	In early stages, lie in bed and bring knees to chin; later, drop objects in a line on floor and pick up singly
Hip or pelvis	Circumduction	In bed, swing extremity in circle; when weight-bearing is permissible, stand on one leg and swing other in a circle
	Abduction and adduction	In bed, carry foot from one corner of bed to other; later, stand on unaffected leg and abduct other
	Flexion and extension	Do not wait for weight-bearing period: in bed, lie on side and kick (with leg); on back, bring knees to chest; "walking horses" when on feet; climb stairs along rail; bring knees to chest, leaning on chair
	Internal and external rotation	In bed, turn foot and leg to left and right; later, pivot on one foot
Leg	Flexion and extension	In bed, bring knee to chest; later, climb stairs along rail; kick leg when reclining
	Internal and external rotation	In bed or chair, simply rotate leg; on weight bearing, pivot on leg
Foot	Flexion and extension	Place bandage on big toe and pull on bandage, as if playing horse. Later, stand on ball of foot and go up on toes
	Eversion and inversion	With ankle on knee, do passively. Place well foot alongside injured foot and then invert and evert together. Move towel sidewise with toes and outer border of foot
Toes	Flexion and extension	Move towel lengthwise by "crabbing" with toes; try to pick up a pencil; go up on toes and down again

[a] All exercises should be prescribed in a definite fashion such as: "Squeeze a sponge or crumple a newspaper three times a day, 5 minutes by the clock or, with well hand resting on table, rotate a pail, half-full of water, twenty times, with pail almost touching floor."

receive particularly careful attention. Men should be encouraged to shave and women to wear cosmetics, for this attention increases one's self-esteem.

SLEEP

Sleeping and waking hours should be regulated by a reasonable schedule. The patient's care must be fitted into the home routine to some extent, but it is best to adjust the daily schedule, as nearly as possible, to the patient's habits. No one who is bedridden misses much by "getting up" late. If early awakening is the rule, however, do not let the patient wait until noon before he gets his bath and breakfast! The hour of retiring is immaterial but should be kept as consistent as possible from day to day to allow formation of a sleeping habit. The patient should be quiet and undisturbed at night, yet know that someone is within calling distance at all times. Small night lights, available in most hardware stores, may add to the peace of mind of sick persons.

SUNLIGHT AND FRESH AIR

Much has been made of fresh air and sunlight. The medical benefits of sun in the presence of adequate vitamin intake are doubtful, and any air with sufficient oxygen is all that is needed. The psychological value of sun and fresh air is such, however, that these factors have been rightly stressed. Whenever it can be managed, they should be made available to bedridden patients. The environment should be free of unpleasant odor and unnecessary equipment. Supplies should be kept in a central place and clearly labeled.

URINARY BLADDER FUNCTION

The management of incontinence from the medical point of view is discussed elsewhere. It is the function of the nurse or of the family to report incontinence immediately, should it occur, and to keep track of all urination so that retention does not go unnoticed.

Beyond this the genitals must be kept dry and clean at all times, and a patient must never be allowed to remain wet with urine. As soon as incontinence is discovered, the sheets must be changed and the patient bathed, massaged, oiled, and powdered. Liberal use of powder around the genitals is indicated.

Incontinence must be remedied, if possible, or, when it is anticipated, a rubber sheet, or preferably a plastic sheet, should be used under the bottom sheet. To include this routinely in all sickbeds, however, is not kind to the patient, since rubber sheets often make the bed uncomfortable. In this respect, plastic vinylite sheets are preferable as long as they are reasonably new and soft.

BOWEL ACTION

Good nursing requires that a record be kept of the patient's bowel movements, including their color and whether they are well formed or liquid. Such constant observation will often indicate trouble before it becomes serious. The physician can be alerted at any change in the schedule of bowel movements or in the quality or quantity of feces. He can often treat effectively the causes of such irregularities. If bowel incontinence occurs, it should be overcome whenever possible and the sooner the better. As with urinary incontinence, soilage by feces cannot be permitted to remain. The patient's bed and clothing must be changed immediately, and the skin must be cleansed and treated. In incontinence of some duration it has been found useful to treat the perianal skin and that of the buttocks with tincture of benzoin, which protects against irritation; many people find that an application of Desitin ointment is helpful and soothing.

NUTRITION

Nutrition is an important part of the patient's care and with the aid of the section in this book dealing with this subject it should be possible to manage this problem. The family should be able to cater within reason to the patient's likes and dislikes, so that nourishment will be taken in sufficient amounts. The importance of making the food appetizing and serving it in an appealing way can never be overemphasized, and variety is always appreciated. A patient generally enjoys his meal more if he has company while eating, and if it is impossible for him to join the family for his meals, care should be taken to visit with him in his room while he is dining, or even a visit while he is enjoying his dessert is appreciated.

ATTITUDE

It is of the utmost importance for all members of the family of the chronically ill and elderly patient as well as others concerned with his care to provide the proper atmosphere for their charge. An attitude of despair or apathy cannot help being transmitted to the patient. Irritation caused by the patient's inability to handle routine tasks speedily or by his refusal to cooperate in all phases of the treatment cannot help him in his efforts to gain the greatest possible degree of independence; on the contrary, it may only serve to discourage him. Members of the family must remember not to do too much for the patient; they must remember that independent activity is the key to his mental, physical, and social well-being; conversely, they must not ignore him and make him feel exiled from family life. The disabled, elderly person needs a sense of achievement, a reason for living. Any routine chores that he can perform, any useful projects that can be suggested, any hobbies that he can manage will make the hours pass in an interesting way. This not only will improve the patient's morale but also will make life more pleasant for all concerned.

The family should be willing to cooperate with the doctor, the nurse, the therapist, and any other medical and paramedical personnel involved in the patient's care. If specific foods are required, they should make certain that the patient eats them and not other foods that have been excluded. If exercises are needed, the family must see that they are performed and help with

them when necessary. If transportation to a clinic or a community agency is required, it is up to the members of the family to see that it is provided. Patients confined to wheelchairs or to their beds should be given a change of scenery when possible. Their bedrooms should not become the worlds of their later lives unless it is necessary.

Responsibilities lie heavily upon the shoulders of those faced with the many problems of caring for chronically ill patients. Family members, too, need a change in their daily activities from time to time. The change can be brief (a day) or extended (3 to 5 days) and will provide them relief from the cares required by the aged or chronically ill person. However, with a healthy, optimistic but practical attitude, patients and their families can learn to accept the handicaps of their respective problems and adapt to them successfully.

TERMINAL CARE

As chronic illness progresses, the time may come when the patient is completely helpless and death is inevitable. This is a period when good nursing becomes a heavy chore, nevertheless it provides the opportunity for true compassion and to show a generous spirit. For a family, it is a most consoling feeling to have been able to sustain a loved one during the terminal phase of illness.

Everything must be done to keep the patient clean, free of bedsores, and as comfortable as possible. The patient may find a semireclining position with a back support to be the most comfortable. Profuse sweating may occur; if so, the skin should be sponged with diluted alcohol and the patient be kept as dry as possible.

While the skin of dying patients may feel cool, they can suffer from elevated temperatures. Open windows, fans, and a cool room temperature are desirable, the patient being kept covered, although lightly. Patients in their dying hours may seem unconscious, but actually their hearing may be quite acute. Nothing, therefore, should be said near these patients which is not intended for their ears.

As the senses fail, there may be a desire for light. The room of the dying patient should be well lighted, well aired, and quiet. If these simple precepts are observed to the last, much of the discomfort associated with dying and death can be prevented.

The opportunity to discuss the impending death must also be given to the patient. The family, the minister, the priest, the doctor— all can play a role in affording the emotional comfort the patient desires. Too often, a feeling of helplessness occurs at the time these important human supports are needed, and shunning the patient during his last hours results.

REFERENCES

Annual Report, 1971. New York: National Council of Homemaker and Home Health Aide Service, 1972.

BLACK, SR., KATHLEEN N. Teaching family process and intervention. *Nurs. Outlook* 18:54–58, 1970.

BRODY, ELAINE M. Serving the aged: Educational needs as viewed by practice. *Social Work Journal of the NASW,* 15: No. 4, October, 1970.

DEUTSCH, SUZANNE Z., and KRASNER, BARRETT. Meeting the needs of the older patient through comprehensive planning. *J. Geriatric Psychiatr.,* 3, #1, 1969.

DUCAS, DOROTHY (Ed.). *National Voluntary Health Agencies of 19 Member Agencies of the National Health Council,* New York, 1969.

Encyclopedia of Social Work. New York: NASW, 1971, pp. 51–71, 433–443.

EVANGELA, SR. M. The influence of family relationships on the geriatric patient. *Nurs. Clin. North America* 3:653–662, 1968.

HARRISON, CHERIE. The institutionally deprived elderly. *Nurs. Clin. North America* 3, December, 1968, pp. 697–707.

HODKINSON, MARY A. *Some clinical problems of geriatric nursing. Nurs. Clin. North America* 3: 675–686, 1968.

Home Health Aide Services. New York: National League for Nursing, Council of Public Health Nursing Services, 1968.

Household and Family Characteristics, Population Characteristics. Bureau of Census, U.S. Department of Commerce, Series p. 20, No. 218, March 23, 1971.

KENNEDY, ROWLAND B. Physician-sponsored home health services: Private delivery profile. *Am. Fam. Physician* 3:151–155, 1971.

KRAMER, CHARLES H., and DUNLAP, HOPE E. Optimal frustration aids recovery, *Geriatric Nurs.* 3:14–18, 1967.

KRUSEN, F. H. *Physical Medicine and Rehabilitation for the Clinician.* Philadelphia: Saunders, 1961.

MANGEN, SR., FRANCIS X. Psychological aspects of nursing the advanced cancer patient. *Nurs. Clin. North America* 2:647–658, 1967.

MANSFIELD, ELAINE. Compensatory behavior in the aging. *Geriatric Nurs.* 3:18–20, 1967.

MOORE, FLORENCE. *Testimony Before the Committee on Finance. U.S. Senate, on H.R.I.* New York: National Council of Homemaker and Home Health Aide Services, 1972.

QUINT, JEANNE. The dying patient, a difficult nursing problem. *Nurs. Clin. North America* 2: 763–773, 1967.

PETERSEN, DREW M. *Home Health Care: Whose Decision?* AMA Ogden, Utah: Council of Medical Services, National League for Nursing, 1970.

Recommendations for Homemaker and Home Health Aide Training and Services. Public Health Service Publication No. 1891, U.S. Department of Health, Education and Welfare, 1969.

Senior Citizens News 3, #125, November 28–December 2, 1971.

SHANAS, ETHEL. Measuring the home health needs of the aged in five countries. *J. Geront.* 20:37–40, 1971.

SHOCK, N. W. *Aging—Some Social and Biological Aspects.* Washington, D.C.: American Association for the Advancement of Science, Publ. No. 65, 1960, pp. 241–260.

WEYMOUTH, LILYAN. The nursing care of the so-called confused patient. *Nurs. Clin. North America* 3:709–715, 1968.

White House Conference on Aging, January, 1972. Report to the Delegates from Conference Sessions and Special Concern Sessions. Washington, D.C.: National Council of Senior Citizens.

18

Tips on Choosing and Using Crutches, Canes, and Walkers*

A lot of patients' money is wasted, and their ability to function is often impaired, by ordering walking appliances they cannot and will not use. This chapter provides the family doctor with a basic guide to early recognition of a patient's need for ambulation aids, patient conditioning, selecting the most appropriate appliances, supervising their fitting, and giving instruction in use. The patient was a 55-year-old teacher who had severe pain in her left hip and knee from osteoarthritis. A succession of well-intentioned doctors had prescribed various drugs and canes—none of which was effective—and she finally had to give up teaching. At last her current (and permanent) family physician referred her to a physical therapist, who gave her two axillary crutches and some instruction in how to use them.

The results read like a Madison Avenue testimonial:

her pain has been relieved;

she has discontinued medications; and

she has returned to her career.

While this example illustrates the wisdom of having a competent physical therapist evaluate and train patients who need walking appliances, it is often more practical for a knowledgeable family physician to offer these services himself. In fact, whether or not you choose to refer, as a family physician you still have at least one major obligation: early recognition of need. Many patients may waste their money or miss important benefits unless you conscientiously seek out those who might gain from short- or long-term use of an appliance.

For example, suppose an overweight patient complains of pain on walking due to moderate degenerative changes in his hip and knee. Instead of automatically prescribing pain medication and a weight-reduction diet, some consideration should be given to relief of weight bearing by ambulation aids. Moderate degenerative changes often improve symptomatically with ambulation aids.

The benefits of a walking appliance for such a patient are subtle. Support of just 20 percent of body weight with a cane can relieve the involved lower extremity joint of nearly 40 percent of total force. This potentiation of effect occurs because the cane, held on the side opposite the painful joint, decreases the pull of the stabilizing muscles on the joint while supporting minimal body weight.

Another patient who may experience dramatic relief of pain with a walking appliance is the individual with senile osteoporosis of the vertebral column. Pain emanates from minimal compression fractures of the vertebrae caused by the center of gravity falling anterior to the thoracic vertebrae whenever the patient stands. Using two crutches anterior to the line of gravity reduces compressing forces on the vertebrae, which not only relieves his pain but also gives him greater physical freedom. Such a patient could be expected to tolerate bracing very poorly.

* Prepared with the assistance of Charles D. Bonner, M.D., physical medicine, Cambridge, Mass.; Jack Hofkosh, R.P.T., physical therapy, New York City; Robert H. Jebsen, M.D., physical medicine, Seattle, Wash.; and Charles Neuhauser M.D., P.T., family medicine, Madison, Wisc. Dr. Jebsen's contribution to this article was supported in part by Social Rehabilitation Services Grant No. RT-3.

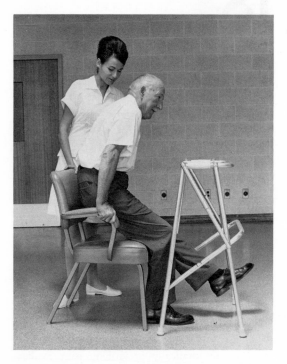

FIG. 88. Patient with fractured hip learning to sit properly onto an armchair.

Therefore, walking appliances are particularly applicable for the osteoarthritic.

The benefits of properly prescribed walking appliances, in addition to support and redistribution of body weight, include:

stability, through a wider base of support and altered center of gravity;

relief of pain;

decreased fear of reinjury and instability;

early return to work or school after injury;

prolongation of ambulation in spite of progressive disease.

Of course, there are some negative factors, too. The patient with spinal osteoporosis may exhibit strong feelings about being labeled a cripple or "handicapped" by society because he uses crutches to relieve pain. But unless you can persuade him to try crutches, the prejudices he shares with society will keep him from a more active, less painful life.

If these benefits are to be achieved, and if you do not refer your patients to a physical therapist, your responsibilities also include patient conditioning, selecting the most appropriate appliances, supervising the fitting of the appliances, ensuring that patients are properly instructed in their use, and follow-up care which includes periodic review of the patient's status. The balance of this article takes up each of these points.

Recognition of a patient's need for ambulation goes beyond seeing the immediate benefits. Deformity and debilitation must be prevented, and muscles strengthened in anticipation of using walking appliances.

If you plan to prescribe a walking appliance for a patient temporarily confined to a bed or chair, be sure to give him basic guidelines for maintaining strength and range of motion. You may need to explain the physiological benefits of activity in ordinary terms to gain his confidence and cooperation.

You might say, for example: "The more you are up and and around the better your circulation will be. Your general health will be better. Your body will heal itself faster. You'll feel better. If you spend most of your time lying down or sitting, you may get fat and your muscles *will* get weak. Walking will be even harder."

Recent experience with military personnel injured in Vietnam has furnished evidence of the benefits to selected patients of early weight bearing after certain fractures of the lower extremities. Weight bearing instituted within 24 hours after cast application is reducing the incidence of nonunion in these young men and resulting in a quicker return to active duty. Almost all patients are achieving full weight bearing within a few days, even though they are not encouraged to bear weight if they experience pain. This military rehabilitation program is individualized since, of course, personality, pain tolerance, anxiety, and coordination are all taken into account.

It may help your debilitated patient to set aside certain times of the day for walking, with gradual increments in time and distance. You'll want to have the patient, his family, physical therapist, or visiting nurse keep a record of his improving performance and, more importantly, to show your patient that you too recognize his gains.

Proper bed positioning can, of course, aid in preventing development of muscle contractures. Foot drop has been largely eliminated by wide use of footboards in hospitals and homes. But make sure that your patient is keeping his heels flat down against the board and that the balls of his feet are carefully inspected each day for red spots that might indicate development of pressure sores. A padded footboard might reduce chances of a pressure sore.

Hip flexion contractures are a greater problem and occur fairly often in long-term bed patients. To prevent them, have your patient lie on his stomach for several 30-minute periods each day, legs together, since hip flexion can occur with external rotation when the legs are abducted.

In addition, hip range-of-motion exercises should be instituted as soon as possible for any long-term bed or chair patient, stressing extension and internal rotation. If your patient cannot lie in a prone position, make sure he doesn't sit up for more than half the day and that he spends at least part of the day with his hips extended, on his back or side.

An exercise program for maintaining muscle strength and promoting circulation also has general application. It's not surprising that patients have wobbly knees when they first get up since the quadriceps diminish in strength after just 24 hours of inactivity.

A good and simple bed exercise is quad setting. Tell the patient to tighten his knee muscles so that the front of his knee wrinkles up. Have him repeat this exercise ten times several times a day. If the patient is a child, you might use a felt-tip pen to draw a face on his knee; ask him to make the little face laugh.

Patients often have trouble isolating muscle groups for this type of isometric exercise, and you might want to try still another teaching technique presented above.

If your patient will be depending on the strength of one leg when he gets up, make sure that the leg will be ready. He may need to strengthen hip and knee extensors against gravity, hand resistance, or weights. He must maintain strength and flexibility in the noninjured as well as the injured extremity.

For the upper extremities, he can strengthen the "push" muscles—shoulder depressors, elbow and wrist extensors—by doing sitting pushups in his bed or an armchair. In bed, he places his hands palm down on two or three thick books at his sides and pushes to straighten his elbows and lift his body from the bed. In the armchair, he pushes down against the arms to raise himself from the seat.

There are dangers to handing out crutches with no thought given to the musculature required to use them. Unless his shoulder and elbow extensors are strong enough, a patient will probably lean on the shoulder bars of his crutches, with the attendant danger of nerve compression. Sustained compression of the radial nerve results in crutch paralysis, an insidious disability. The median and ulnar nerves are also affected occasionally. Sensation is rarely affected, and as the triceps and wrist extensors become weaker, the patient leans ever more heavily on the shoulder bar, increasing the injury.

Crutch paralysis is more common in women because of their comparatively weaker upper extremities and is always a potential danger in patients who have upper extremity involvement. This should not limit the prescribing of crutches, but rather, points out the need for proper instruction and followup. Be sure to check the strength of the triceps and wrist extensors regularly. Do not rely on sensory changes; muscle atrophy or wrist drop may be the first sign of paralysis due to nerve pressure.

Proper fit is, of course, another factor in prevention of crutch paralysis. It is discussed in the text on page 25.

Beware the pitfall of underprescribing walking appliances. Your own awareness of the cultural view that walking appliances label a man as a cripple may lead you to prescribe the appliance which has the least stigma to image,

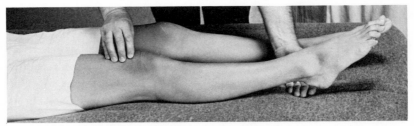

A

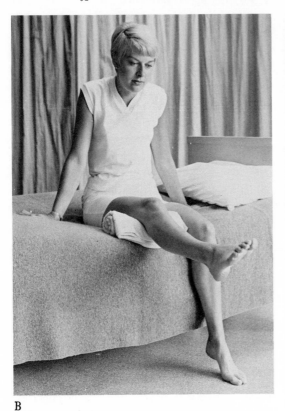

B

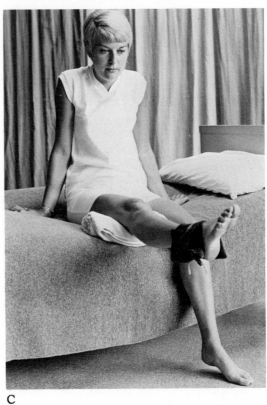

C

FIG. 89. KNEE EXTENSORS. A. "Just start to lift your heel off my hand," the physician tells his patient. He places first his fingertips then the patient's along the proximal edge of the patella and asks her to feel the tightening of the quadriceps. B. Here, the patient straightens her knee against the force of gravity. The rolled-up towel under her knee helps stabilize the leg while sitting on the soft bed. C. She now progresses to resistance against weights, having sewn this bag and bought some one-pound lead weights from a plumber's shop. The patient gradually increases the weights. (With a bigger bag, she could use various sized canned goods for progressive weights, i.e., a one-pound can of peas.)

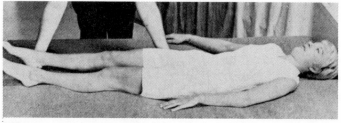

90A

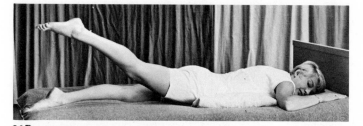

90B

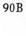

FIG. 90. HIP EXTENSORS. A. "Push your heel down against my hand and feel your hip muscles tighten against my other hand." The patient then tries to tighten gluteal muscles on both sides, pushing both feet down into the bed. B. The patient exercises her hip extensors by raising her leg against the force of gravity. Resistance can be gradually increased by having someone in the family push against the thigh gently or by adding weights at the ankle if the knee is stable.

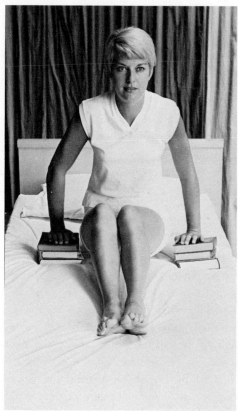

91A

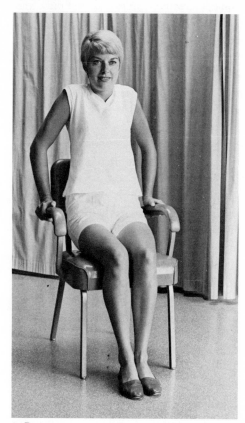

91B

FIG. 91. SHOULDER DEPRESSORS, ELBOW AND WRIST EXTENSORS. A. To strengthen her shoulder depressors and elbow and wrist extensors, patient uses several books to substitute for the blocks ordinarily used for sitting push-ups in physical therapy departments. She pushes down, straightening her elbows, to lift her body from the bed. B. Now the patient sits in an armchair to practice sitting push-ups. She pushes down against the arms of the chair to lift her body from the seat.

rather than the one greatest in therapeutic value. When you recognize that a patient needs to relieve weight bearing on a joint, for instance, consider the advantages of crutches before you suggest that he try out a cane.

Selection of the appropriate appliance—as well as the gait to be used with it—requires neat tailoring. Some patients—perhaps having sustained a fracture, amputation, or laceration—improve. Others, those suffering from chronic or debilitating illnesses, such as arthritis or multiple sclerosis, regress; they present a continuing need for evaluation; they require ever more stability as their strength, balance, or coordination becomes increasingly impaired, and the walking appliance must be changed accordingly.

Walkers (also called walkerettes) are the most stable walking appliances, followed in descending order by a pair of axillary crutches, two forearm crutches, one forearm crutch, two canes, and then, one cane. There are also special adaptations for each. See Table 7.

The way a patient walks with his appliance also affects his stability; thus, you should also prescribe his gait sequence.

Some gaits are designed to support one lower extremity, others to support both legs having independent motion, and still others to support both extremities having no independent motion. For example, the gaits used for supporting one lower extremity are, in descending order of stability: three-point nonweight bearing, three-point partial weight bearing, one crutch, and then one cane. Gaits supporting both extremities which move independently are, in descending order of stability: walker or crutch gait, four-point, and then two-point. Swing-to or swing-through gaits are employed when a patient must move both legs as a unit, with no independent leg motion.

Selection of the appliance and gait is complicated by the type, degree, and location of the disability, along with any involvement of the upper extremity, ataxia, or visual disturbance—all affecting the degree of stability needed. Keeping in mind the need to tailor the appliance and

gait to the patient, rather than vice versa, it may be useful to examine typical appliance-gait choices.

Lower-extremity conditions which require progressively less ambulation support include:

Amputation. Without prosthesis, prescribe swing-through or swing-to gait with walker or crutches. With prosthesis, start with a three-point crutch gait progressing to one forearm crutch, then one cane. Some patients progress to walking with prosthesis alone. A physical therapist can evaluate possibilities according to the amputation site and length of the stump.

Hemiplegia. Prescribe a cane or single forearm crutch. With the unaffected arm, a patient should advance the cane, step with the weak leg, then step with the strong leg. He should progress rapidly to the faster pace of advancing the cane and weak leg at the same time; some patients progress to walking without an aid. If the patient has a problem with balance, he may do well with a three- or four-legged cane, or two ambulation aids.

Fracture. A swing-through three-point gait with crutches or walker is indicated for nonweight bearing and a three-point gait for partial weight bearing. Your initial recommendation will depend on the site of the fracture, stage of healing, and amount of weight bearing allowed. If the patient may take more than 50 percent of his weight on the broken leg, a four-point gait is the choice, progressing quickly to a two-point if possible. *Caution:* Hip flexion contracture is a potential hazard of the unilateral nonweight-bearing three-point gait because the patient usually holds his affected hip and knee in a flexed position. Be certain the patient understands the danger and maintains range of motion through exercise and prone-lying.

Paraplegia. Prescribe crutches with a swing-to or swing-through gait. The latter is faster. A paraplegic uses aids primarily for therapeutic ambulation unless the lesion is low enough to leave voluntary hip flexion. In this case, the patient can use a four-point or alternate two-point gait with axillary or forearm crutches.

Table 7. Guidelines for Selecting Walking Appliances

Typical Patient Profile	Appliance	Advantages	Disadvantages	Precautions
Elderly, apprehensive, generally debilitated, and/or brain damaged, or any condition where balance is poor. He requires support of more than 50% of his body weight. *Example:* Amputation, early training; severe arthritis; fracture of hip or lower extremity (elderly or fearful); multiple sclerosis, sprains (elderly or fearful).	Walker (Walkerette)	1. Most stable of walking appliances. 2. Sequence relatively easily learned by geriatric and/or brain-damaged patient. 3. Older and apprehensive patients feel safer with walkers. 4. Does not require normal balance.	1. Cannot be used on stairs (unless of special stair-climbing type). 2. Wobbly on uneven ground. 3. Difficult to maneuver in a small room or among furniture. 4. Imposes slow pace. 5. Promotes stooped-over posture. 6. Natural walking sequence cannot be used, making transition to cane difficult, and often creating a limp because of irregular timing of stride.	Never place wheels on a walker. Although allowing a faster pace and easier maneuverability, wheels are hazardous because they negate stability.
Any patient who requires support of more than 50% of his body weight; has adequate shoulder depressors, triceps and hand grip. *Example:* Amputation; moderate arthritis; fracture of hip or lower extremity; muscle disease; multiple sclerosis; paraplegia; sprains; various injuries such as lawn-mower lacerations; etc.	Axillary crutches	1. Patient can move at a fast pace. 2. Can be used on stairs, in a small room or amid clutter, and on uneven ground. 3. Require little space to store or transport. 4. Greater stability than cane or forearm crutch. 5. Can be used with good posture. 6. Patient develops good coordination between sides of body and between arms and legs because reciprocal action of arms and legs is possible.	1. Sequences too complicated for some patients to learn. 2. Require fairly good balance. 3. Older patients tend to be apprehensive with crutches. 4. Possible to develop crutch paralysis of the triceps from bearing weight on the axillary bar. Patients who are debilitated or have pain and weakness in the upper extremities are likely candidates for crutch paralysis.	Instruct the patient not to lean into the shoulder bar. Crutch paralysis may develop. Sensation is rarely affected; muscle atrophy may be the first sign of paralysis. Make sure the crutches have large rubber suction tips.

TABLE 7. (*Continued*)

Typical Patient Profile	Appliance	Advantages	Disadvantages	Precautions
Patient has weak triceps, wrist extensors, or hand grip but requires support of more than 50% of his body weight.	Adapted axillary crutches. 1. For weak wrist: extend strap across dorsum of wrist between two uprights of crutch. 2. For weak handgrip: sew a glove onto the hand grip; a gripper snap at the wrist will keep the hand in place.	Same as axillary crutches	Same as axillary crutches	Call patient in for frequent checks on strength of his triceps and wrist extensors. This patient is a prime candidate for crutch paralysis.
Usually an adult who requires support of no more than 40–50% of his body weight. The patient must have a strong hand grip unless the crutch is adapted for forearm weight bearing, as with the shelf-crutch (see below). *Example:* Arthritis, all stages.	Forearm crutch	1. Impossible to develop crutch paralysis. 2. More stable than cane because there are two points of contact, forearm and hand.	1. Less stable than axillary crutches.	When using a single forearm crutch, the patient should always hold it in the hand opposite the involved extremity, for three reasons: 1. The center of gravity stays evenly between the two legs, improving balance and eliminating a lurching gait. 2. A wide base of support improves balance. 3. Reciprocal motion is the normal walking pattern. The right hand swings forward with the left leg, and vice versa.

Indication	Device	Stability/Advantages	Comparison	Use/Precautions
Requires support of no more than 40–50% of his body weight but cannot bear weight on hands because of flexion contractures of the elbow, wrist fracture requiring a cast with elbow held at right angle, severe hand deformity, or below-elbow amputation.	Shelf-crutch, an adapted forearm crutch	More stable than cane because the entire forearm serves as the point of contact.	Same as forearm crutch	Same as forearm crutch
Can walk without support but needs appliance to improve balance or to relieve weight bearing stresses on osteoarthritic hip or knee. Requires support of no more than 20–25% of body weight.	Cane	1. A small amount of weight borne on a cane can widen the base of support and eliminate lurch in the patient's gait. 2. Partially unloads the pull of hip stabilizing muscles, cuts in half the total force upon a diseased hip or knee. 3. Accepted by patients to whom appearance is very important. 4. Restores the patient's confidence in his sense of balance.	1. Least stable of walking appliances because there is only one point of contact with upper extremity.	When using a single cane, the patient should use it in the hand opposite the leg to be supported (see precautions under forearm crutch).
Patient with poor balance and slow gait, usually hemiparetic. An elderly patient who requires improvement in his balance and perhaps mild support for his stability.	Three- or four-legged cane	1. *With slow gait*, it provides more stability than the standard cane. 2. The cane can stand by itself if patient wishes to use that arm for some activity.	1. With faster walking there is a rocking action from the rear legs which eliminates any stability advantage. 2. Some authorities feel the three-legged cane is no more stable than a regular cane. 3. The protrusion of the multi-legged base makes it easy to hit door jambs and furniture.	The patient should use it in the hand opposite the leg to be supported.

Most physicians refer paraplegics for the inclusive training offered by physical therapists.

Sprain. In most cases, a nonweight-bearing three-point gait would be indicated, with crutches or walker, to prevent stress on the joint.

Various injuries, such as lawn-mower lacerations. If weight bearing is not a factor, the four- or two-point gaits would be indicated to retain natural walking rhythm, promote venous return, prevent edema, and to exercise a normal range of motion in the ankle, knee, and hip.

Regressive conditions likely to require more appliance support include:

Arthritis. Lower extremity, unilateral—prescribe a cane gait with a cane or forearm crutch; if it is more severe, prescribe a weight-bearing three-point gait with forearm or axillary crutches. Lower extremity, bilateral—prescribe a two- or four-point gait with forearm or axillary crutches,

or a walker if the problem is severe. Fitted hand grips, wrist straps, or shelf-crutches might be considered for patients with upper-extremity involvement.

Multiple sclerosis and muscle disease. Needs are variable. M.S. may present primarily as paraplegia or hemiplegia. Patients with muscle disease often cannot use walking aids effectively when muscles of the shoulder girdle and triceps are weak. If the problem is primarily lack of coordination rather than weakness, however, a cane or crutch may prove very helpful.

Use the tables in this chapter to help you select the most appropriate appliances for your patients. The charts describe the comparative advantages and disadvantages of walkers, crutches, forearm crutches, and canes for a given patient.

It is dangerous to provide patients with ambulation aids if they are not fitted properly. The aids may not provide needed support and may be

TABLE 8. GUIDELINES FOR SELECTING THE GAIT

Typical Patient Profile	Gait	Advantages	Disadvantages
Requires maximum support and stability. Possibly upper extremity involved.	Four-point	1. Patient feels safe. 2. Basic pattern of reciprocal arm and leg motion. 3. Easier to learn than the alternate two-point.	1. Slow pace 2. Many elderly patients find the sequence hard to master.
Requires intermediate support and stability.	Alternate two-point	1. Normal walking pattern.	1. Fast pace 2. Difficult sequence to learn.
Unilateral involvement, nonweight bearing.	Three-point nonweight bearing		
Requires maximum support and stability	Swing-to		1. Very slow
Requires intermediate support and stability	Swing-through	1. Fast pace	
Unilateral involvement, weight bearing. Requires intermediate to maximum support and stability	Three-point partial weight bearing	1. Exercises the injured leg, improves circulation, maintains range of motion.	
Spinal injury			
Requires maximum support and stability	Swing-to		1. Very slow
Requires intermediate support and stability	Swing-through	1. Fast pace	

more of a hazard than a help. In addition, a walker or cane of inappropriate height for the patient may produce more strain than relief.

Though most patients have an inner desire for independence, many may seem poorly motivated; the task of walking with the aid of appliances strikes them as formidable.

For these two reasons—the need for proper fit and the necessity for motivation-oriented training in the aid's use—your assistant should familiarize herself with the measurement, fitting, and use of ambulation aids. Once she grasps the subject, she should be able to fit and instruct a patient in less than 15 minutes under your guidance and supervision.

To gauge roughly the correct crutch height, subtract 16 inches from the patient's height. With the crutches situated five inches in front of and five inches to the side of the patient's feet, which are together, you should be able to insert three fingers between the shoulder bar and the patient's anterior axillary fold.

When the elbow is bent 15 to 30°, the position of the hand indicates the level of the hand grip. The triceps muscle, as it straightens the elbow, can then not only support body weight, but also act as a shock absorber.

Try to fit the patient with an adjustable model, to compensate for individual variations. Once the correct fit is obtained, you can then advise the patient to buy the less expensive, non-adjustable crutches of the correct size. With a cane, simply saw the tip off to get the correct length, allowing for the height of the rubber suction tip.

Rubber suction tips are an essential part of

TABLE 9. LEARNING TO WALK WITH SUPPORT

Appliance: Walker_____Crutches_____Forearm crutch_____Cane_____

Weight bearing: Right leg_____lbs. Left leg_____lbs.

(Test your feeling for weight by placing your foot on a bathroom scale and gently increasing weight to the amount specified here.)

		Weight bearing	Nonweight bearing
Crutch gait: 4-point_____	2-point_____	3-point_____	3-point_____
swing-to_____	swing-through_____		

HERE ARE SOME SUGGESTIONS YOU MAY FIND HELPFUL

1. Hold self-closing doors open with one crutch.
2. Attach a crutch-holder on a wheelchair for convenient storage.
3. To carry things when using crutches, keep a small bag in your hand or use a pouch-type shoulder bag.
4. To carry things when using a walker, attach a bicycle basket on the front of the walker.
5. If you are using a cane in one hand and cannot hold things with your other hand, use an arm sling to carry small items.
6. For kitchen work, use a cart to transport things around the kitchen. Assemble everything you'll need on a table and then work while sitting down.
Use a high stool when doing dishes.
7. If you are going back to work or on a shopping trip, call the buildings you'll be entering to locate a door you can enter easily (revolving doors are difficult) and the elevator. Practice the distances you'll need to cover, as well as going up and down double steps if you'll travel by bus.
8. Remove all throw rugs from your home, or use extreme caution.
9. Practice going backward as well as forward on crutches, to develop your balance for crowded surroundings.

all walking appliances. Use the large type, one and a half inches in diameter, on crutches, forearm crutches, and canes. The smaller type about one inch in diameter is adequate for a walker. Never use metal gliders on these appliances.

While some experts feel that shoulder pads may encourage leaning on the crutches, others believe they prevent the crutches from slipping out from under the arm and also are more comfortable against the ribs. Foam-rubber hand grips help reduce pressure on the heels of hands in people just starting out on crutches. Once their hands have hardened, however, most people prefer to do without the grips since they cause considerable perspiring and often deteriorate with heavy use.

Of course, you'll still need to give your patient individual counsel to make his experience with walking appliances safer and more comfortable. Does the patient's home have stairs? Railings? Will he have to climb aboard a bus? To illustrate: On his first day back at work after breaking a leg, a New York executive telephoned his physician (who is also a personal friend): "Oh, Great Healer," he jeered, "why didn't you think of having me practice walking the equivalent of the two city blocks from my train to my office before I tried it for real?" "I thought you'd be smart enough to think of it yourself," the doctor retorted, but admitted later that the idea had never occurred to him.

It is essential to make a follow-up appointment within 2 to 3 weeks, for *any* patient on a walking appliance. Your evaluation should review the patient's needs, appropriate selection and proper fitting of the appliance, and training which ensures his continuing safety and comfort.

Figures 92–106 on the following pages are presented as a teaching aid for your assistant, and for self-instruction and reminders for your patients.

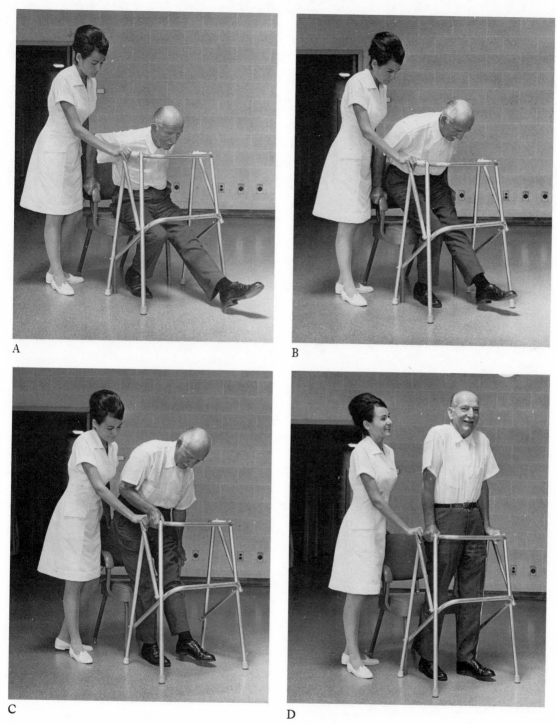

Fig. 92. Standing up. A. After surgery for a broken left hip, this man is learning how to stand with his walker. He sits on the front edge of the chair, which will help him bring his center of gravity over his right foot. Notice that his right foot is slightly under the chair, which helps him straighten his knee. B. He leans forward, bringing head forward, and pushes down on the armrests with his hands. C. He moves the hand opposite the injured leg to the walker and shifts his weight forward onto his strong leg. D. He stands erect.

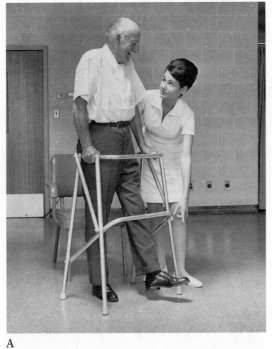

A

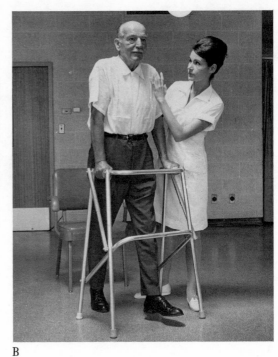

B

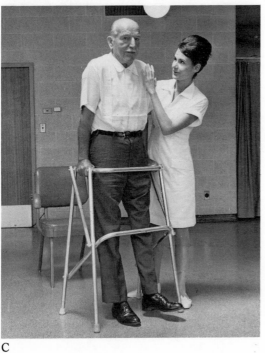

C

FIG. 93. WALKING. A. "Keep your heel off the floor as you stand up," the nurse cautions the patient. Notice that his elbows are slightly bent when he stands in one place. B. He places the walker 8 to 10 inches ahead. C. He straightens his elbows to swing himself forward to the walker.

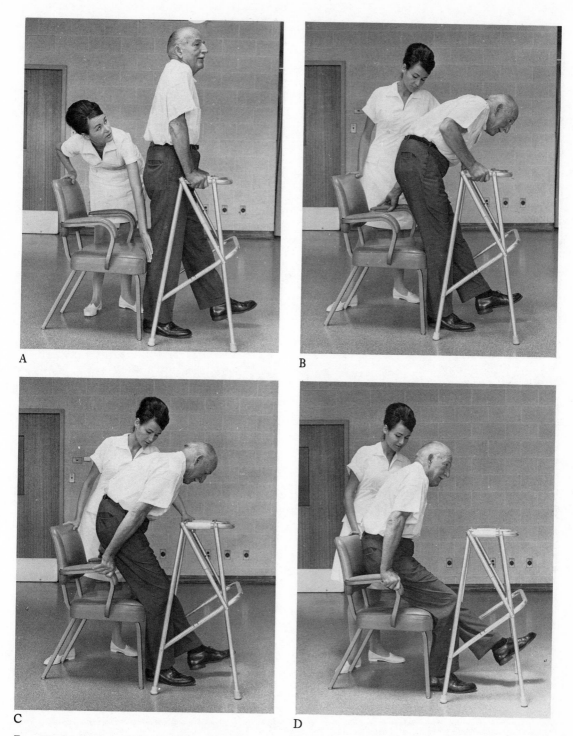

FIG. 94. SITTING DOWN. A. "Be sure that the back of your strong leg is against the chair before you sit down," warns the nurse. B. With his strong leg against the chair, he puts his opposite hand on the chair arm. C. Then he places his right hand on the right chair arm and leans forward as . . . D. He gently lowers himself onto the chair. He is instructed to avoid low chairs and to use chairs with arms whenever possible.

261

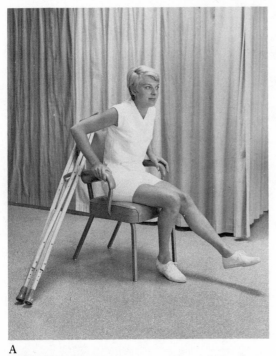

A

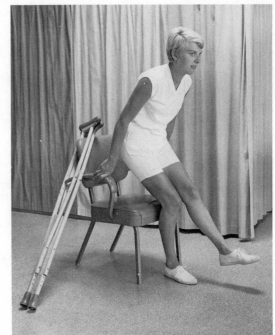

B

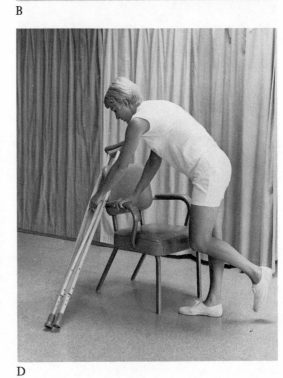

C

D

262

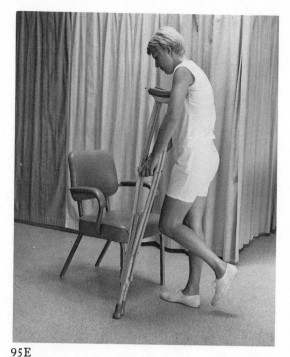

95E

Fig. 95. Standing with axillary crutches. A. This young woman keeps her crutches handy by hooking them onto the back of the chair. To stand she slides forward in the chair, with the foot of her strong leg slightly under the chair. B. She pushes down against the armrests and leans slightly forward as she stands. C. She pivots on her strong right foot. D. Placing both hands on the armrest, she picks up both crutches with the one hand. E. She then places both crutches under one arm before shifting one crutch to the other arm.

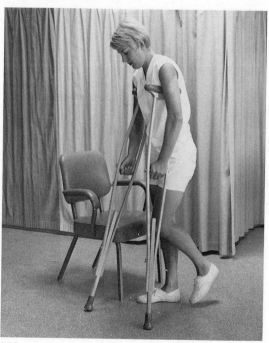

96A

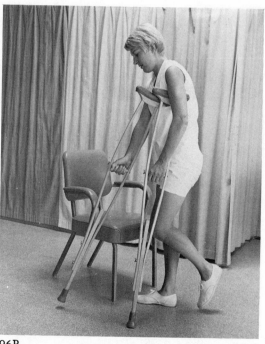

96B

Fig. 96. Sitting down in chair with crutches. A. As the young woman approaches the chair she moves her strong leg in close to the chair. B. She then places both crutches under her left arm.

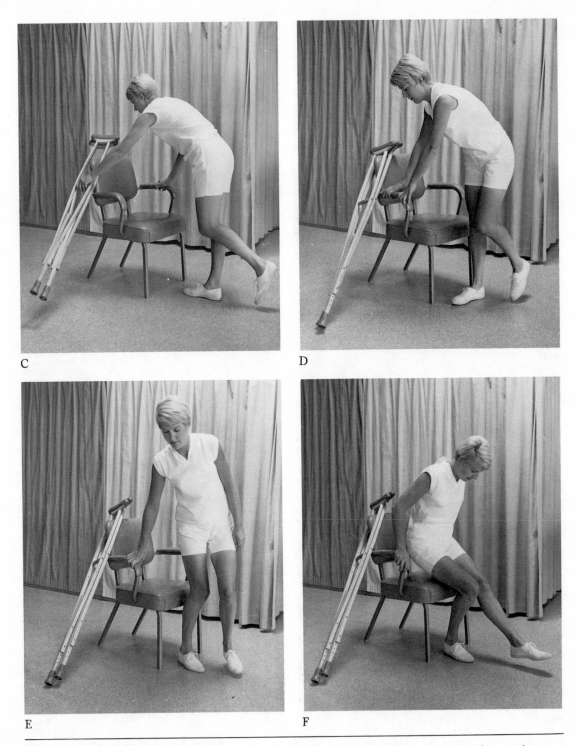

D

E

F

FIG. 96 (*Continued*). C. Placing her right hand on the left arm of the chair, she hooks the crutches onto the back of the chair. D. Now she pivots on the right foot. E. Placing her right leg against the chair, she brings her right hand around to the right chair arm. F. She gently lowers herself into the chair.

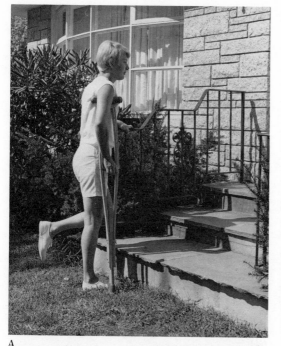

A

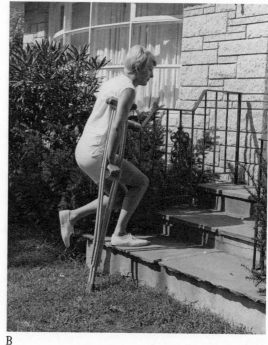

B

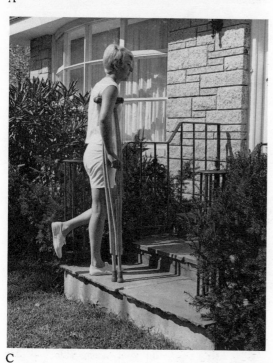

C

FIG. 97. GOING UPSTAIRS WITH CRUTCHES. A. "Up with the good leg, down with the bad." Since she cannot put any weight on her left leg, she uses her crutches and the handrail to support her weight. B. She swings her strong leg up a step. C. Then she lifts her body weight by straightening her strong hip and knee, as she would for normal stair climbing. Leaning forward helps in straightening a weakened "strong knee."

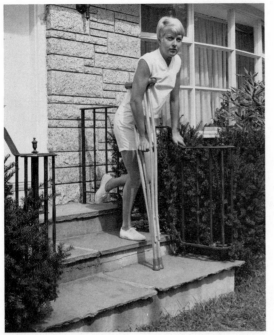
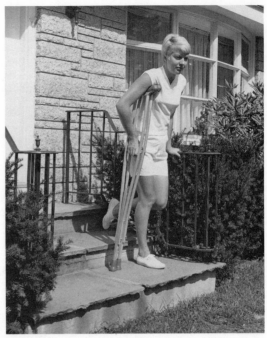

98A

98B

Fig. 98. Coming downstairs with crutches. A. "Up with the good leg, down with the bad—for going down too." With her crutches on the strong side going down, she keeps the stronger left leg on the step above as she moves her crutches down a step. B. Then she brings her leg down. Notice that she keeps her head and shoulders back to keep her center of balance and thus keep from pitching forward. The rule "up with the good leg, down with the bad" holds for curbs too. Two crutches are used instead of crutch and rail.

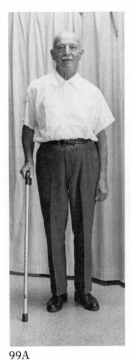
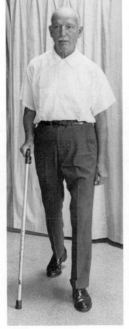
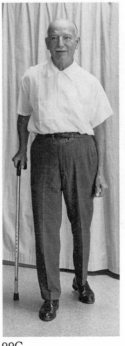

99A

99B

99C

Fig. 99. Standing with a cane. A. This patient remembers: "Always hold your cane on your strong side." B. He moves the cane and weak leg ahead together. C. He then brings his strong leg forward. Holding the cane on the strong side improves balance and promotes a smoother, more normal walking pattern.

266

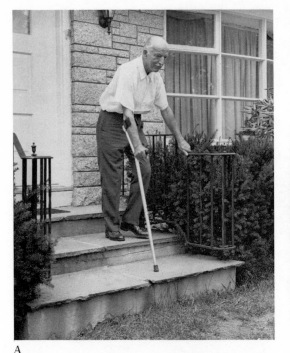

A

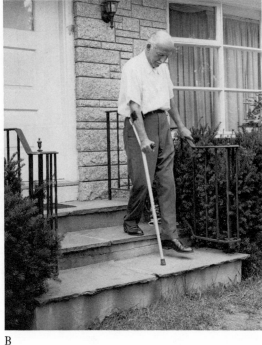

B

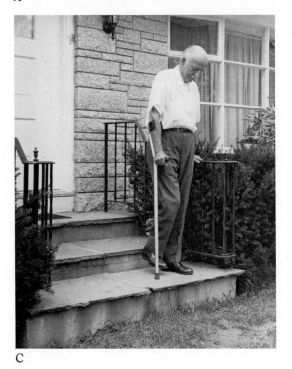

C

Fig. 100. Walking on stairs with a forearm crutch. A. "Move your crutch with your bad leg." Up with the good, down with the bad applies to canes and forearm crutches, too. He places his crutch down on the next step and his opposite hand ahead on the railing. B. He steps down with his weaker leg. C. Then he brings his strong leg down. If the patient had the use of only one hand, he would need handrails in his home on both sides of the stairs so that he could ascend and descend independently.

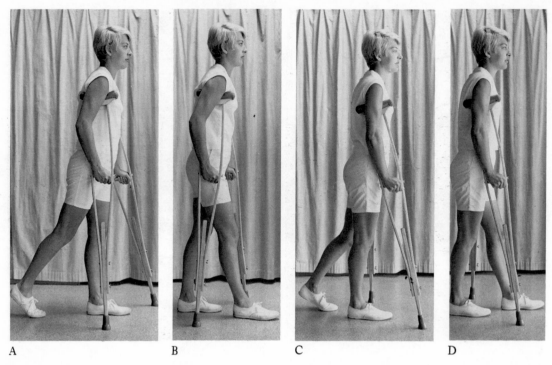

A   B   C   D

FIG. 101. FOUR-POINT GAIT. A. Only one crutch or one foot moves at a time. Here, the left crutch moves. B. Right foot moves. C. Right crutch moves. D. Left foot moves.

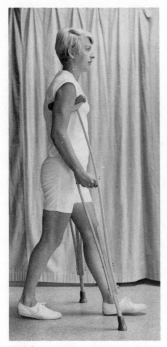
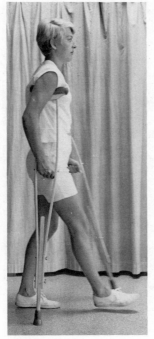

102A   102B

Fig. 102. ALTERNATE TWO-POINT GAIT. A. Opposites move together. As with the swinging of arms in normal walking, the opposite crutch moves with the leg. Right crutch *and* left foot move. B. Left crutch *and* right foot move.

Fig. 103. WEIGHT-BEARING THREE-POINT GAIT. A. "Don't put more than 20 pounds on the left leg," his doctor has cautioned. Here, this patient takes weight and strain off his broken left hip by moving both the crutches and the injured left leg forward as a unit. B. He then takes most of his body weight on his crutches as . . . C. He brings the right foot forward by itself.

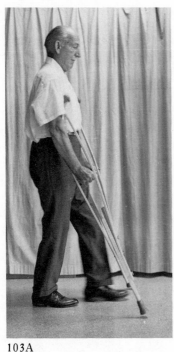

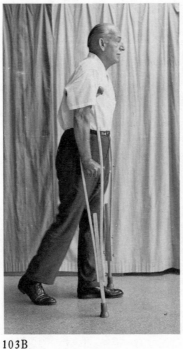
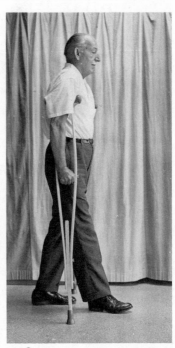

103A   103B   103C

269

Fig. 104. Nonweight-bearing three-point gait (swing-through). A. "Keep your knee bent to keep your foot off the floor." When the doctor prescribes no weight bearing for the left leg, she holds her injured foot off the floor and places both crutches ahead. B. Then she swings both legs through the crutches, while keeping the injured leg bent and bearing weight only on the crutches. She moves at a fast pace. For a slower, more stable pace, she would swing her leg to a point just behind her crutches as in the swing-to gait.

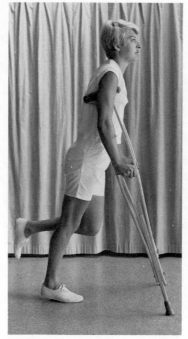
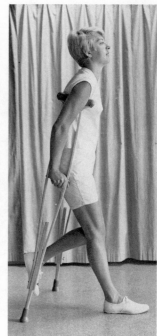

104A

104B

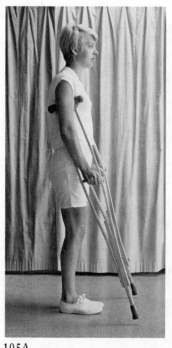
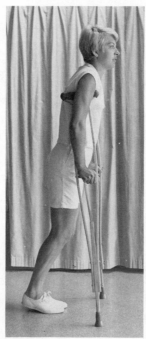

105A

105B

Fig. 105. Swing-to gait. A. "Swing your legs up to a point just behind your crutches." She places her crutches 8 to 10 inches ahead. B. She then uses her arm and shoulder muscles to swing her legs up to her crutches.

270

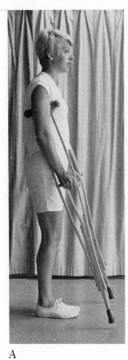
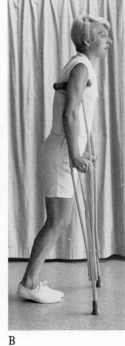
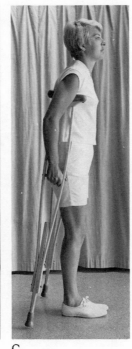

Fig. 106. Swing-through gait. A. "Swing right through." When the patient with paralyzed legs has good balance, she places her crutches 8 to 10 inches ahead of her feet. B. She uses her arm and shoulder muscles to swing her body through her crutches. C. She brings her feet 8 to 10 inches ahead of her crutches, thus achieving a very fast pace.

A   B   C

19
Home Evaluations

The old adage "there is no place like home" still has merit in dealing with the placement of the elderly. Going home is a major rehabilitation goal. There are practical situations to be met and decisions to be made, however, before home placement can be realistically accepted as the best living arrangement for the person concerned. Many times, there are insurmountable social factors that mitigate against the home as being the best place for the elderly person to go.

A not uncommon contraindication to home placement is the elderly individual who could go home, even to his own apartment, but in essence needs 24-hour supervision 7 days a week. Because of the modern way of life, it is almost impossible to find help that can meet these needs and also be within the range of reasonable financial reimbursement. In other instances, the patient may have a devoted family, but a residual difficulty with incontinence of bladder and bowel may remain. This is a particular problem if it takes place at night and requires family members to break their rest and get up and pan the patient two or three times. Unless appropriate help can be obtained to assist in sharing this responsibility, it can become an impossible situation.

There are other impediments to home placement as well. Many times the closest relative can be a daughter or a son with a spouse who has very little interest in, and even hostility toward, providing care for the in-law. The family may have a number of young children who are already taxing the capabilities of the parents involved, and taking on the elderly grandparent may foster adolescent emotional problems. The premorbid situation may have been one where the patient and the family never got along personally together anyway, because of personality problems, alcoholism, drug addiction, or lack of communication, and these situations usually do not wash themselves away so that the postmorbid situation can become an acceptable change. Frequently, the patient, as seen in the hospital, is an entirely different individual than when he is in his own home milieu; and this too must be taken into consideration.

If all these things are irrelevant and the patient does have the opportunity to go home, then the physical environment can be a problem. It became evident that many patients in a rehabilitation institute, who developed abilities of a functional nature while in the hospital, utilizing various assistive devices, aids, and equipment there, often regressed when they returned home because the same types of assistive devices were not available. Therefore, programs have been developed whereby selected team members go into the home, evaluate problems, and make recommendations that ensure the patient's being able to continue his functional abilities once he returns to this environment.

The home evaluation is best done by the team of experts who have been working with the patient during his disability and who have a good, basic knowledge of his assets and liabilities. It is done in order to give various team members the opportunity to assess what modifications and equipment may be needed in the home so that the patient can return there and maintain or improve the gains made in rehabilitation. The primary attention is focused upon the physical features of the home, including factors such as safety, accessibility, and energy conservation, plus modifications that will allow normal home activities in spite of residual disability. Other factors to be assessed include family attitudes, their understanding of the patient's abilities or degree of disability, the needs of the returning family member, opportunities for diversion, recreation, and social interaction, as well as a chance for resumption of former family role, and the possibility for follow-up. Visits can also, occasionally, be made to the patient's place of employment to advise on aspects such as accessibility, safety, and modification of equipment.

Whenever possible, the patient should be present, so that his abilities, difficulties, equipment needs, etc., can be checked in situ. Vital information can be obtained from this practice; for instance, a person may be checked out in the center as a wheelchair independent, but he returns to a home where hallways and doorways are too narrow to allow access in turning in the wheelchair. A patient may have good endurance in level walking, and he returns to a first-floor apartment which turns out to be in a section of the city where the first floor is actually reached by a steep flight of outside steps to the front door, or a steep, sloping walk to two steps at the back door. His endurance may not be equal to this.

Professional members of the team go to provide the following expertise:

1. The house physician goes so that he is available to answer any medical questions the family might raise.

2. The social worker goes if social factors are predominant and need clarification in the home setting.

3. The nurse participates if nursing procedures are especially pertinent, such as turning, bed positioning, and dressing of wounds.

4. The physical therapist goes if there is some residual deficit in motor function.

5. The occupational therapist goes if there is some residual difficulty in the activities of daily living or adjustment to perceptual handicaps or homemaking.

6. The speech therapist usually goes on follow-up visits only if it is indicated that there are significant changes in communication abilities noted by the family, in particular with stroke patients.

Once the home visit is considered, it is necessary to inform the patient and family and discuss this thoroughly for its acceptance. Though most associations with a discharge home are happy ones for the patient, such a concrete step as suggesting a home evaluation may have other implications that disturb him. For instance, it may make the patient realize that he will have to face residual disability, a society less understanding of handicaps than the secure environment of the rehabilitation center, and a permanent change in life style. The team member who has the closest relationship to the patient is often the appropriate one to inform him of the proposal and its purposes. Some patients require the reassurance that the staff members are not coming to pronounce judgment on the decor of their home or to completely rearrange it.

Prior to the actual evaluation, any obstacles expected to be faced, such as curbs, stair climbing, etc., should be practiced beforehand with the patient. Transportation is provided for the patient by the family or by public transportation. The physical and occupational therapists share the responsibility for assessing the following areas: (1) access to the dwelling, for instance, need for rails for any outside steps, selection of the easiest entrance, need for ramps; (2) requirements for safe ambulation, such as enough space for walking aids, if used, elimination of scatter rugs, putting fragile or unsteady furniture in locations where there is no temptation to use it for balance, elimination of trailing electrical cords; painting or taping thresholds for visibility, if they cannot be removed; (3) requirements for wheelchair mobility, such as space for turning, access to bed, toilet, and bath; sufficiently wide doorways, absence of thresholds or such that the wheelchair can roll over them, if wheelchair homemaking is contemplated (the occupational therapist performs this assessment); (4) requirements for transfers, such as access, sufficient height and firmness of bed, assistive devices, such as rails, bathtub seat, safety treads, safe, comfortable easy chair is also an alternative to wheelchair; (5) general mobility needs, such as accessibility of telephone, windows, light switches, a table to eat or work at; (6) safety at night, such as lights, transfers possibly without prosthesis or need for a bedpan at the bedside; (7) the taking of measurements where these are critical, such as the bathtub height; (8) demonstrations of transfers given to the family members if pertinent. Sometimes, these may also be done at the hospital before the visit. The occupational therapist also checks accessibility of clothes, placement of food and utensils in the kitchen, availability of storage space, the need for ADL and housekeeping aids. He will also observe the patient's practical and functional behavior to ascertain safety judgment, basic problem-solving skills, and carry-over of newly learned techniques in familiar surroundings.

Experience has shown that it is probably important to follow up this procedure, once recommendations have been made for change, because many patients and families will be more conscientious about making these changes if they know that someone is going to come back and check up on them. The follow-up visit also serves to show whether the patient has improved or deteriorated in his previous functional abilities since discharge.

Recommendations are divided into five categories: bedroom adaptations, bathroom adaptations, kitchen adaptations, personal care and safety, and general safety. In all, 149 items are included in these five categories. See Table 10. The most frequently *suggested* recommendations are: removal of scatter rugs, installation of grab bars for the toilet, installation of railings on staircases, installation of grab bars for the bath-

tub, placement of slipex strips on the bottom of the bathtub, and securing the edges of large rugs. The recommendations most frequently *followed* are: removal of scatter rugs, installation of grab bars for the toilet, installation of railings on staircases, removal of thresholds or painting them white, and securing the edges of large rugs.

In the author's rehabilitation center, all personnel who have been associated with home evaluations realize their extreme value to the therapeutic team as well as to the patient and his family. Most patients and their relatives accept the opportunity gladly, although a few consider it an invasion of privacy. Some lived in substandard housing facilities and obviously feared that the staff would think less of them after the visit. It was found that the incorporation of home evaluations was definitely instrumental in promoting collaboration and coordination between therapist, hospital, and other community services interested in the welfare of the patient.

Therapists learned a great deal about the importance of understanding patient and family attitudes and how these may affect the reaction of patients to authority. Some team members learned that their sincere efforts to advise the patient could be wasted if they did not understand the patient and his responses to changes of routine or long-standing habit. In a few cases, the extent of the poverty, inadequate facilities, and excessive burden of care could not have been fully comprehended without a home evaluation. Old patients pouring water from a bucket to flush a nonfunctioning toilet and the absence of bathtubs (which was rarely divulged even while going through the painstaking training of bathtub transfer) are good examples.

Another benefit involved the patient's family. Only on a home visit, with the family present, is the role of the patient in the home really discovered. Clarified for the therapists, at last, are the duties and responsibilities and expected future functions which the patient will fulfill. Many times, when it is obvious that the patient

TABLE 10. CHECKLIST OF ITEMS WHICH MAY PRESENT PROBLEMS DURING TIME OF HOME EVALUATION

BEDROOM ADAPTATION
1. Bed against wall
2. Bedboard
3. Bed rails
4. Bedside commode
5. Chair next to bed
6. Extra mattress
7. Firm mattress
8. Grab bar or trapeze by bed
9. Humidifier
10. Hospital bed
11. Higher bed
12. Lower bed
13. Low bed with railings
14. Night light
15. Night table
16. Rearrange bureau drawers
17. Rearrange furniture
18. Remove castors from bed
19. Remove wheels from bed
20. Rubber sheet for bed
21. Single bed with railing
22. Single bed with firm mattress
23. Single bed in single room
24. Urinal and/or bedpan
25. Wash basin in room

BATHROOM ADAPTATION
26. Bathtub seat
27. Chair or stool in bathroom
28. Commode downstairs
29. Grab bar for bathtub
30. Grab bar for toilet
31. Grab bar near towel rack
32. Lower mirror
33. Mirror on sink
34. Rearrange bathroom set-up
35. Raised toilet seat
36. Reinforce towel rack
37. Remove hamper
38. Remove scale
39. Remove vanity table
40. Rubber tips on footstool
41. Sanitary chair with toilet armrest
42. Slipex strips in bathtub
43. Slipex strips on floor
44. Shower attachment
45. Sliding bathroom door
46. Washbowl adaptation

KITCHEN ADAPTATION
47. Armchair in kitchen

48. Carrier basket
49. Cutting board
50. Electric oven
51. Electric can opener
52. Faucet extension or hose
53. High stool
54. Install shelf
55. Lower shelf
56. Rearrange food in refrigerator
57. Rearrange kitchen furniture
58. Rearrange utensils
59. Sharp knife
60. Specific utensils
61. Use hot plate rather than stove
62. Utility cart

PERSONAL CARE AND SAFETY
63. Adjustment of clothing
64. Adjustment of hearing aid
65. Cane
66. Daily exercise
67. Driving lessons with hand controls
68. Elastic stockings
69. Electric shaver
70. Elevation of legs
71. Frequent hair washing
72. Hand splint and/or sling
73. Lifted shoe
74. Lofstrand crutches
75. Lotion for skin
76. No driving
77. Postural drainage
78. Shoulder bag
79. Space shoe
80. Supervision at night
81. Supervision of VNA
82. Supervision of aide, homemaker, or family member
83. Supervision in ADL
84. Supervision in ambulation
85. Supervision on stairs
86. Supervision in transfers
87. Visiting physical therapist
88. Wash stump
89. Walker
90. Walker tips
91. Wheelchair
92. Wheelchair armrest
93. Wheelchair leg rest
94. Wheelchair restraining strap
95. Wheelchair table
96. Zipper shoelace

GENERAL SAFETY

97. Adjust closet bar and/or drawer handle
98. Adjustment of electric fixture
99. Adjustment of front door
100. Adjustment of venetian-blind cords
101. Adjustment of wheelchair brakes
102. Adequate lighting
103. Bell to ring for assistance
104. Captain's chair with raised seat
105. Castors on chairs
106. Chair back to wall
107. Convert first-floor closet into a bathroom
108. Cover exposed pipes
109. Cover radiators
110. Change of dwelling
111. Crutch hook
112. First-floor apartment
113. First-floor toilet
114. First-floor sleeping quarters
115. Foam-rubber cushion
116. Footstool for dressing
117. Gate at top of stairs
118. Handle on window frame
119. Install steps
120. L-shaped desk
121. Lengthening light cord
122. Leveling front-porch steps
123. Mat in front of couch
124. Ramp construction
125. Raised car seat
126. Rearrange furniture for more wheelchair and/or walking space
127. Rearrange apartment set-up
128. Rearrange rugs
129. Remodeling stairs
130. Remodeling stair railing
131. Remove door mat
132. Remove scatter rugs
133. Remove loose stair treads
134. Remove thresholds and/or paint white
135. Remove wax from floor
136. Replace kitchen flooring
137. Rubber tips on chairs
138. Secure electric wiring
139. Secure banister knobs
140. Secure edges of carpet
141. Secure loose boards on porch
142. Secure rocking chair
143. Secure screen door
144. Secure stairway
145. Secure telephone cord
146. Sturdy chair with raised seat
147. Telephone adaptation
148. Use back stairway
149. Wax bureau drawers

will not be allowed to maintain independence in a certain area, the therapist can begin to try to change attitudes by immediately demonstrating the patient's achieved level of independence in the actual environment he will be in after discharge. For some unexplained reason, the patient can demonstrate his independence in dressing to his family on the rehabilitation ward, but it is not real to the family until the patient is seen actually dressing independently at home. This most concrete and realistic situation is the most persuasive and effective plea that can be made to change family attitudes, which if unchanged, can result in the obliteration of all ADL training. Also of great help is an exact demonstration of the amount of actual assistance the patient needs, followed by a discussion of the techniques and equipment to be utilized. The family's confidence in the patient's abilities grows in response to their greater understanding of the simple routines he can follow. It is apparent that the predischarge evaluation, made, ideally, a month before discharge, is of major value to the comprehensive physical restoration of the patient.

An unforeseen problem which required solution was the rigid meal-preparation habits of many housewives. A surprising number of patients turned out to be can-opener or delicatessen cooks. Not only is this type of meal easily prepared, but many patients prefer to eat this kind of food. Others were quite contented with their husband's or children's cooking.

The concept of home evaluations being an extension of comprehensive restorative services has really been effective. Both staff and patients demonstrated the value of the procedure. It was possible to make many suggestions for the safety and better management of patients, and those who accepted and followed them did well in maintaining their functional goals. Critical things, such as changing sleeping quarters from the second to the first floor or having a visiting nurse come in, were usually done; in fact, many structural changes were even accomplished. Simpler things did not always occur because of resistance to having a familiar way of life changed. Probably the greatest asset was the significant, mutual exchange in communication by all parties concerned in the restorative process, which enhanced the goal of providing better and continuing patient care.

REFERENCES

BONNER, C. D., and YU, Y. H.   Home evaluation— an extension of comprehensive restorative care. *Geriatrics* 27:59–66, 1972.

Protocol from Department of Physical Medicine and Rehabilitation. Cleveland: Highland View Hospital. No authors cited. 1961.

20
The Nursing Home

The aged or chronically ill may require care and assistance that exceed anything available in the home yet may not require the elaborate services of a modern hospital. In some cases, a person may be only moderately incapacitated, sufficiently well to remain at home, but there may be no one there to provide the little care needed to make this possible. Such patients need a type of home which may vary from a kind of staffed boardinghouse to an institution akin to a chronic-disease hospital. Institutions of this nature have sprung up and range from sheltered homes, supplying only the most basic services, to specialized nursing homes, with skilled, intensive nursing care. Intermediate types of such institutions give personal care and some skilled nursing, or personal care without professional nursing. Such institutions have carried varied names, such as *convalescent homes, rest homes, homes for the aged,* and so forth. The qualities of their facilities and services have also varied from excellent to substandard.

Much has been said about the inadequacy of nursing homes both on the national and local level. Probably no other industry has been subject to criticism and investigation, both formal and secret, as frequently as the nursing-home industry. Exposés by newspapers in particular have been common, and even President Nixon has expressed his feelings as follows: "Many of our nursing homes are outstanding institutions. But altogether too many are not. That is why many of these, the substandard ones, are described as little more than warehouses for the unwanted, dumping grounds for the dying.

"I have even heard of doctors who refuse to visit some nursing homes because they get too depressed. Too often it seems that nursing homes serve mainly to keep older people out of sight out of mind, so that no one will notice their degradation and despair."

In spite of this, nursing homes have multiplied and become big business. From 1966 to 1969, the number of nursing homes in this country has doubled. Previously it had taken twelve years to double the number of homes. Much of this increase was triggered by Medicare and Medicaid, which poured federal money into the business.

There are now approximately 900,000 beds available in 22,000 nursing homes throughout the United States. This is an average of about 43 beds per institution, and the trend has been toward fewer but larger facilities.

Contrary to ownership patterns in hospitals, about 85 percent of nursing homes and related facilities and 60 percent of the beds are owned by proprietary organizations; about 11 percent of the homes and 26 percent of the beds belong to nonprofit organizations; and 4 percent of the beds are sponsored by government agencies.

Most newer homes are now being built in larger sizes and specifically as nursing homes. There are still too many converted private residences being used, but many are closing or adding modern wings. Women outnumber men three to one in resident population.

Because of the enormous pressures to improve the quality of care which have come from within as well as from without the industry, rules and regulations for nursing homes have become more stringent. An attempt has been made to designate levels of care to be provided by the homes as well as to define the type of patient who belongs at each level. In many ways this has failed and perhaps can never be achieved, because patients are not inanimate objects made to fit into preshaped holes. Further, it is extremely difficult to keep each level of care unit filled with only that type of patient. Not only do patients vacillate in their nursing needs, which would require moving them from home to home or unit to unit, but also the type of patient who is present in the highest number is relegated to the type of nursing home which lacks sufficient numbers and are reimbursed by few insurance plans, and usually at an unreasonably low fee. This situation has a tendency to make patients, families, and referring agencies upgrade the patient's nursing-care needs so that some third party will pay the bill. Medicaid, which many consider welfare, is about the only reimburser that still covers all nursing homes. However, many people shun welfare because of its stigma to them; and, on the other hand, many nursing homes shun welfare recipients because they feel the payment formula is too low and the payment too long in coming. In Massachusetts, the State Welfare Department has owed nursing homes millions of dollars for several years. This makes it difficult to place such patients, with the result that they back up and occupy high-cost hospital beds. Further confusion is caused by the fact that the standards are set and supervised by the Department of Public Health; the bills are paid, in all welfare instances, by the Department of Public Welfare, but the formula for reimbursement is established by the Rate-Setting Commission. All are independent agencies, and better coordination and cooperation could be established.

Guidelines for levels of care and criteria for classification of patients according to levels of care have been developed. The following have been circulated by the Division of Medical Care, Department of Public Health of the Commonwealth of Massachusetts, dated 1971:

CRITERIA FOR CLASSIFICATION OF PATIENTS ACCORDING TO LEVEL OF CARE

The determination of Patients' Level of Care will be based on the following:
1. Assessment of the individual's needs for a specific level of care.
2. Evaluation of the capability of a facility to meet the individual's need.
3. Implementation of the most appropriate plan to meet the individual's need in planning for continuity of care.

The above criteria may serve as a guideline to health-team members, but the exercise of professional judgment must inevitably determine the individual's appropriate placement.

CONCEPT OF LEVELS I AND II CARE

Level I, Intensive Rehabilitative Care and Skilled Nursing Care and Level II, Skilled Nursing Care require knowledge of the physical and psychosocial needs of the individual and the measures necessary to attain and to maintain a state of optimum health. Skilled Nursing and Rehabilitative care has as its scope, the treatment of disease, prevention of illness, prevention of complication of illness, and restoration of health. It requires a systematic method of assessment of total individual needs and the development of a patient-care plan in collaboration with other health team members. The patient-care plan continually undergoes reevaluation and revision and is coordinated by the professional nurse who is responsible for the individualized care of each patient, whether she does this directly or through delegation. Levels I and II further necessitate the rendering of direct service by a professional staff required to have specialized training and skills in teaching, in communication, and in comprehension of individual behavioral response to illness and to disability.

Facilities providing Level I Care to Medicare recipients will meet the Conditions of Participation for Extended Care Facilities.

Extended Care Facilities (ECF's) have been defined by the Joint Commission on Accreditation of Hospitals as establishments with medical staffs and continuous professional nursing service, designated to provide comprehensive inpatient care of relatively short duration and to serve convalescent patients who are not acutely ill.

Level of Care Guidelines for Extended Care Facilities, compiled by Massachusetts Blue Cross, Inc., February, 1970, provides the following excerpts:

DEFINITIONS
A. Concept of Extended Care
The concept of extended care is one which is re-

lated to the provisions of continuity of care in modern medical practice. Therefore, the term *extended* refers to a facility *which provides an extension of hospital care, not to a facility for care over an extended period*. The overall goal is to provide an alternative to hospital care for patients who still require general medical management and skilled nursing care on a continuing basis but do not require constant availability of physician service ordinarily found only in a hospital setting.

All extended-care facilities participating in the program are considered capable of rendering the skilled nursing care which constitutes extended care. However, many ECF's provide care for a much wider range of medical conditions than those conditions which require the type of continuous skilled nursing services which are reimbursable under the Medicare program. For this reason, personnel who prepare ECF claims should be particularly familiar with those factors which distinguish the need for extended care from the need for other less intensive levels of institutional care.

B. Skilled Nursing Services

A skilled nursing service is one which must be furnished by or under the supervision of licensed nursing personnel to achieve the medically desired result. However, a service which could be safely and adequately performed by a person without special training is not a skilled service even though it may be performed by licensed nursing personnel.

C. Medical Necessity

The determination of medical necessity is a medical judgment to which the physician certifies the need for skilled nursing services prescribed for a given patient. A medical need may exist, but, if no skilled nursing services are required, the care is not covered.

Facilities providing Level II or Skilled Nursing Care have the following distinctions:

1. Care and services will meet individual needs under the general direction of a physician and will emphasize nursing direction, observation, assessments, skills, and nursing judgments.
2. Laboratory services that are justified in the management and control of certain medical conditions.
3. Nursing care will be directed by a registered nurse; a registered nurse or qualified licensed practical nurse will be in charge of each unit throughout a 24-hour period.

4. Physician attendance for each individual in the facility will be required at least every 30 days and more often when medically necessary.
5. The individual stay will vary and may be short- or long-term, dependent upon individual needs, goals, and the therapy necessary to achieve those goals.

A regular and continuing need for the provision of the following services is characteristic of skilled nursing care:

1. Administration of injectable medications, periodic intravenous and hypodermoclysis solutions. Intravenous therapy will be administered by the physician and/or registered nurses with special preparation and training in the technique.
2. Rehabilitative nursing activities for patients who have been determined to have a higher functional level (e.g., activities of daily living; ambulation regime; bowel and bladder program; range-of-joint motion, and good body alignment).
3. Teaching rehabilitative nursing techniques and management care (e.g., diverting of body functioning, as in a colostomy, ileostomy, nephrostomy, and ureterostomy).
4. Patients who have reached their maximal level of functioning but who require continued skilled nursing care to maintain this level.
5. Nasopharyngeal suction as required for the maintenance of a clear airway.
6. Maintenance of tracheotomy, gastrostomy, bladder catheters, and other indwelling tubes.
7. Administration of tube feedings.
8. Administration of oxygen on an intermittent or continuous basis.
9. Treatment of excavating ischemic ulcers.
10. Assisting the teachable brain-damaged patient to function more independently.

RESTORATIVE THERAPY SERVICES

Restorative therapy services are professional services that include physical therapy, occupational therapy, and speech therapy. Such services may be required by any individual regardless of the level of care. The emphasis is placed upon helping the patient to achieve some degree of self-actualization; to utilize remaining abilities, and to develop new abilities, which are possible within the scope of the disability. Restorative therapy services shall always be ordered by the physician and provided or directed by a qualified therapist. The need for or provision of therapy is not an indication in itself of a need for a specific level of care.

CONCEPT OF LEVEL III OR SUPPORTIVE CARE

Level III, or Supportive Care, provides the ambulatory and semiambulatory individual with services beyond room and meals but is below the level of skilled care. Level III, therefore, will be provided to those individuals whose physical needs can be met and maintained with a minimum of medical and nursing supervision and to individuals with mild behavioral symptoms of brain damage.

GUIDELINES FOR LEVEL III

Facilities providing Intermediate or Supportive Nursing Care have the following distinctions:
1. Care and services emphasize basic nursing care and those services which are under the direction of a physician.
2. Physician attendance for each individual is provided at least every 90 days and more often when indicated.
3. Nursing care is under the direction of a registered or licensed practical nurse. A R.N. or L.P.N. is required during the day and evening tour of duty, and additional nursing services are provided sufficient to meet patient needs.
4. The average stay is usually long-term, but in each case, according to individual needs.

A regular and continuing need for provision of the following services is characteristic of supportive nursing care:
1. Aid or supervision in bathing and personal hygiene, including bed baths.
2. Prevention and treatment of skin irritation and treatment of uncomplicated decubitus ulcers.
3. Routine observation of vital signs and recording of findings in the patient's record.
4. Supervision of individuals with behavioral problems and those socially unable to cope with the environment.
5. Supervision in self-care activities of daily living such as: feeding, grooming, ambulation, and toilet activities.
6. Continued restorative nursing measures to aid patient's mobilization activities and management of self-care devices (wheelchair, commode, walkers, prosthesis, splints, etc.).
7. Administration of topical, oral, and routine injectable medications by licensed nursing personnel.
8. Simple daily dressings and routine care of patients with temporary casts, braces, splints, or other appliances requiring nursing care or direction.
9. Use of protective restraints (bed rails, posey belts, etc.) as ordered by a physician, supervised

and applied in accord with written patient-care policies and procedures.

CONCEPT OF LEVEL IV OR RESIDENT CARE

Level IV or Resident Care is required primarily for social and/or economic reasons that prevent an individual from remaining in the setting of a private home. The services emphasize minimum basic care and the provision of room and meals to residents who are otherwise independent.

GUIDELINES FOR LEVEL IV

Facilities (Level IV) providing Resident Care have the following distinctions:
1. Care and services emphasize supervised protection, care, and assistance.
2. Physician services are provided on an emergency basis or as arranged for individual residents either in or out of the facility.
3. Care and services throughout each 24-hour period may be directed by licensed nurses or may be directed by nonprofessional individuals with experience in providing care and services to meet the physical, social, and emotional needs of aged individuals and others with limited capacities not requiring continuing nursing care.
4. The average stay is usually long-term but, in each case, according to individual needs.

A regular and continuing need for or provision of the following services is characteristic of resident care:
1. Personal supervision and protection from environmental and other hazards.
2. Regular diets, including modifications as specified in A.D.A. Manual.
3. Supervision and administration of medications will follow the Licensure Regulations for Level IV established by the Department.
4. Assistance in personal care when required.
5. Stimulation and encouragement in activities of daily living and mobility, according to individual capabilities and needs.
6. Diversional and motivational activities.
7. Emergency care and medical care is arranged in accord with written policies and procedures of the facility.

CONDITIONS FOR BENEFITS
IN EXTENDED-CARE FACILITIES

Certain requirements must be met before Medicare payments can be made:
1. The patient must have been transferred to the ECF from a hospital in which he was a patient

for *not less than three consecutive days*. (In counting the three days, count the day of admission but not the day of discharge.)

The hospital discharge must occur after June 30 or on or after the first day of the month in which the beneficiary attains age 65, whichever is later.

II. The transfer from a hospital to the ECF must come *within* 14 days of the individual's discharge from the hospital.

In some cases if the person has not already exhausted his 100-day coverage in an ECF, he may be eligible if he has been in an ECF and transferred to another within 14 days of his discharge from the previous ECF. Such a stay in a previous ECF is called an *intervening stay*.

III. If resumption of skilled nursing care is necessary within 14 days of the patient's discharge from the extended-care facility, and no bed is available in an extended-care facility, he may be placed in a hospital for less than three days and then transferred to a participating extended-care facility.

IV. Payment may be made for covered extended-care services only if a physician makes the required *certification* and *recertification* or recertifications, depending on the length of stay of the beneficiary.

The extended-care facility is responsible for obtaining the required physician certification and recertification statements and for retaining them in file for verification by the intermediary or by the Social Security Administration. Also, the ECF determines the method by which certifications and recertifications are made. They may be included in forms, notes, or other records a physician normally signs in caring for a patient or on separate forms designed for this purpose. Except as otherwise specified, each certification and recertification statement is to be separately signed by a physician.

The *certification* must state that skilled nursing care is necessary on a continuous basis for any of the conditions for which the patient was receiving inpatient hospital services. It must be signed by the physician at the time of admission or shortly thereafter.

Recertification

A. Must state that continued skilled nursing care is necessary for the condition(s) for which the patient received hospital care, or for any condition(s) which arose after the patient transferred to the ECF while still being treated for one of the conditions for which he was previously hospitalized.

B. Must contain an adequate written record of the following unless the required information is included elsewhere, for example, in the patient's medical record:

1. Written record of the reasons for continued care.
2. The estimated period of time the patient will need the care of the ECF.
3. Plans for post-ECF care.

The first recertification must be signed by the physician not later than the 12th day of stay, and subsequent recertifications must be signed by the physician or utilization review committee not later than at 30-day intervals thereafter.

The initial certification may be included on the patient transfer form if it is properly documented and signed by the responsible physician. A Health Care Referral Form (#2626) has been designed for this purpose and is available from Blue Cross upon request.

Beginning with the second recertification, the utilization review committee may perform the function of the attending physician in recertifying the need for continued care. This requires amending the utilization review plan for the ECF to include this procedure and also filing the amended plan of review with the Massachusetts Department of Public Health.

Special forms for certification (2332) and recertification (2333) on single sheets are available for the initial certification and each subsequent recertification, as well as on a single sheet (958) for combined certification and recertification. Blue Cross will supply these on request.

The selection of the appropriate nursing home for a loved one can be most difficult. The physician in charge of the case may be able to offer constructive suggestions. In many localities, various agencies and organizations stand ready with information and advice for those who search for a suitable nursing home. Social workers and coordinators of continuing care units are particularly knowledgeable.

In the average community, for instance, the Department of Public Welfare or the local Board of Health, or both, will undoubtedly be able to supply not only a list of licensed homes in the area, but also other pertinent data, such as *who is eligible, in which homes,* and so on. If no such organization is within easy reach, the State Department of Public Health can probably be of help. In the case of a patient suffering from mental confusion or illness, there may be a State Department of Mental Health. Also, some societies have home-placement agencies which, for a fee, furnish information and arrange assistance.

The National Geriatrics Society, a nonprofit organization of institutions caring for the aged, maintains a list of approved and accepted facilities. This list is available to physicians, hospitals, and individuals and includes public, proprietary, and voluntary hospitals, sanitariums, nursing homes for the aged, and similar institutions which care for the aged. The Department of Health, Education and Welfare in Washington, D.C., can furnish listings of homes in the individual states.

If information is obtained from a local council of social agencies, one should determine whether the data are merely taken from a directory or whether a visiting service is maintained for the purpose of verification. (Because it is hard to find adequate personnel and financial support for such a project, it is extremely difficult to keep these data current.)

While nursing homes are primarily located in urban or suburban areas, they may also be found in small towns, villages, or rural districts. However, skilled-nursing homes are more often situated in or near the more heavily populated areas.

When the choice has been narrowed down, following inquiries to appropriate sources, it remains to select the best suited institution, and this must be done by personal contact with the management of the available institutions and by inspecting prospective homes. In doing this, one must be prepared first to ascertain whether the home is properly licensed by the state authorities as a nursing home meeting basic requirements* and whether it is accredited with the Nursing

* *Basic Requirements for Nursing Homes* from State Department of Public Health.

Home Association. Also, one must ascertain whether the home provides the precise level of care for which the patient qualifies.

The staff of the nursing home should include a physician and a registered nurse, on duty or on call 24 hours a day. The exact number of professionals, such as physicians and registered nurses, involved depends on the size of the home and new rules and regulations in one's area. A small nursing home may need to share such a person with several other small establishments. There should also be enough practical nurses and aides or orderlies, or both, for round-the-clock nursing care. There must be an adequate supporting staff to assure cleanliness, properly prepared food, and a generally homelike atmosphere.

Once these basic questions have been answered, one must then ascertain by direct inquiry from the administration and by personal inspection whether certain other essential and desirable features are present. The following constitute some of the items of interest that must be studied. Hardly any nursing home will provide all these features, but the more of them that are present, the better the home.

CHECKLIST OF DESIRABLE FEATURES IN A GOOD NURSING HOME

PLANT

SIZE
Ideally, a nursing home should accommodate about 25 beds per unit.

AGE
A modern brick or concrete structure built for its current purpose, or at least a modernized plant, is preferable. Beware of improvised, ramshackle, or even condemned buildings.

FLOORS
Preferably, there should be only one floor level or, if necessary, only a few stairways, at least

3 feet, 8 inches wide, with no more than three steps per flight, and handrails. Second floors are not desirable, but if they exist, all safety precautions must have been taken, especially with a direct exit to the outside with a wide door.

SPACE

Lounges, living rooms, and recreational areas are a must. Easy chairs, reading lamps, and television ought to give homelike atmosphere. Areas for occupations (hobbies, crafts) are desirable. Dining rooms should be available to those able to sit at tables.

Space must be adequate to assure each patient's privacy and to allow him to live among his personal belongings. If private rooms are not available, privacy must be given by means of curtains with ceiling tracks. Private places must be available for entertaining visitors.

Space must be available for exercise and comfortable ambulation (watch for overcrowding!). All rooms, including toilets, must be large enough to accommodate wheelchairs.

Space must be available to permit the segregation of the severely ill, disoriented, dying.

SAFETY DEVICES

An adequate sprinkler system, fire extinguishers, emergency exits, fire escapes of noncombustible material are musts. These must be in good condition and clearly marked.

The following questions must be answered affirmatively: (1) Are fire drills conducted periodically? (2) Are standard fire precautions observed? (3) Is the electric wiring properly installed and in good condition? (4) Are exits free and unblocked at all times? (5) Is trash removed from attics, closets, and out-of-the-way places?

The following safety devices are musts: (1) Grab bars on the walls adjacent to the toilets, to assist the patient in transferring himself from chair to toilet and vice versa; (2) handrails for sinks and showers and two sets of fixtures, so that water can be turned on either from a seated or standing position; (3) seats, benches, and mats in the bathrooms; (4) thermostatically controlled water in all fixtures used by the patients (the temperature should never exceed 110° F); (5) slip-resistant floors; and (6) adjustable closet rods and shelves for the convenience of wheelchair patients. If obese patients are cared for, especially if paralyzed, a Hoyer lift should be available.

FACILITIES AND PROGRAM FOR CARE

PERIODIC REEVALUATION

In addition to 24-hour medical and registered-nurse coverage, the home should provide a periodic reevaluation of all patients from a medical point of view to determine whether they might be improved enough to permit more activity or discharge, worsened to require hospitalization, or in need of specialized medical or rehabilitation care. For this and other medical needs, there ought to be access to a clinical laboratory and portable x-ray and electrocardiogram machines. There should be adequate provisions to treat acute illnesses that arise, and a well-organized plan of cooperation with a nearby hospital in case transfer to a hospital becomes necessary.

PHYSICAL AND OCCUPATIONAL THERAPY

Adequate programs and personnel for physical and occupational therapy are desirable, even on a consultation basis. It is most important that the value of therapy and rehabilitation be recognized by the administrative personnel, so that appropriate referral of a patient to a center where these services are available might be carried out. Because in most nursing homes extensive physical therapy cannot be accomplished because of the scarcity of these specialists, use of rehabilitation centers should be encouraged, or a number of homes might share a therapist for some of the simpler procedures. An extensive array of equipment is not necessary. Again, it should be pointed out that the therapist must work under the direction of a physician. An occupational-therapy program to complement the physical-therapy program is equally desirable. These services must be strictly controlled by rigid guidelines and adequate supervision. In a number of instances, therapists have incorporated and made excessive income at the expense of the federal programs. This happens when patients are treated indefinitely without setting and achieving specific goals.

RECREATION PROGRAM

Another desirable feature is a recreational program, with a staff member responsible for this activity. If no such person is available, it should be ascertained whether or not outside volunteer help is solicited or encouraged by the home. This may come from Boy or Girl Scout groups, the American Red Cross, church groups, women's clubs, service organizations, and so forth. Additionally, when the patients are invited by these groups to participate in community activities, they should be encouraged to do so, as a means of promoting their sense of belonging, and consequently, their self-respect.

FOOD

Another important aspect of care in a nursing home is the provision of food. This must be well-balanced, adequate in quality and quantity, and served in an appetizing way. A dietitian should be available, at least on a part-time basis, to provide the necessary planning and supervision of dietary management which can only be given by a professional.

SOCIAL WORKER

The availability of a trained social worker is another important factor in an adequate nursing-home-care team. Such a worker will be especially appreciated by patients without family, or those whose families neglect them.

MANAGEMENT

A trained director often offers advantages. An advisory board of three or more licensed physicians can give the home medical guidance and assure good care and standards.

OTHER TYPES OF HOMES

Many of the foregoing points will also pertain to the homes offering fewer services than do the skilled nursing homes. These are the *sheltered homes* and *personal-care homes* mentioned earlier as Level IV. Generally speaking, these homes give room and board and various other kinds of home services, which might include laundry and some help with personal activities, such as shopping, correspondence, and so forth. Personal-care homes, with either little or no skilled nursing, may include such personal services as help in walking, getting in and out of bed, general bathing, dressing, and feeding. They may also prepare special diets for the patient and supervise medication (provided the latter can be self-administered).

OTHER FACTORS IN THE SELECTION OF A NURSING HOME

TLC

Of paramount importance in any type of nursing home is one aspect of care that is governed by no law, that is seldom, if ever, mentioned in a brochure or prospectus, and that can be measured by no yardstick of man's making—*tender, loving care* (TLC). Although it constitutes the most significant factor of all in the life of a patient, this is a "commodity" that has no price, and its presence or absence is in no way contingent upon the cost of care. Here, only close personal observation can give the answer, since one could hardly expect satisfactory replies to the questions: "Does this home give TLC? Aside from their professional qualifications, are the people most intimately associated with the patients the kind of people that I myself would like to depend on? Do they have warmth, compassion, outgoing personalities, and can they be described as good, substantial citizens?"

The single answer to these questions lies not in the administrative office or on the lips of the attendants, but rather on the faces of the patients —in their general appearance and their apparent attitudes toward themselves and their fellow patients. If the majority of the patients seem apathetic, dull, and lifeless, if many of them are seen in their rooms listening to radio or TV, both of which are, after all, only passive entertainment, or, even worse, if they are doing nothing at all—then the observer can only conclude that the humane element is missing and this is not the right place for his loved one!

If, on the other hand, the home itself is bright and cheerful, the patients apparently happy and busy at something, no matter how inconsequential, it might be well to allow this to be the decisive factor in a final choice, since it can, depending on the patient's physical condition and needs, far outweigh some, but not all, of the more tangible specifications.

COSTS

The costs of stays in nursing homes are high and, for most people, create serious financial problems. Financial aid, in the form of state, federal, or local assistance, is obtainable in many areas. The scope of subsidies for medical care provided for the aged varies from state to state, starting with hospital care, which is limited to emergency situations, and continuing on through comprehensive medical care. While hospitalization is the type of service for which the largest expenditure is made in old-age assistance, the second largest portion of such payments is for nursing and convalescent care.

Regardless of the fee quoted, and before coming to any formal agreement, it must be ascertained exactly what the stated price includes, because some contracts exclude certain extras, such as physicians' fees, medication, hospitalization, or special diets. It is also important to have a thorough understanding of the specific accommodations the patient will have and the extent of nursing and medical care covered by the contract. There should also be a definite commitment concerning laundry and other incidentals and, more important, concerning fixation of responsibility in case the patient needs a change of care or facilities.

It should be remembered that price alone is no criterion of the quantity or quality of the care given, and once again the reader is reminded that his own personal observations, weighed in relation to the verbal assurance he receives, must be the decisive factor.

While there is room for great improvement in the average nursing home, it is encouraging to note that the operation of a nursing home is increasingly regarded as "good business." Increased competition will result in improved services and facilities, to the benefit of those who must depend on nursing homes for all or a portion of their declining years.

21

The Dilemma of Health Insurance

To state that the financial reimbursement for the medical care of the elderly and chronically ill is a dilemma is probably a gross understatement. It is almost impossible to put into words the magnitude of this problem and the horrendous reality of the actual situation.

Everyone is cognizant of the skyrocketing costs of medical care today. Hospitalization in particular has been costing more each year, so that in many instances, in certain hospitals, a semiprivate room can cost even more than $100.00 a day. Such costs make it practically impossible for the average citizen to spend any long periods of time in a hospital or nursing home for any chronic illness without losing all his life's savings.

There are probably many reasons for the high cost of medical care. Some of these are as follows: through the actions of labor unions, there has been a marked increase in salaries at almost all levels of job categories in the hospital. This includes even those who receive the minimum wage. Many hospitals have also, each year, incorporated a cost-of-living wage increase in addition to merit increases, a fact that creates further spiraling of costs. In recent years, there have been many innovations in patient care. Such things as open-heart surgery and cardiac transplants require highly skilled teams and are very expensive. Coronary-care units or intensive-care units, where acutely ill individuals are cared for with nurses, doctors, and highly expensive electronic equipment around the clock, are also very expensive. Cobalt bombs for cancer irradiation are costly. There are also many new laboratory techniques and newer laboratory equipment which increase the cost of operation to the hospital. Many hospitals have required expansion, new buildings, or refurbishings of old buildings, and the cost of labor has increased each year, requiring a large outlay of funds. Basic cost of food, equipment, linen, and all the staples which are involved in the daily routine of the hospital have increased. In many instances, more physicians, or physician's assistants, and more clerical help have had to be employed because of the massive influx of forms which have to be filled out for Medicare and insurance companies before claims are paid.

More and more time is demanded for this administrative red tape, which allows many physicians less time to spend with and care for their patients. There are also problems of under or poor utilization of beds, low hospital census, and poor administration to be considered.

The cost reached such alarming proportions that in 1965 an attempt was made by the federal government to establish programs which would be helpful, particularly, to those two groups which needed it so desperately—the elderly and poor—taking into consideration that most elderly persons are also poor.

Medicare was one of the first governmental health insurances to be established. This was to provide payment for medical care for all citizens over age 65, regardless of income. It is divided into two parts: Part A is hospital insurance only, and Part B is medical insurance which also helps to pay doctors' bills and bills for certain other types of medical services that a person might need.

Probably one of the first problems with Medicare was that it required individuals to register in the program on their own behalf, instead of its being set up automatically on their 65th birthday. Since there was a certain amount of confusion with the program, there are still a number of elderly individuals who have not realized that they should register for Medicare at age 65; and many have lost out on some of the benefits which they might have received.

When first introduced, it was stated that the hospital insurance would help to pay for "covered services." Unfortunately, these covered services have been vaguely defined and, as time has gone on and the cost of the program has increased, the covered services have diminished and become more restricted.

Part A of Medicare pays for "covered services" received as a bed patient in a hospital up to 90 hospital days for each benefit period. It will also pay for a bed patient in an extended-care facility up to 100 days for each benefit period for the same illness which prompted the hospital admission. If a patient needed home health services, he could receive up to 100 home health visits for each benefit period. Medicare, however, has always been written as a coinsurance policy so that the individual also assumes responsibility in paying part of the bill. Many individuals did not realize this and were upset when they received bills from hospitals for services that they thought should have been completely covered by Medicare.

The patient is responsible, in Part A, for paying the first $72.00 of services rendered. This is applied toward the first 60 days of hospitalization, after which the insurance will pay for all covered services. From the 61st day through the 90th day, however, again the patient has to pay $18.00 a day toward his expenses and Medicare pays the difference. The services which are paid for are: a bed in a semiprivate room (2 to 4 beds in the room); all meals, including special diets; operating-room charges; regular nursing services, including intensive-care nursing; drugs furnished by the hospital; laboratory tests; x-ray and other radiological services; medical supplies, such as splints

and casts; use of appliances and equipment furnished by the hospital, such as wheelchairs, crutches, braces, and medical social services.

Medicare will not pay for: personal comfort or convenience items, such as charges for telephone, radio, television, private-duty nurses, extra charge for use of a private room (unless needed for medical reasons), noncovered levels of care, or doctor's services.

In an extended-care facility, hospital insurance pays for all covered services for the first 20 days, and for the next 80 days the patient contributes $9.00 a day toward the bill. The service paid for includes: a bed in a semiprivate room; all meals, including special diets; regular nursing services; drugs furnished by the extended-care facility; physical, occupational, and speech therapy; medical supplies, such as splints and casts; use of appliances and equipment furnished by the facility, such as wheelchair, crutches, braces; medical social services. It, too, does not pay for personal comfort or convenience items, such as telephone, radio, or television; private-duty nurse; any extra charges for use of a private room (unless medically needed); noncovered levels of care; or doctor's services.

If a patient requires home care after having been in a hospital or extended-care facility, and this is confirmed by the doctor, Part A insurance will pay for all "covered services" for as many as 100 visits. These visits must be medically necessary and furnished by a participating home health agency. Benefits may be paid for up to a year after the most recent discharge. The condition being treated must be a continuation of the condition for which the patient was hospitalized or in the extended-care facility.

Part A Medicare will pay for part-time nursing care; physical, occupational, or speech therapy; part-time services of home health aides; medical social services; medical supplies furnished by the agency; and use of medical appliances. It will not pay for: full-time nursing care; drugs and biologicals; personal comfort or convenience items; noncovered levels of care; or meals delivered to the home. It is important to note that in all three levels of care that have been indicated, one of the items not paid for is "noncovered levels of care," which, again, is a very vague statement and leaves a very weak link in the chain. It should also be noted that Medicare does not pay in regular nursing or convalescent homes at all.

Each individual of age 65 does have the possibility of also participating in Part B of Medicare, which is medical insurance. For this, it is necessary for each person to pay a monthly premium. This premium is subject to change. The four dollars a month, required through 1970, was increased to $5.30 starting in July 1971, and the premium continued to rise to $5.80 in 1972, $6.30 in 1973, and $6.70 in 1974. Part B provides, in addition to hospitalization, extended-care facility, and home health care services, the following: doctor's services; outpatient hospital services; medical services and supplies; home health services; outpatient physical therapy; and certain health-care services. Again, this is written as a coinsurance, so that for each calendar year, the patient must pay the first $60.00 of allowable charges. Once the Medicare record shows that the patient has paid the first $60.00 for the calendar year, Medicare will pay 80 percent of the allowable charges for the rest of the year. This is very important to understand, because, again, this has led to a great deal of friction between patient and provider, because the patient has thought that Medicare was paying all the bills. As each calendar year rolls around, the coinsurance deductibles are applicable again.

Medicare is mediated through certain fiscal intermediaries, such as Blue Cross/Blue Shield, Aetna Insurance Company, Travelers Insurance Company, and others. They usually provide excellent records to the individual to keep them abreast of benefits which have been paid. An example of this is shown in Figure 107. The Explanation of Medicare Payments form is labeled very clearly at the bottom so that the patient can see that it is not a bill. It shows the provider number of the individual providing the

services, the date when the service was provided, the charge that the doctor made, and the charge that Medicare allows. Many times, patients look at this and feel that Medicare has paid this allowable charge. They should follow the explanation further down, however, where they will see how much of the total allowable charges documented went toward the $60.00 deductible and how much has been applied to the deductible for this year. At the end, it shows the actual payment to the doctor which, in this case, was 0. Many patients only add up and see the allowable charges and wonder why the doctor keeps billing. In effect, the intermediary keeps the record of all charges, adds them up toward the $60.00 deductible, and once the $60.00 deductible has been met, then Medicare begins paying their 80 percent of the bill. Until that time, it is necessary for the patient to pay his own expenses—unless the deductibles are covered by some other type of program, such as Medex or Medicaid, if a person so qualifies.

Keeping in mind the deductibles described above, Part B Medicare would pay for the following when a doctor treats the patient: medical and surgical services by a doctor of medicine, or a doctor of osteopathy; certain medical and surgical services by a doctor of dental medicine or a doctor of dental surgery; services of podiatrists when they are legally authorized to perform by the state in which they practice; other services which are ordinarily performed in the doctor's office and included in his bill, such as diagnostic tests and procedures, medical supplies, services of his office nurse, and drugs and biologicals which cannot be self-administered. Part B does not pay for (and this is very important): routine physical checkups; routine foot care, treatment of flat feet, sprains, or partial dislocations of the feet; eye refractions and examinations for prescribing, fitting, or changing eyeglasses; hearing examinations for prescribing, fitting, or changing hearing aids; immunizations, unless directly related to an injury or if there is immediate risk of infection, such as an antitetanus shot given after an injury; services of certain

EXPLANATION of MEDICARE PAYMENTS
(THIS IS NOT A BILL)

FOR THE CLAIM RECEIVED ON 04-15-71

MASSACHUSETTS MEDICAL SERVICE
P.O. BOX 2194, BOSTON, MASS. 02106 TELEPHONE ▶ 617/357-8000

THIS IS A STATEMENT OF THE ACTION TAKEN ON YOUR MEDICARE CLAIM.
KEEP THIS NOTICE FOR YOUR RECORDS.

PATIENT'S NAME

DATE 04-22-71

HEALTH INSURANCE CLAIM NUMBER
011-12-0142-A

CONTROL NUMBER
00-71-105-152-02-0

ALWAYS USE INFORMATION IN BOX WHEN WRITING ABOUT THIS CLAIM

SERVICES WERE PROVIDED BY	WHEN	CHARGES SUBMITTED	CHARGES ALLOWED	REASON CHARGES NOT ALLOWED: MEDICARE DOES NOT PAY FOR	SERVIC PLACE TY
01 M02961 9004	04 06 71	10 00	10 00		1 1

ASSIGNED	TOTALS ▶	10 00	10 00	MEDICARE PAID	BE SURE TO READ IMPORTANT INFORMATION ON THE BACK OF THIS NOTICE.
Total allowed charges subject to the $50 deductible & 20% coinsurance	▶		10 00		
This went toward the $50 deductible	▶		10 00		
Medicare pays 80% of the allowed charges over the deductible	▶		0 00	0 00	YOU HAVE MET $ 20.00 OF YOUR DEDUCTIBLE FOR 19 71.
Inpatient radiology & pathology physicians' charges not subject to a $50 deductible & 20% coinsurance	▶		0 00	0 00	
TOTAL MEDICARE PAYMENT	▶			0 00	PAID TO CHARLES D BONNER M

REMARKS:

THIS IS NOT A BILL

FIG. 107. Sample of Medicare record sent to patient so that he may know his own and Medicare's financial liability.

practitioners, for example, Christian Science practitioners, chiropractors, or naturopaths. It pays for ambulance transportation by an approved ambulance service to a hospital or skilled nursing home *only* when it means other transportation may endanger the patient's health and the patient must be taken to the nearest facility that is equipped to take care of him. Under certain restrictions, it will pay for ambulance services from one hospital to another; from a hospital to a skilled nursing home; from a hospital or skilled nursing home to the patient's home, if his home is in the same locality.

As far as outpatient hospital benefits are concerned, Part B Medicare will pay for: laboratory and other diagnostic services; medical supplies, such as splints and casts; other diagnostic services. It will not pay for tests given as part of a routine checkup; eye refractions and examinations for prescribing, fitting or changing eyeglasses; immunizations unless directly related to an injury, or if there is immediate risk of infection, such as an antitetanus shot given after an injury; hearing examinations for prescribing, fitting, or changing hearing aids. Outpatient physical therapy services are covered by medical insurance when they are furnished under the direct supervision of a doctor or when furnished as part of a covered home health service.

Under home health benefits, Part B will pay for part-time nursing care; physical, occupational, or speech therapy; part-time services of home health aids; medical social services; medical supplies furnished by the agency; use of medical appliances. It will not pay for: full-time nursing care; drugs and biologicals; personal comfort or convenience items; noncovered levels of care; meals delivered to the home.

There are a number of other medical services and supplies which will be paid for by Part B of Medicare: diagnostic tests, such as x-rays and laboratory tests furnished by approved, independent laboratories; radiation therapy; portable diagnostic x-ray services furnished in the home under a doctor's supervision; surgical dressing, splints, casts, or similar devices; rental or purchase of durable medical equipment prescribed by a doctor to be used in the home, for example, wheelchair, hospital bed, or oxygen equipment; devices other than dental to replace all or part of an internal body organ; this includes corrective lenses after a cataract operation. Part B does not pay for prescription drugs and drugs you can administer yourself, for example, insulin injections for diabetes, hearing aids, eyeglasses, false teeth, orthopedic shoes, or other supportive devices for the feet, except when shoes are a part of a leg brace.

Under the hospital insurance, Part A, one should note that each individual also has a lifetime reserve of 60 additional days. This is like a bank account of extra days to draw upon if needed. They can be utilized if more hospitalization is needed beyond the 90-day benefit period. The patient, however, during these days, must pay $36.00 a day toward the daily hospital bill.

Blue Cross/Blue Shield has a plan which can be purchased along with Medicare; this reduces the patient's out-of-pocket liability. This plan is called *Medex* and comes in three packages.

Medex I pays the initial $68.00 deduction that the person would have to pay himself and also full semiprivate less the $17.00 per day that the patient is contributing toward his hospital stay during the 61st to the 90th day. It would extend the hospital benefit period to 120 days and pay full semiprivate rates. In the case of physician benefits or out-of-hospital benefits, again, Medex I would pay the initial $50.00 deduction and the 20 percent liability which the patient has for his continued expenses.

Medex II extends the hospital coverage for an additional 275 days, bringing this type of coverage to a total of 365 days, for which it pays the full semiprivate rate after the 91st day. It also pays the deduction for physician benefits and out-of-hospital benefits plus the 20 percent of continued expenses. It also adds benefits for extended-care facilities, paying the $8.50 per day the patient would pay from the 21st to the

100th day, and paying $10.00 per day from the 100th to the 365th day. The patient would have to pay the balance. In other nursing homes, Medex II would pay $8.00 a day toward the daily rate, and the balance would have to be paid by the patient.

Medex III, in addition to the above, will pay 80 percent of charges up to $300.00 for inpatient, private-duty nursing care, after $100.00 deductible per benefit period. It will also pay 80 percent of the charges for drugs requiring prescription used outside the hospital after a $25.00 deduction per calendar year.

It is obvious that depending upon whether one chooses Medex I, II, or III, the monthly premium which the patient pays for this coverage will be higher.

Medicaid, which is primarily a medical assistance program, was developed soon after Medicare. Its aim, basically, was to provide better health-care services to the poor, regardless of age. In many ways, it was doomed before it got started, because it allowed many alternatives to be accepted by the various states. It was a program which would require a contribution from both the federal government and the state as well as depending upon the option taken. Many states did not choose the maximum options available and therefore did not implement very meaningful programs. Two states did not adopt Medicaid at all, because they felt that the state's share of providing the medical services to the large underprivileged population they happened to have would bankrupt their state's treasury. On the other hand, certain states, such as Massachusetts, chose all the options available and found that their welfare costs spiraled markedly.

To qualify for this medical assistance program, the individual must also meet a means test which allows him to possess only a limited amount of money or earthly goods. Payments to hospitals are usually made by a per diem fee which has been designated by a local rate-setting commission after annual audit of the institution's books. Fees for private providers have to be

reasonable and customary. Any exceptional expenditures must be approved by the state before they can be purchased.

If a state accepted all the options available, it would be able to provide quite extensive medical coverage, including the services of dentists, allied health personnel, equipment, nursing-home payments, and other services. The decreasing covered services of Medicare are still being covered in this program. The biggest problem with the Medicaid program is the lack of adequate numbers of qualified individuals and social workers to mediate the program in the various local offices. Fees paid to private providers as well as to institutional providers are frequently six months to a year behind schedule. This has made it necessary for many hospitals to borrow huge sums of money to maintain their current budget expenditures. This, in turn, means payment of large sums of interest and, paradoxically, this increases the hospital daily fee, which one is desperately attempting to curtail.

The main complaint of nursing homes is that the Medicaid reimbursement is inadequate; and many nursing homes will set aside only a small number of beds for Medical Assistance patients, which again, in effect, means that many of these patients become backed up in hospitals at much higher rates and thus Medicaid costs spiral because of improper placement.

Medical Assistance is set up so that if the patient is over 65 and on Medicare, and if he also qualifies for Medicaid, the initial deductible and all other deductibles, including the 20 percent on Part B, will be paid for by Medical Assistance.

It should be noted, however, that the greater part of the health care of the American public is financed through private health insurances. The 26th annual report of the Health Insurance Council showed that over nine out of every ten Americans below age 65, or about 92 percent, were covered by a private hospital-expense insurance. Of those covered for some or all of their hospital expenses, 92 percent also had surgical-expense protection, and 81 percent had nonsurgical medical expense coverage. Major medical expense policies covered over 78½ million persons under age 65. This form of protection, which reimburses the insured for both in and out of hospital expenses, was held by seven out of every ten persons below age 65.

Dental-expense insurance offered by the insurance companies covered 7.8 million persons, which is more than 20 times the number of individuals who were insured just seven years prior to this report. Benefits paid by private health-insurance companies totaled 1.73 billion dollars during 1971.

It is interesting to note that practically all the statistics available concerning private health-insurance coverage apply to individuals under the age of 65, which again emphasizes the fact that it is most difficult for anyone over age 65 to get adequate coverage, whether in the private sector or the government sector.

It should also be noted that there are major differences between insurance policies and insurance companies, and the individual must check closely to know whether or not he is getting what he is actually paying for. One area to be closely studied is that which applies to what coverages are available for long-term chronic illnesses, because it is these with which we are dealing. Again, the cost of medical care has risen to such an extent that private insurances, as well as Medicare, are trying to see how they can reduce their expenditures, and thus their coverages are becoming less.

There are several gimmicks which are being used. In essence, certain insurance companies say they will not pay for custodial care; then they will make their own definition of *custodial care*—in some instances, the definition being as ridiculous as that "custodial care is any situation in which the patient is not improving." Other insurance companies are writing into their policies that they will only pay for services or calls in a hospital; then they make their definition of *hospital* rule out chronic-care facilities, rehabilitation centers, and any facility that does not

do major surgery. In effect, the patient may find himself getting excellent medical or rehabilitative care in a facility without an operating room that performs major surgery; and the insurance company will not pay his bill under the plea that he is not in a *hospital*. These are some of the problems to which the elderly and the poor have to address themselves at the present time.

There has been much effort among various groups and the federal government to conceive of a representative, adequate, and acceptable health-care insurance plan. There are a number of these under study at the present time, which are here briefly described. The number of plans proposed is a testament to the marked complexity of this problem and the diversity of opinions.

The Nixon administration has proposed a plan called the *National Health Insurance Partnership Act*. This would provide mandatory insurance for the employed and federally financed coverage for the poor. Private insurance companies would underwrite and administer the plan subject to government regulations. Subscribers to this plan would receive unlimited hospital and physician services, laboratory and x-ray services, subject to deductibles and coinsurance. Employees and employers would pay for the general plan; the insurance for the poor would be paid out of tax revenue. This insurance for the poor is limited to thirty hospital days, all inpatient doctor services during those days, and eight outpatient visits a year. Federal officials estimated that the government's share of the cost would be 5.5 billion dollars. The employer-employee contribution would be a compulsory 20 million dollars by 1974.

Senator Edward Kennedy has suggested a plan called the *Health Security Plan*. It seeks to set up a cradle-to-the-grave nationalized insurance coverage for every state's citizens. The plan would provide all physician and institutional services, drug treatment, nursing-home care, and private psychiatric services with some limitations. Fifty percent of the cost of this plan would be paid for from general income from a series of payroll taxes. Cost estimates of this program are from 53 billion to 77 billion dollars a year.

The American Medical Association endorsed a plan called *Medicredit,* in which the federal government would pay insurance premiums for the poor and would allow income-tax credits to all others toward purchase of approved private insurance. Benefits would include 60 days of hospitalization, all emergency and outpatient services, all physician services, dental and ambulance services, drugs, psychiatric services, and physical therapy, all subject to deductibles and coinsurance. Catastrophic illness coverage would also be available. Everyone under age 65 would be eligible, their eligibility being based on their tax liability. The estimated cost of this plan is 14.5 billion dollars a year.

The Health Insurance Assocation of America proposed a plan called *National Health Care Act.* This would provide a standard of health insurance through private carriers paid by direct payment to insurance companies, income tax deductions, and government contributions. The poor and previously uninsurable would be covered by state assigned-risk pools. Medicaid and Medicare would remain. By 1976, everyone would be entitled to 120 days hospitalization and six outpatient doctor visits a year as well as all inpatient physician services, nursing-home care, well-baby care, dental services for children, but subject to deductibles and coinsurance. The estimated cost of this to the government would be 3.3 billion dollars in the first year.

The American Hospital Association proposed *Ameriplan.* This is based upon the formation of health-care corporations. Each corporation would cover a particular area and together they would supervise and oversee health care for the entire population. Benefits have not been clearly defined and the cost has not been estimated.

Senator Jacob Javits in New York sponsored the National Insurance and Health Services Improvement Act. This would make health insurance universally available by expanding Medicare to include the general population. As with Medicare, the federal government would collect the money and provide coverage through private carriers. The subscribers would choose either an approved private or employer plan. Subscribers would be entitled to 90 days hospitalization, posthospital care, and all physician-related services—again, with appropriate deductibles and coinsurance. Insurance would be paid through employer-employee contributions and general tax revenue. The government would share the cost to be estimated at $10.5 billion the first year, rising to $68.1 billion by the fifth year.

Senator Russell Long has proposed a catastrophic health-insurance bill. Under this bill, up to age 65, one would have to pay the cost of the first 60 days in the hospital, plus 25 percent of hospital cost thereafter. The patient would also pay the first $2000 in doctors' bills plus 20 percent of the amount above that. To finance this, a new tax of .3 percent would be added to the first $9000 of all workers' wages on top of the .8 percent Medicare tax now being paid, or an initial maximum $22.00 a year. It was estimated that this bill would help only one person in every 300 to 400 people who get large hospital bills for protracted stays in the institution.

During the 92nd Congress, there were more than 2000 health-related bills proposed. This is four times the number proposed six years before. None of these health bills was passed during the 92nd Congress, and if the 93rd Congress is less liberally inclined, it may be many a year before a suitable bill is available. It must be emphasized that in almost all the bills under consideration, no real mention of comprehensive assistance to the chronically ill, the disabled, the elderly (all those requiring long-term hospitalization and medical care) is made.

It is obvious that any national health-insurance program which provides all the features required such as: (1) coverage for all people, regardless of age; (2) coverage for all diseases, regardless of whether short or long; (3) coverage for all expenses, whether for hospital or doctors' bills, for allied health personnel, drugs, or nursing homes, etc., will be a very costly package. It cannot be undertaken without marked support from the federal government, the state governments, and private industry. Further, in spite of fantasied reductions in war expenditures, space exploration, and administrative waste, it will require a huge contribution from the average tax payer. Medicare and Medicaid programs have shown that the United States is not yet ready to spend this kind of money, because the minute these costs, even though realistic, become too high, programs begin to be cut back, and, as always, the patient is the one who suffers. It is, therefore, important, as one views his own health-care situation, that even though he has Medicare, Medex, etc., until a foolproof bill is passed which pays for all the patient's expenses regardless of the problem, one should maintain as much health insurance as he can financially afford, because the time may come when coverage additively may be needed to pay a catastrophic long-term bill. Any plan one decides to participate in should be thoroughly surveyed to make sure that the benefits that are needed, such as rehabilitation services, chronic-disease hospital services, nursing-home services, home-care services, etc., are mentioned and covered, because, again, one might find himself with a piece of paper, which, when the chips are down, becomes quite worthless.

REFERENCES

Annual Survey. *Private Health Insurance Coverage.* New York: Health Insurance Council, 1971.

Major Health Plans. *Boston Herald Traveler.* August 9, 1971.

Medicare Extension Plan I, II, and III. Boston: Blue Cross/Blue Shield, 1972.

Rules for the Medical Assistance Program. Boston: Department of Public Welfare, 1966.

Your Medicare Handbook. Baltimore: Department of Health, Education and Welfare. Social Security Administration, 1970.

Index

Index